PLANTS OF THE GODS

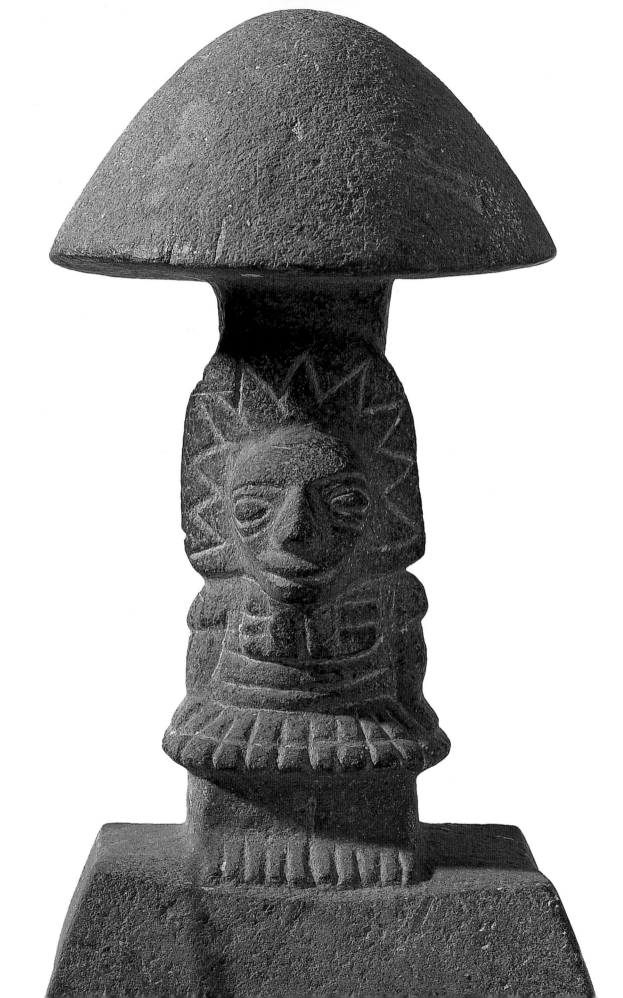

Richard Evans Schultes

Albert Hofmann

Christian Rätsch

PLANTS OF THE GODS

Their Sacred, Healing, and Hallucinogenic Powers

"The more you go inside the world of Teonanacatl, the more things are seen.
And you also see our past and our future, which are there together as a single thing already achieved,
already happened. . . . I saw stolen horses and buried cities, the existence of which was unknown,
and they are going to be brought to light. Millions of things I saw and knew. I knew and saw God:
an immense clock that ticks, the spheres that go slowly around, and inside the stars, the earth,
the entire universe, the day and the night, the cry and the smile, the happiness and the pain.
He who knows to the end the secret of Teonanacatl can even see that infinite clockwork."

—María Sabina

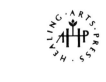

Healing Arts Press
Rochester, Vermont

Healing Arts Press
One Park Street
Rochester, Vermont 05767
www.InnerTraditions.com

First published by Healing Arts Press in 1992

A production of EMB-Service for Publishers,
Lucerne, Switzerland

Library of Congress Cataloging-in-Publication Data
Schultes, Richard Evans.
  Plants of the gods : their sacred, healing, and hallucinogenic powers / Richard Evans Schultes, Albert Hofmann, Christian Rätsch.—2nd ed.
      p. cm.
  Includes bibliographical references
    ISBN 978-0-89281-979-9
    1. Hallucinogenic plants. 2. Hallucinogenic plants—Utilization. 3. Ethnobotany. I. Hofmann, Albert, 1906- II. Rätsch, Christian, 1957- III. Title
    QK99.A1 S39 2001
    394.1'4—dc21   2001004425

13
Healing Arts Press is a division of Inner Traditions International
***

Picture on title page: Mayan "mushroom stone" from El Salvador, late formative period (300 B.C.–A.D. 200); height 13 ¼ in. (33.5 cm).

Original concept and design: Emil M. Bührer, Franz Gisler, Joan Halifax, and Robert Tobler
New material translated by: Annabel Lee and Michael Beasley
Composition: SatzWeise, Föhren, Germany
Photolithography: Pesavento AG, Zurich, Switzerland
Printed and bound in India by Replika Press Pvt. Ltd.

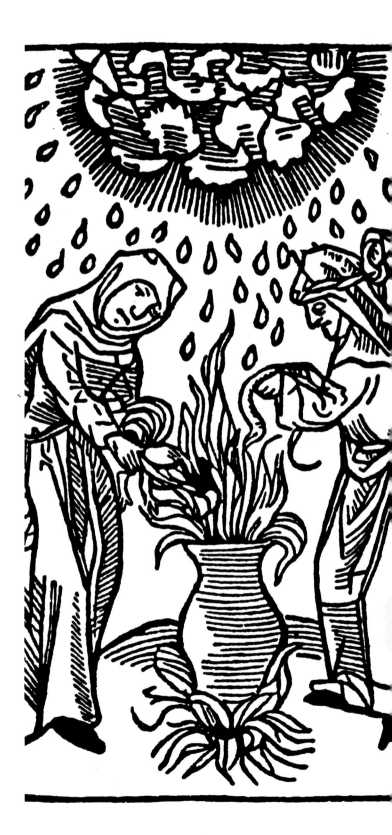

CONTENTS

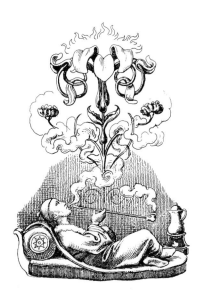

The dreaming smoker stretched out comfortably on his chaise enjoys visions induced by Hashish. This engraving is from M. von Schwind's *Album of Etchings,* published in 1843.

Page 4 left: The witches of medieval Europe induced inebriation with a great variety of brews, most of which had at least one of the Nightshades as a psychoactive constituent. During their intoxications, they engaged in many aspects of hexing, both malevolent and benevolent. This illustration, a woodcut, published in 1459, portrays two witches calling for rain and thunder, possibly during a dry spell, and preparing a brew to help them achieve this goal.

For the Huichol Indians of Mexico, the Peyote cactus *(Lophophora williamsii)* (see page 7) is not a plant but a god, a gift from the Earth Goddess to humans to assist them in attaining a connection to her in the mystical realms. The Huichol celebrate a great Peyote festival every year *(below),* at which all members of the tribe partake in eating the freshly harvested Peyote cactus.

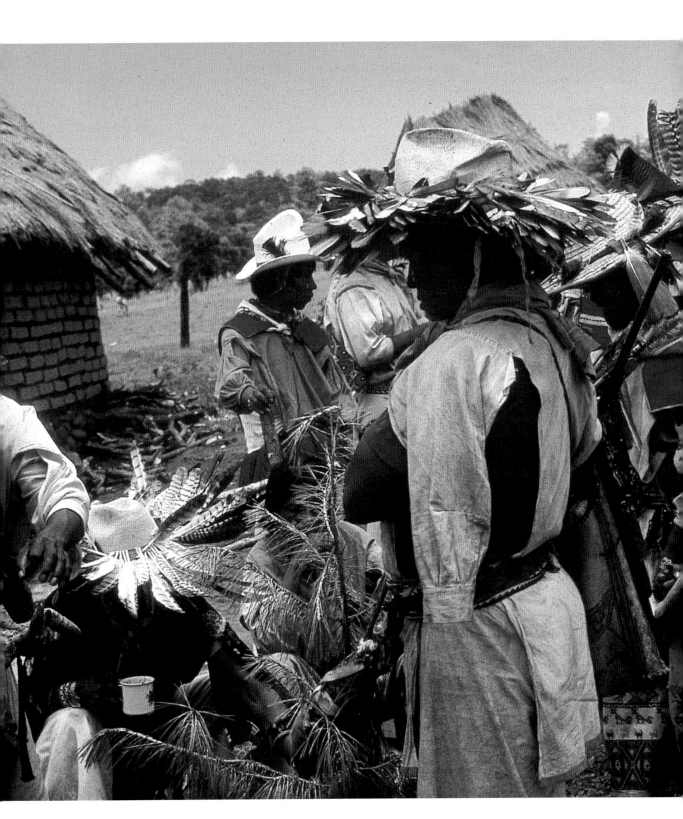

PREFACE

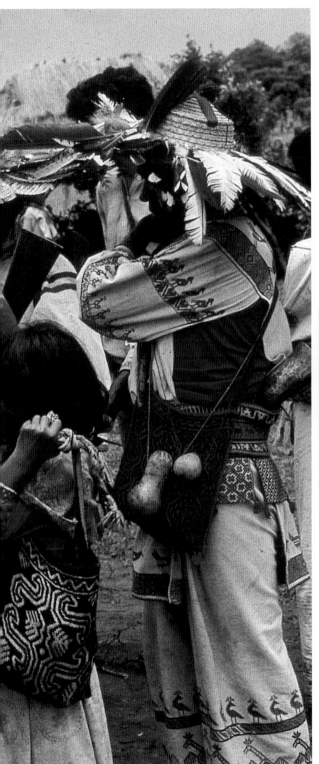

The earliest forms of life on Earth were plants. Remarkably preserved plant fossils have recently been discovered dating back 3.2 billion years. These early plants provided the foundation for the development of all later forms of plants and indeed of animals, including that most recent of creatures, the human being. The green plant cover of the earth has a marvelous relationship with the sun: chlorophyll-bearing plants absorb solar rays and synthesize organic compounds, the building materials for both plant and animal organisms. In vegetable matter, solar energy is stored in the form of chemical energy, source of all life processes. Thus the Plant Kingdom provides not only body-building foods and calories but also vitamins essential for metabolic regulation. Plants also yield active principles employed as medicines. The intimate relationship between the human and plant

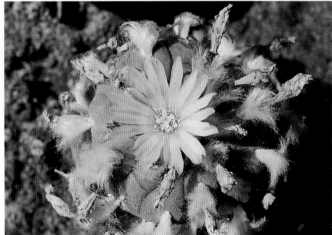

world is easily discerned, but the production of substances profoundly affecting the mind and spirit is often not so easily recognized. These are the plants that make up the substance of *Plants of the Gods*, focusing attention on the origin of their use and the effect that they have had on man's development. Plants that alter the normal functions of the mind and body have always been considered by peoples in nonindustrial societies as sacred, and the hallucinogens have been "plants of the gods" *par excellence*.

"In consciousness dwells the wondrous,
with it man attains the realm beyond the material,
and the Peyote tells us,
where to find it."
—Antonin Artaud, *The Tarahumars* (1947)

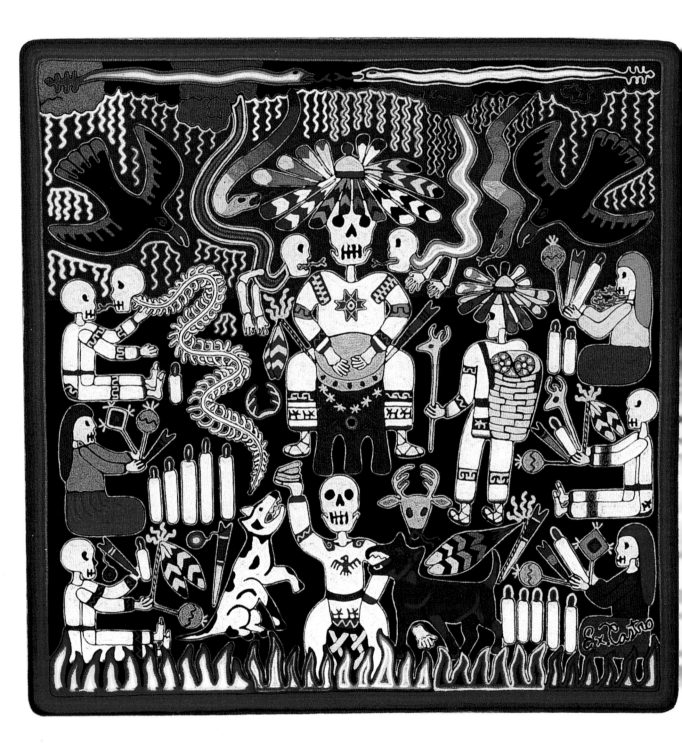

The shamans of the Huichol Indians use the sacred Peyote cactus so that they may attain a visionary state of consciousness in the alternate reality, which is causal to occurrences in mundane reality; what affects the former will change the latter. The shaman in the middle of the yarn painting is depicted with a skull because he is a "dead man" and thus has the ability to travel into the nether realms.

INTRODUCTION

The use of hallucinogenic or consciousness-expanding plants has been a part of human experience for many millennia, yet modern Western societies have only recently become aware of the significance that these plants have had in shaping the history of primitive and even of advanced cultures. In fact, the past thirty years have witnessed a vertiginous growth of interest in the use and possible value of hallucinogens in our own modern, industrialized, and urbanized society.

Hallucinogenic plants are complex chemical factories. Their full potential as aids to human needs is not yet fully recognized. Some plants contain chemical compounds capable of inducing altered perceptions, such as visual, auditory, tactile, olfactory, and gustatory hallucinations, or causing artificial psychoses that, without any doubt, have been known and employed in human experience since earliest man's experimentation with his ambient vegetation. The amazing effects of these mind-altering plants are frequently inexplicable and indeed uncanny.

Little wonder, then, that they have long played an important role in the religious rites of early civilizations and are still held in veneration and awe as sacred elements by certain peoples who have continued to live in archaic cultures, bound to ancient traditions and ways of life. How could man in archaic societies better contact the spirit world than through the use of plants with psychic effects enabling the partaker to communicate with supernatural realms? What more direct method than to permit man to free himself from the prosaic confines of this earthly existence and to enable him to enter temporarily the fascinating worlds of indescribably ethereal wonder opened to him, even though fleetingly, by hallucinogens?

Hallucinogenic plants are strange, mystical, confounding. Why? Because they are only now beginning to be the subject of truly scientific study. The results of these investigations will, most assuredly, increase interest in the technical importance of the study of these biodynamic plants. For man's mind, as well as his body and the organs of the body, need curative and corrective agents.

Are these nonaddictive drugs of interest as "mind-expanding agents," as media for attaining "the mystic experience," or as agents to be employed merely as aids in hedonistic adventure?

There is, however, another aspect that engages the scientist's attention: Can a thorough understanding of the use and chemical composition of these drugs not lead to the discovery of new pharmaceutical tools for psychiatric treatment or experimentation? The central nervous system is a most complex organ, and psychiatry has not advanced so rapidly as many other fields of medicine, mainly because it has not had adequate tools. Some of these mind-altering plants and their active chemical principles may indeed have far-reaching positive effects when they are fully understood.

An educated public must be an integral part in such development of scientific knowledge, especially in so controversial a field as hallucinogenic drugs. It is for this reason that we offer the present volume—directed neither to the scientists who are deeply involved in research in this field nor to the casual reader, but to the concerned public. It is our belief that scientists—for the sake of humanity itself and its advancement—must make technical knowledge available to those able to take advantage of its presentation. It is in this spirit that we wrote *Plants of the Gods,* hoping that it may, in one way or another, further the practical interests of mankind.

Richard Evans Schultes
Albert Hofmann

THE REVISION

When the book *Plants of the Gods* first appeared in 1979, it was a milestone in ethnobotany and ethnopharmacology. The book inspired and influenced many young researchers around the world and encouraged them to continue in their own work. Because of this there have been some new discoveries about the plants of the gods. Many questions about the activity and constituents of psychedelic plants have been clarified. I have tried to incorporate the new information in a way that preserves the original character of the book and reflects the current state of knowledge. I hope that the plants of the gods retain their valuable position in our world and that they reach the many people upon whom the sacredness of nature is dependent.

Christian Rätsch

WHAT ARE PLANT HALLUCINOGENS?

Many plants are toxic. It is no accident that the etymological origin of the word *toxic* stems directly from the Greek word τοξικον *(toxikon)*, for "bow," referring to the use of arrow poisons.

Medicinal plants are useful in curing or alleviating man's illnesses because they are toxic. The popular interpretation tends to accept the term *toxic* as implying poisoning with fatal results. Yet, as Paracelsus wrote in the sixteenth century: "In all things there is a poison, and there is nothing without a poison. It depends only upon the dose whether something is poison or not."

The difference among a poison, a medicine, and a narcotic is only one of dosage. Digitalis, for example, in proper doses represents one of our most efficacious and widely prescribed cardiac medicines, yet in higher doses it is a deadly poison.

We all realize the meaning of the term *intoxication,* but it is popularly applied primarily to the toxic effects from overindulgence in alcohol. In reality, however, any toxic substance may intoxicate. Webster defines *toxic* as "Of, pertaining to, or caused by poison." It might be more specific to state that a toxic substance is a plant or animal substance or chemical ingested for other than purely nutritional purposes and which has a noticeable biodynamic effect on the body. We realize that this is a broad definition—a definition that would include such constituents as caffeine: while employed in its usual form as a stimulant, caffeine does not evoke truly toxic symptoms, but in high doses it is a very definite and dangerous poison.

Hallucinogens must be classed as toxic. They induce unmistakable intoxications. They are likewise, in the broad sense of the term, narcotics. The term *narcotic,* coming from the Greek ναρκουν *(narkoyn),* to benumb, etymologically refers to a substance that, however stimulating it may be in one or more phases of its activity, terminates its effects with a depressive state on the central nervous system. Under this broad definition, alcohol and tobacco are narcotics. The stimulants such as caffeine do not fall under the definition of *narcotic,* since in normal doses, they do not induce a terminal depression, though they are psychoactive. English has no term that, like the German *Genußmittel* ("medium of enjoyment"), includes both narcotics and stimulants.

But the term *narcotic* has popularly been inter-

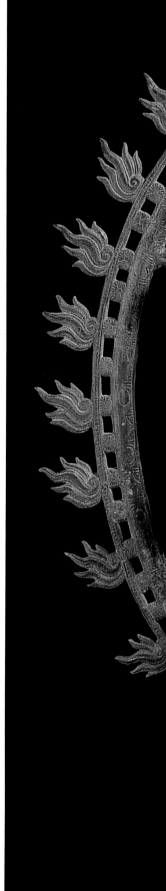

Datura has long been connected to the worship of Shiva, the Indian god associated with the creative and destructive aspects of the universe. In this extraordinary bronze sculpture from Southeast India of the eleventh or twelfth century, Shiva dances the *Ānandatān-dava,* the seventh and last of his dances, which combines all inflections of his character. Under his left foot, Shiva crushes the demon *Apasmāra-purusa,* who is the personification of ignorance. In Shiva's upper right hand, he holds a tiny drum that symbolizes Time by the rhythm of his cosmic dance in the field of Life and Creation. His lower right hand is in the *abhaya-mudrā,* expressing Shiva's quality of safeguarding the universe. In his upper left hand, he holds a flame that burns the veil of illusion. His lower left hand is held in the gajahasta and points to his raised left foot, which is free in space and symbolizes spiritual liberation. Shiva's hair is bound with a band, and two serpents hold a skull as a central ornament, thus showing Shiva's destructive aspects of Time and Death. On the right is a *Datura* flower. Garlands of *Datura* blossoms are woven among the locks of his whirling hair.

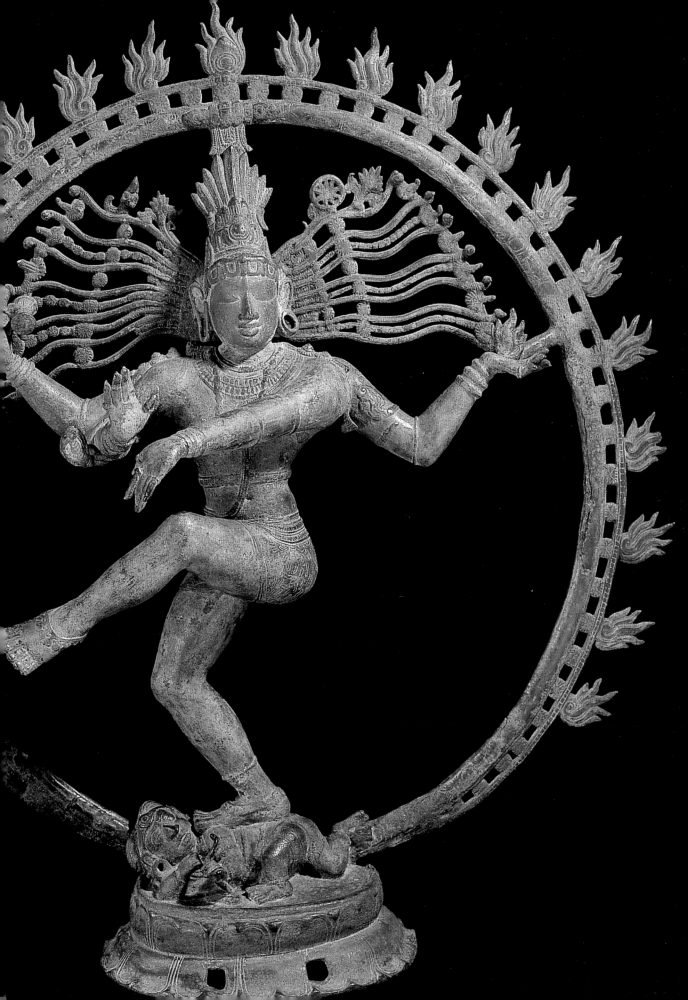

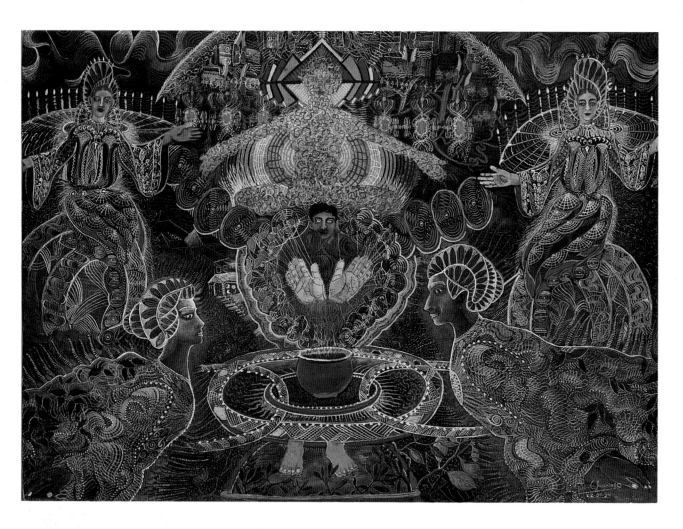

preted as referring to dangerously addictive agents, such as opium and its derivatives (morphine, codeine, heroin) and cocaine. In the United States a substance must be included in the Harrison Narcotic Act to be considered legally a narcotic: thus Marijuana is not legally a narcotic, although it is a controlled substance.

Hallucinogens are, broadly speaking, all narcotics, even though none is known to be addictive or to have narcotic effects.

There are many kinds of hallucinations: the most common and popularly recognized is the visual hallucination, often in colors. But all senses maybe subject to hallucinations: auditory, tactile, olfactory, and gustatory hallucinations can occur. Frequently a single hallucinatory plant—as in the case of Peyote or Marijuana—may induce several different hallucinations. Hallucinogens may likewise cause artificial psychoses—the basis of one of the numerous terms for this class of active agents: *psychotomimetic* ("inducing psychotic states"). Modern brain research has shown, however, that hallucinogens trigger brain activity entirely different from that apparent with true psychoses.

Modern studies have demonstrated such a complexity of psychophysiological effects that the term *hallucinogen* does not always cover the whole range of reactions. Therefore, a bewildering nomenclature has arisen. None of the terms, however, fully describes all known effects. The terms include *entheogens, deliriants, delusionogens, eidetics, hallucinogens, misperceptinogens, mysticomimetics, phanerothymes, phantasticants, psychotica, psychoticants, psychogens, psychosomi-*

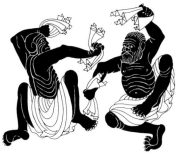

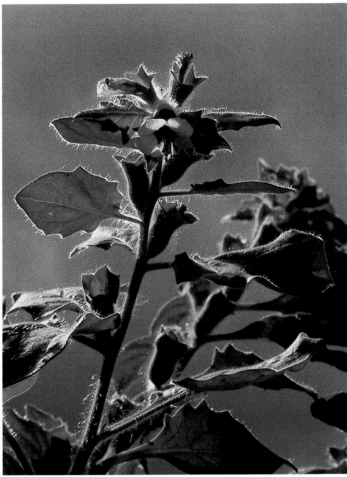

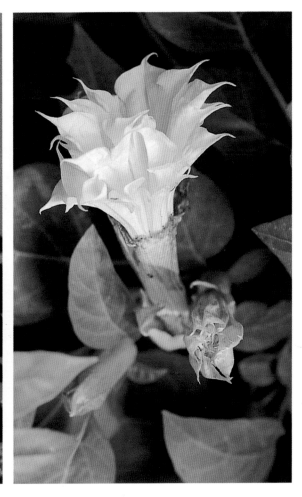

metics, psychodysleptics, psychotaraxics, psychotogens, psychotomimetics, schizogens, and *psychedelics,* among other epithets. In Europe, they are frequently called *phantastica.* The most common name in the United States—*psychedelics*—is etymologically unsound and has acquired other meanings in the drug subculture.

The truth is that no one term adequately delimits such a varied group of psychoactive plants. The German toxicologist Louis Lewin, who first used the term *phantastica,* admitted that it "does not cover all that I should wish it to convey." The word *hallucinogen* is easy to pronounce and to understand, yet not all of the plants induce true hallucinations. *Psychotomimetic,* while often employed, is not accepted by many specialists because not all the plants in this group cause psychotic-like states.

But since these two terms—*hallucinogen* and *psychotomimetic*—are easily understood and widely used, we shall employ them in this book.

Among the many definitions that have been offered, that of Hoffer and Osmond is broad enough to be widely accepted: "Hallucinogens are . . . chemicals which, in non-toxic doses, produce changes in perception, in thought and in mood, but which seldom produce mental confusion, memory loss or disorientation for person, place and time."

Basing his classification of psychoactive drugs on the older arrangements of Lewin, Albert Hofmann divides them into analgesics and euphorics (Opium, Coca), sedatives and tranquilizers (Reserpine), hypnotics (Kava-kava), and hallucinogens or psychedelics (Peyote, Marijuana, etc.). Most of these groups modify only the mood,

13

either stimulating or calming it. But the last group produces deep changes in the sphere of experience, in perception of reality, in space and time, and in consciousness of self. Depersonalization may occur. Without loss of consciousness, the subject enters a dream world that often appears more real than the normal world. Colors are frequently experienced in indescribable brilliance; objects may lose their symbolic character, standing detached and assuming increased significance since they seem to possess their own existence.

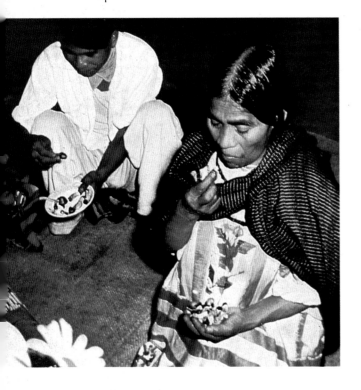

The psychic changes and unusual states of consciousness induced by hallucinogens are so far removed from similarity with ordinary life that it is scarcely possible to describe them in the language of daily living. A person under the effects of a hallucinogen forsakes his familiar world and operates under other standards, in strange dimensions and in a different time.

While most hallucinogens are of plant origin, a few are derived from the Animal Kingdom (toads, frogs, fish) and some are synthetic (LSD, TMA, DOB). Their use goes back so far into prehistory that it has been postulated that perhaps the whole idea of the deity could have arisen as a result of the otherworldly effects of these agents.

Indigenous cultures usually have no concept of physically or organically induced sickness or death: both result from interference from the spirit world. Therefore, hallucinogens, which permit the native healer and sometimes even the patient to communicate with the spirit world, often become greater medicines—the medicines *par excellence*—of the native pharmacopoeia. They assume far more exalted roles than do the medicines or palliatives with direct physical action on the body. Little by little, they became the firm basis for "medical" practices of most, if not all, aboriginal societies.

Hallucinogenic plants owe their activity to a limited number of types of chemical substances acting in a specific way upon a definite part of the central nervous system. The hallucinogenic state is usually short-lived, lasting only until the causative principle is metabolized or excreted from the body. There would seem to be a difference between what we might call true hallucinations (visions) and what perhaps could be described as pseudo-hallucinations. Conditions for all practical purposes apparently very similar to hallucinations may be induced by many highly toxic plants which so upset the normal metabolism that an abnormal mental condition may develop. A number of the plants (for example, *Salvia divinorum*) experimented with by members of the so-called drug subculture and which were considered as newly discovered hallucinogens by their users belong to this category as well. Pseudo-hallucinogenic conditions may be induced without the ingestion of toxic plants or substances; high fevers are known to cause such reactions. Fanatics of the Middle Ages who went without food or water over long periods finally induced such alterations in normal metabolism that they did actually experience visions and hear voices through pseudo-hallucinogens.

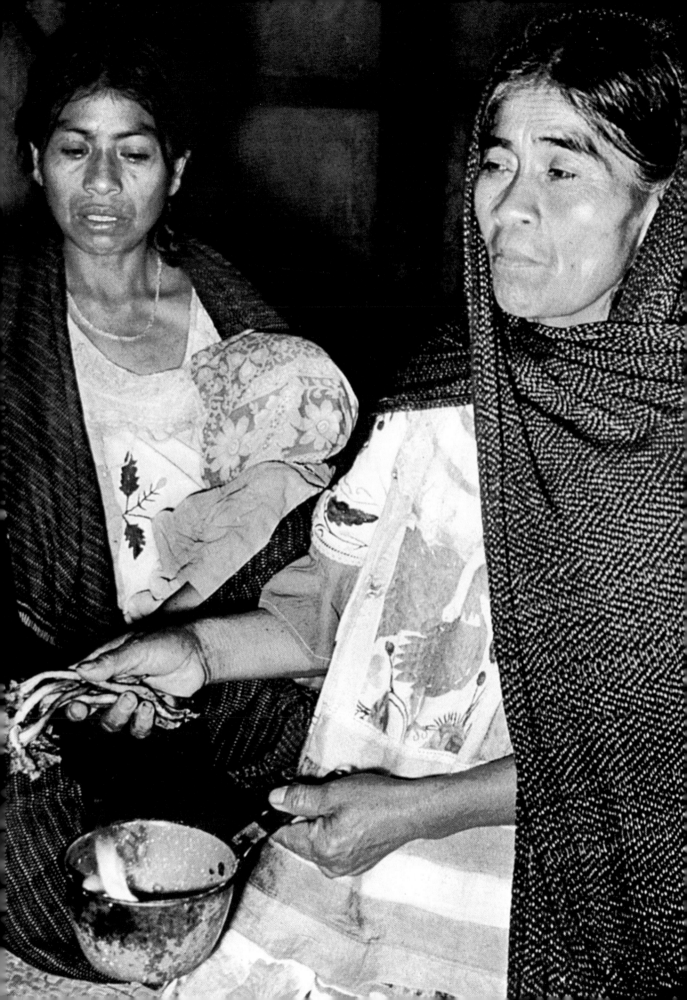

THE PLANT KINGDOM

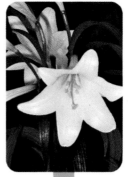

Madonna Lily
Lilium candidum

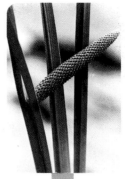

Sweet Flag
Acorus calamus

Before the eighteenth century, there was really no logical or widely accepted classification or naming of plants. They were known in Europe by the vernacular names current in the various countries and were referred to technically in Latin by cumbersome descriptive phrases, often several words long.

The invention of printing and movable type in the middle of the 1400s stimulated the production of herbals—that is, botanical books—mainly on medicinal plants. The so-called Age of Herbals, from about 1470 to 1670, led to the freeing of botany and medicine from the ancient concepts of Dioscorides and other classical naturalists that shaped Europe for some sixteen centuries. These two centuries saw more progress in botany than had taken place during the previous millennium and a half.

Yet it was not until the eighteenth century that Carolus Linnaeus, or Carl von Linné, a Swedish naturalist-physician and professor at the University of Uppsala, offered the first comprehensive and scientific system of classification and nomenclature for plants in his monumental, 1,200-page book *Species Plantarum,* published in 1753.

Linnaeus grouped plants according to his "sexual system"—a simple system of twenty-four classes based primarily on the number and characteristics of the stamens. He gave each plant a generic and a specific name, resulting in a binomial nomenclature. Although other botanists had used binomials, Linnaeus was the first to employ the system consistently. While his sexual classification—highly artificial and inadequate from the point of view of an evolutionary understanding of the Plant Kingdom (which was to come later)—is no longer followed, his binomial nomenclature is now universally accepted, and botanists have agreed on the year 1753 as the starting point of current nomenclature.

Believing that he had classified most of the world's flora in 1753, Linnaeus calculated the size of the Plant Kingdom as 10,000 or fewer species. But Linnaeus's work and the influence of his many students had stimulated interest in the flora of the new lands that were being opened to colonization and exploration. Consequently, nearly a century later, in 1847, the British botanist John Lindley increased the estimate to nearly 100,000 species in 8,900 genera.

MONOCOTYLEDONEAE

Hallucinogenic species occur among the highest-evolved flowering plants (angiosperms) and in the division fungi of the simpler plants. Angiosperms are subdivided into monocots (one seed leaf) and dicots (two seed leaves).

Sweet Flag, Hemp (Marijuana), and Deadly Nightshade *(above, right)* as well as Fly Agaric *(below, right)* are representative psychoactive species.

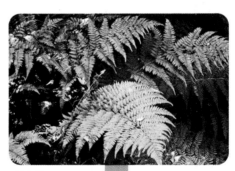

Male Fern
Dryopteris filix-mas

PTERIDOPHYTA

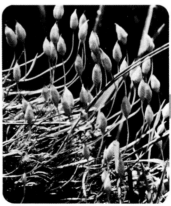

BRYOPHYTA

Haircap Moss
Polytrichum commune

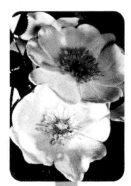

Scotch Rose
Rosa spinosissima

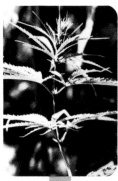

Hemp; Marijuana
Cannabis sativa

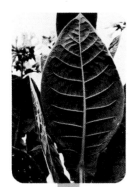

Tobacco
Nicotiana tabacum

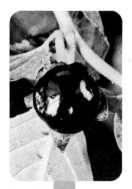

Deadly Nightshade
Atropa belladonna

Archichlamydeae

Metachlamydeae

DICOTYLEDONEAE

Angiospermiae

Dicots (flowering plants with two seed leaves) are separated into Archichlamydeae (petals absent or separate) and Metachlamydeae (petals joined).

Spermatophytes are the seed plants, subdivided into cone-bearers (gymnosperms) and flowering plants (angiosperms).

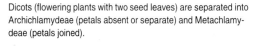

Gymnospermae

SPERMATOPHYTA

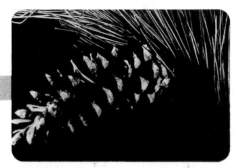

White Pine
Pinus strobus

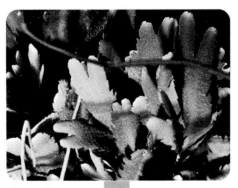

Seaweeds
Algae

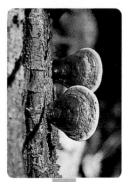

Polyporales
Ganoderma lucidum

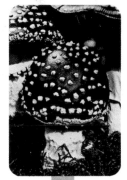

Fly Agaric
Amanita muscaria

ALGAE

FUNGI

THALLOPHYTA

Mushrooms and molds (fungi), seaweeds (algae), mosses and liverworts (bryophytes), and ferns (pteridophytes) are simpler plants.

17

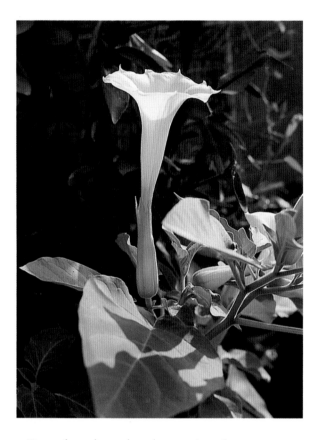

Even though modern botany is only two centuries old, estimates have greatly increased. They vary from some 280,000 to 700,000 species, the higher figures being generally accepted by botanists whose research is centered in the still only superficially explored tropical regions.

Modern specialists estimate the fungi at between 30,000 and 100,000 species. The great variance is due partly to lack of comprehensive studies of many groups and partly to inadequate means of defining some of the unicellular members. One contemporary mycologist, realizing that the fungi are very sparsely collected in the tropics, where they abound, suggests that the total figure might reach 200,000.

All of the algae are aquatic, more than half being marine. This most varied group of plants is now believed to comprise from 19,000 to 32,000 species. Algae have been found in pre-Cambrian fossils dating from one to more than three billion years of age. These procaryotic blue-green algae *(Collenia)* represent the oldest known form of life on Earth.

Lichens—a curious group of plants comprising a symbiotic union of an alga and a fungus—number from 16,000 to 20,000 species in 450 genera.

The bryophytes comprise two groups: mosses and liverworts. They are primarily tropical, and many new species are to be expected from the tropics with increased field investigations. That they are not an economic group may be in part responsible for our lack of understanding of their extent.

Present calculations assign 12,000 to 15,000 species to the pteridophytes: the ferns and their allies. An ancient group of plants, it is best represented today in tropical regions. The seed-bearing plants, or spermatophytes, clearly dominate the land flora of the present time. The gymnosperms, or cone-bearing plants, constitute a small group of some 675 species; dating back into the Carboniferous Age, this group is apparently dying out.

The principal group of plants today—the plants that dominate the earth's flora and which have diversified into the greatest number of species and which, in the popular mind, comprise the world's flora—are the angiosperms. Angiosperms are seed plants in which the seed is covered or protected by ovarian tissue, in contrast to the gymnosperms, which have naked seeds. They are commonly called flowering plants. Economically the most important group of plants today, they have dominated the several terrestrial environments of the earth. Consequently, they may have a right to be known as the "most important" plants.

Estimates of their extent vary. Most botanists hold that there are 200,000 to 250,000 species in 300 families. Other estimates, probably more realistic, calculate 500,000 species.

There are two major groups of angiosperms: the monocotyledons, plants with one seed leaf; and those with usually two seed leaves. The monocotyledons are usually credited with one quarter of the total.

Some sections of the Plant Kingdom are of great importance from the point of view of biodynamic species with compounds of significance to medicinal or hallucinogenic activity.

The fungi are of increasing interest: almost all antibiotics in wide use are derived from fungi. They are also employed in the pharmaceutical industry in the synthesis of steroids and for other purposes. Hallucinogenic compounds may be

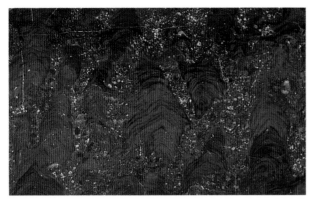 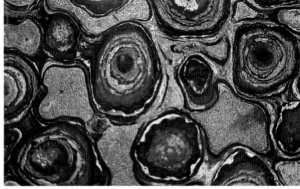

widespread in the fungi, but those that have been of importance in human affairs belong to the ascomycetes (Ergot) and the basidiomycetes (various mushrooms and puffballs). The importance of fungi as sources of aflotoxins of foods has only recently been recognized.

Algae and lichens, interestingly, have as yet not yielded any species reported as hallucinogens. An impressive number of new biodynamic compounds, some of possible medical value, have already been isolated from algae. Recent research has heightened the promise of isolation of active principles from lichens: they have yielded a large number of bacteria-inhibiting compounds and have been shown to be rich in chemovars. There are persistent reports of hallucinogenic lichens employed in northwesternmost North America, but as yet no identifiable specimens or reliable information has been forthcoming. In South America, a lichen *(Dictyonema)* is used as a psychoactive. The bryophytes have been phytochemically neglected; the few that have been studied have given little hope as sources of biodynamic compounds. Similarly, in ethnomedicine, the mosses and liverworts seem to have been ignored.

Some ferns appear to be bioactive and psychoactive. However, phytochemical investigation has been far from exhaustive. Very recent investigations have indicated a hitherto unsuspected wealth of biodynamic compounds of potential interest to medicine and commerce; sesquiterpinoid lactones, ecdyosones, alkaloids, and cyanogenic glycosides. A recent survey for antibacterial activity of extracts from 44 Trinidadian ferns indicated the surprising fact that 77 percent were positive. No hallucinogenic constituents have yet been discovered in laboratory research or by indigenous societies, although several ferns are employed in South America as additives to hallucinogenic drinks (Ayahuasca).

Of the spermatophytes, the gymnosperms exhibit few biodynamic elements. They are known primarily as the source of the sympathomimetic alkaloid ephedrine and the very toxic taxine. Many are of economic importance as sources of resins and timber. This group of seed plants is rich also in physiologically active stilbines and other compounds that act as protective agents against heartwood decay (essential oils).

From many points of view, the angiosperms are the important plants: as the dominant and most numerous group and as the elements basic to man's social and material evolution. They represent the source of most of our medicines of vegetal origin; most toxic species are angiospermous; and almost all hallucinogens used by man, as well as other narcotics, belong to this group. It is easy to understand why angiosperms have been chemically more assiduously studied; but what is not fully recognized is the fact that the angiosperms themselves have been merely superficially examined. It is clear that the Plant Kingdom represents an only partially studied emporium of biodynamic principles. Each species is a veritable chemical factory. Although indigenous societies have discovered many medicinal, toxic, and narcotic properties in their ambient vegetation, there is no reason to presume that their experimentation has brought to light all the psychoactive principles hidden in these plants.

Undoubtedly new hallucinogens are lurking in the Plant Kingdom and, in them, possible constituents of extreme interest to modern medical practice.

PHYTOCHEMICAL RESEARCH ON SACRED PLANTS

Plants of the gods interest various disciplines: ethnology, religious studies, history, and folklore. The two major scientific disciplines that concern themselves with these plants, however, are botany and chemistry. This chapter describes the work of chemists who analyze the constituents of plants used in religious rites and in the magic of medicine men and discusses the potential benefits from such research.

The botanist must establish the identity of plants that in the past were used as sacred drugs or which are still employed for that purpose today. The next step to be explored by scientists is: What constituents—which of the substances in those plants—actually produce the effects that have led to their use in religious rites and magic? What the chemist is looking for is the active principle, the quintessence or *quinta essentia,* as Paracelsus called the active compounds in plant drugs.

Among the many hundreds of different substances that make up the chemical composition of a plant, only one or two (occasionally up to half a dozen) compounds are responsible for its psychoactive effects. The proportion by weight of these active principles is usually only a fraction of 1 percent, and frequently even of one part per thousand of the plant. The main constituents of fresh plants, usually more than 90 percent by weight, are cellulose (which provides the supporting structure) and water (as the solvent and transport medium for plant nutrients and metabolic products). Carbohydrates (such as starch and various sugars), proteins, fats, mineral salts, and pigments make up several more percent of the plant. Together with these normal components, they constitute practically the whole plant, and they are common to all higher plants. Substances with unusual physiological and psychic effects are found only in certain special plants. These substances as a rule have very different chemical structures from those of the usual vegetal constituents and common metabolic products.

It is not known what function these special substances may have in the life of the plant. Various theories have been offered. Most psychoactive principles in these sacred plants contain nitrogen, and it has therefore been suggested that they may be waste products of metabolism—like uric acid

in animal organisms—their purpose being the elimination of excess nitrogen. If this theory were true, one would expect all plants to contain such nitrogenous constituents: that is not the case. Many of the psychoactive compounds are toxic if taken in large doses, and it has therefore been suggested that they serve to protect the plants from animals. But this theory likewise is hardly convincing, because many poisonous plants are in fact eaten by animals that are immune to the toxic constituents.

It remains, therefore, one of the unsolved riddles of nature why certain plants produce substances with specific effects on the mental and emotional functions of man, on his sense of perception, and actually on his state of consciousness.

Phytochemists have the important and fascinating task of separating the active principles from the rest of the plant materials and of producing them in pure form. Once active principles are thus available, it is possible to analyze them to determine the elements of which they are composed; the relative proportions of carbon, hydrogen, oxygen, nitrogen, etc.; and to establish the molecular structure in which these elements are arranged. The next step is the synthesis of the active principle: that is, to make it in the test tube quite independently of the plant.

With pure compounds—whether isolated from the plant or synthetically produced—exact pharmacological assays and chemical tests can be made. This is not possible with whole plants because of the varying content of the active principles and interference from other constituents.

The first psychoactive principle to be produced in pure form from a plant was morphine, an alkaloid present in the opium poppy. It was first isolated by the pharmacist Friedrich Sertürner in 1806. This new compound was named for the Greek god of sleep, Morpheus, because of its sleep-inducing properties. Since then, enormous strides have been made in developing more efficient methods for the separation and purification of active principles, with the most important techniques evolving only during the last decades. These include the techniques of chromatography: methods of separation based on the fact that different substances adhere in varying degrees on absorbent materials or are more or less readily

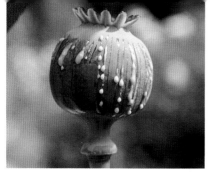

The psychoactive latex of the Poppy *(Papaver somniferum)* emerges white and turns to a resinous brown substance, raw opium. In 1806 morphine was successfully isolated out of the poppy, the first time in history that a single constituent was isolated.

Below: Papaver somniferum from Köhler's *Medizinal-Pflanzen-Atlas,* 1887. This atlas is one of the outstanding plant books of the twentieth century. Morphine is not hallucinogenic; it has been classified as a euphoric drug.

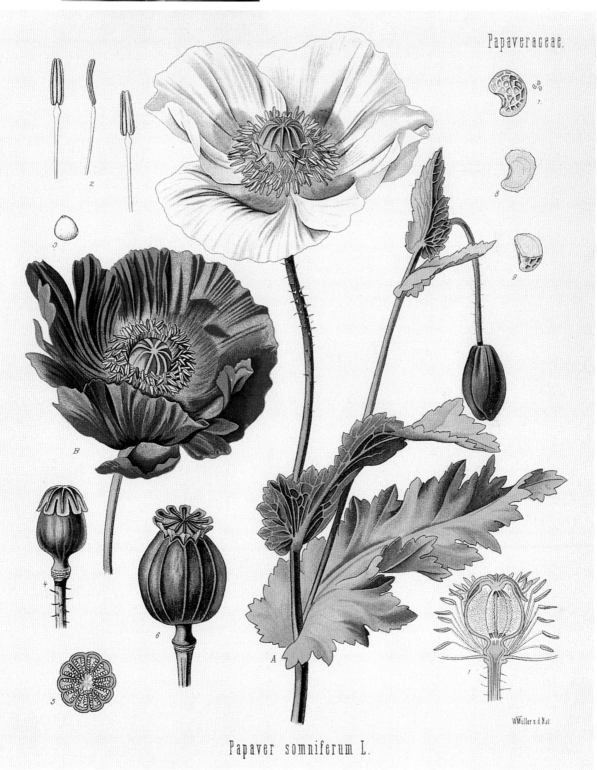

Papaveraceae.

Papaver somniferum L.

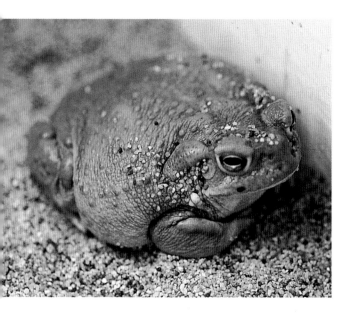

Some psychoactive compounds are also produced by animals. The Colorado River toad *(Bufo alvarius)* secretes considerable amounts of 5-MeO-DMT.

taken up in solvents that do not mix. The methods used in qualitative analysis and to establish the chemical structure of compounds have also undergone fundamental changes in recent years. Formerly, several generations of chemists would be needed to elucidate the complex structures of natural compounds. Today, it takes just a few weeks or even only days to determine them with the techniques of spectroanalysis and X-ray analysis. At the same time, improved methods of chemical synthesis have been developed. The great advances made in the field of chemistry, and the efficient methods now available to plant chemists, have in recent years made it possible to gain appreciable knowledge of the chemistry of active principles found in psychoactive plants.

The contribution made by chemists to the study of sacred plant drugs may be illustrated with the example of the Magic Mushrooms of Mexico. Ethnologists had found Indian tribes in the southern parts of Mexico using mushrooms in their religious ceremonies. Mycologists identified the mushrooms used in these rituals. Chemical analyses showed clearly which species were psychoactive. Albert Hofmann tested one species of mushroom on himself; he discovered that it was psychoactive, that it could be grown under laboratory conditions, and he was able to isolate two active compounds. The purity and chemical homogeneity of a compound can be demonstrated by its ability to crystallize, unless of course it be a liquid. The two hallucinogenic principles now known as psilocybine and psilocine, found in the Mexican Magic Mushroom *Psilocybe mexicana,* were obtained in the form of colorless crystals.

Similarly, the active principle of the Mexican cactus *Lophophora williamsii,* mescaline, had been isolated in pure form and crystallized as a salt with hydrochloric acid.

With the active principles of the mushrooms available in pure form, it became possible to extend research into various fields, such as psychiatry, with useful results.

By determining the presence or absence of psilocybine and psilocine, an objective method was now available for distinguishing true hallucinogenic mushrooms from false ones.

The chemical structure of the hallucinogenic principles of the mushrooms was determined (see structural formulas in the next chapter), and it was found that these compounds were closely related chemically to substances (serotonin) occurring naturally in the brain that play a major role in the regulation of psychic functions.

As the pure compounds can be given in exact doses, their pharmacological actions could now be studied under reproducible conditions in animal experiments, and the spectrum of their psychotropic actions in man determined. This was not possible with the original mushrooms, because their content of active principles tends to vary, between 0.1 and 0.6 percent of the dry weight of the plant tissue. The greater part of this content is psilocybine, with psilocine present usually only in traces. The median effective dose for humans is 8 to 16 milligrams of psilocybine or psilocine. Instead of swallowing 2 grams of the dried mushrooms, which have a rather unpleasant taste, one merely needs to take about 0.008 gram of psilocybine to experience the hallucinogenic effects, which generally last for several hours.

Once the active principles were available in pure form, it was possible to study their use and effective application in medicine. They were found to be particularly useful in experimental

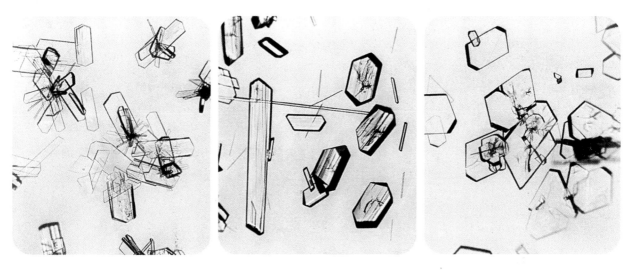

Mescaline—HCl
(mescaline-hydrochloride, crystallized from alcohol)

Psilocybine
(crystallized from methanol)

Psilocine
(crystallized from methanol)

psychiatry, as valuable aids to psychoanalysis and psychotherapy.

One might think that with the isolation, structural analysis, and synthesis of psilocybine and psilocine, the mushrooms of Mexico had lost their magic. Substances that because of their effects on the mind had led Indians to believe for thousands of years that a god dwelt in those mushrooms can now be synthetically produced in the chemist's retort. It should be remembered, however, that scientific investigation has merely shown that the magic properties of the mushrooms are the properties of two crystalline compounds. Their effect on the human mind is just as inexplicable, and just as magical, as that of the mushrooms themselves. This also holds true for the isolated and purified active principles of other plants of the gods.

Many alkaloids crystallize poorly as free bases. They will separate as a crystallized salt, however, when neutralized with a suitable acid, either by cooling the saturated solution or by evaporation of the solvent. Crystallization of substances from solutions is carried out mainly for purification, since by-products remain in the solvent.

As each substance has its own specific crystalline form, this form serves for identification and characterization of a substance. A modern method for the elucidation of chemical constitutions is the X-ray structure analysis. For the application of this method, alkaloids and other substances must be available in crystallized form.

"The largest river in the world
runs through the largest forest . . . By little and little,
I began to comprehend
that in a forest which is practically unlimited—
near three millions of square miles
clad with trees and little else but trees,
and where the natives
think no more of destroying the noblest trees,
when they stand in their way, than we the vilest weed,
a single tree cut down
makes no greater a gap, and is no more missed,
than when one pulls up a stalk of groundsel
or a poppy in an English cornfield."
—Richard Spruce

Below: The photograph depicts an aerial view of the Kuluene River, the southernmost tributary of the Xingú River, a main affluent of the Amazon.

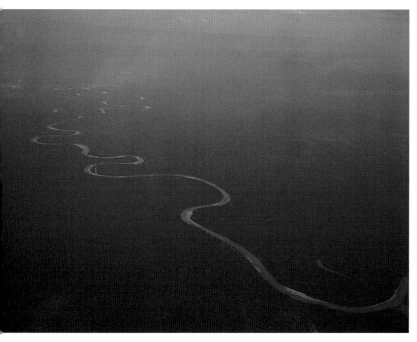

Right: "There were enormous trees, crowned with magnificent foliage, decked with fantastic parasites, and hung over with lianas, which varied in thickness from slender threads to huge python-like masses, were now round, now flattened, now knotted and now twisted with the regularity of a cable. Intermixed with the trees, and often equal to them in altitude, grew noble palms; while other and far lovelier species of the same family, their ringed stems sometimes scarcely exceeding a finger's thickness, but bearing plume-like fronds and pendulous bunches of black or red berries, quite like those of their loftier allies, formed, along with shrubs and arbuscles of many types, a bushy undergrowth, not visually very dense or difficult to penetrate . . . It is worthy to be noted that the loftiest forest is generally the easiest to traverse; the lianas and parasites . . . being in great part too high to be much in the way . . ."
—Richard Spruce

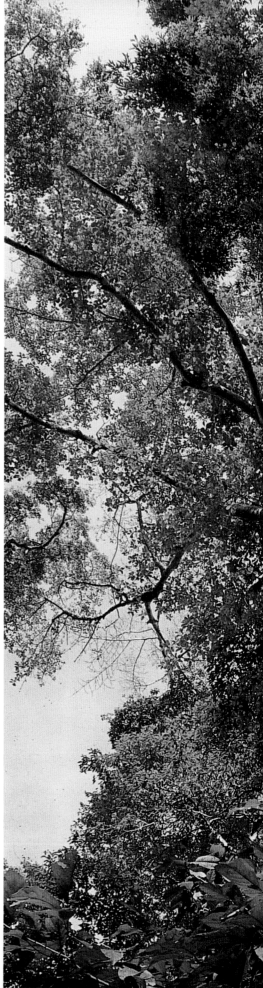

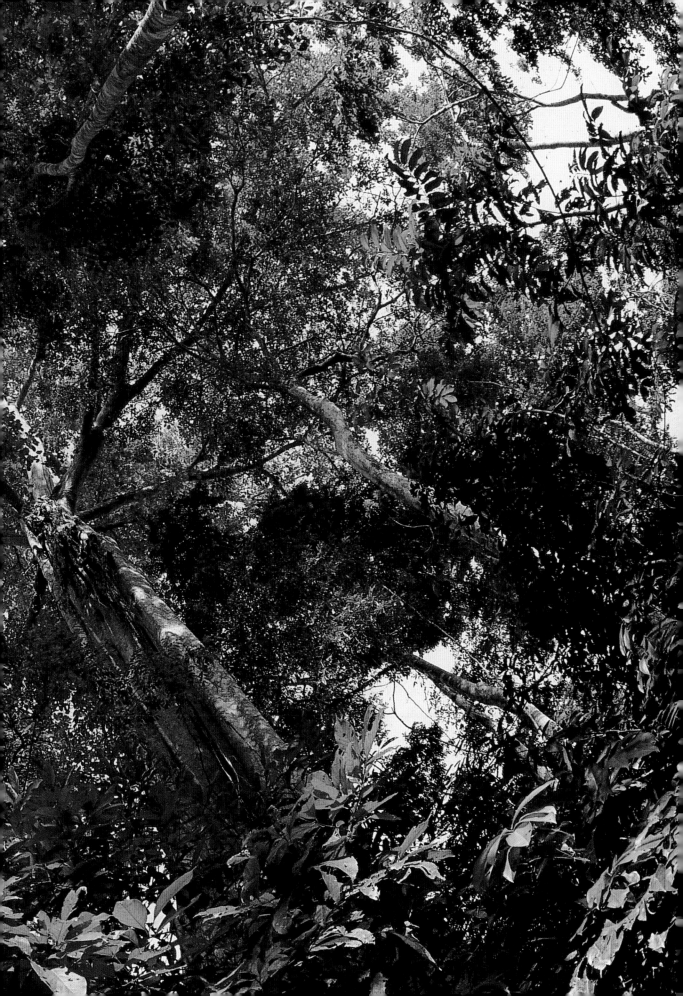

GEOGRAPHY OF USAGE AND BOTANICAL RANGE

Many more hallucinogenic plants exist than those that man has put to use. Of the probable half-million species in the world's flora, only about one thousand are known to be employed for their hallucinogenic properties. Few areas of the globe lack at least one hallucinogen of significance in the culture of the inhabitants.

Despite its size and extremely varied vegetation, Africa appears to be poor in hallucinogenic plants. The most famous, of course, is Iboga, a root of the Dogbane family employed in Gabon and parts of the Congo in the Bwiti cult. The Bushmen of Botswana slice the bulb of Kwashi of the Amaryllis family and rub it over scarifications on the head, allowing the active principles in the juice to enter the bloodstream. Kanna is a mysterious hallucinogen, probably no longer used: the Hottentots chewed the plant material from two species of the Ice Plant family that induced gaiety, laughter, and visions. In scattered regions, relatives of Thorn Apple and Henbane were used for their intoxicating properties.

In Eurasia there are many plants employed for their hallucinatory effects. Most significant, it is the home of Hemp, today the most widespread of all narcotics: as Marijuana, Maconha, Daggha, Ganja, Charas, etc., the drug and its use have spread nearly throughout the world.

The most spectacular Eurasiatic hallucinogen is the Fly Agaric, a mushroom consumed by scattered tribesmen in Siberia and possibly the sacred god-narcotic Soma of ancient India.

Datura was employed over wide areas of Asia. In Southeast Asia, especially in Papua New Guinea, sundry poorly understood hallucinogens are used. The rhizome of Maraba, a member of the Ginger family, is believed to be eaten in New Guinea. In Papua, natives ingest a mixture of leaves of Ereriba of the Arum family and bark of a large tree, Agara, to produce a sleep during which visions occur. Nutmeg may once have been taken in India and Indonesia for its narcotic effects. Tribesmen in Turkestan drink an intoxicating tea made from the dried leaves of a shrubby mint, *Lagochilus*.

The heyday of the use of hallucinogens in Europe occurred in ancient times, when they were used almost exclusively in witchcraft and divination. The major plants involved—Thorn Apple, Mandrake, Henbane, Belladonna—belong to the Nightshade family. The fungus Ergot, a parasite on rye, frequently poisoned entire regions if accidentally milled into the flour. Such attacks led hundreds of citizens to go mad and suffer hallucinations, often causing permanent insanity, gangrene, or death. This plague was known as St. Anthony's fire. Although Ergot was apparently never purposefully used in medieval Europe as a hallucinogen, there are suggestions that the Eleusinian mysteries of ancient Greece were associated with this fungal genus.

The famous and widely employed Kava-kava is not a hallucinogen but has been classified as a hypnotic narcotic.

It is in the New World that the number and cultural significance of hallucinogenic plants are overwhelming, dominating every phase of life among the aboriginal peoples.

There were some hallucinogenic species in the West Indies. In fact, the early indigenous populations used mainly the snuff known as Cohoba; and it is believed that this custom was imported by Indians invading the Caribbean Islands from the Orinoco regions of South America.

Similarly, North America (north of Mexico) is quite poor in hallucinogens. Various species of *Datura* were employed rather widely, but most intensely in the Southwest. The Indians of the region of Texas and adjacent areas used the Red Bean or Mescal Bean as the basis of a vision-seeking ceremony. In northern Canada, Indians chewed the roots of Sweet Flag as medicine and supposedly also for the hallucinogenic effects.

Mexico represents without a doubt the world's richest area in diversity and use of hallucinogens in aboriginal societies—a phenomenon difficult to understand in view of the comparatively modest number of species comprising the flora of the country. Without any question the Peyote cactus is the most important sacred hallucinogen, although other cactus species are still used in northern Mexico as minor hallucinogens for special magico-religious purposes. Of almost equal religious importance in early Mexico and surviving until today in religious rituals are mushrooms, known to the Aztecs as Teonanácatl. At least twenty-four species of these fungi are employed at the present time in southern Mexico. Ololiuqui, the seeds of Morning Glories, repre-

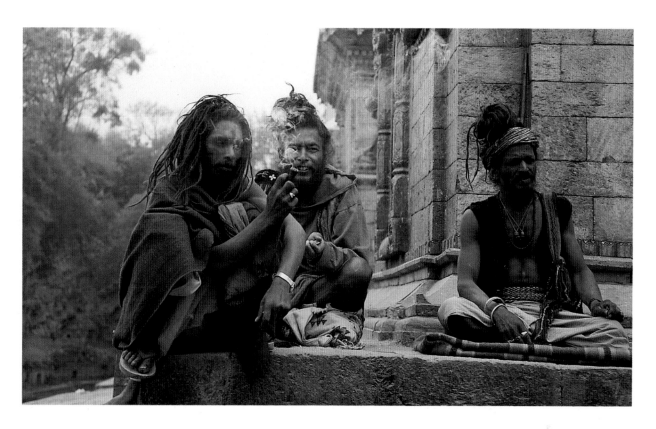

sents another hallucinogen of great importance in Aztec religion and is still employed in southern Mexico. There are many hallucinogens of secondary importance: Toloache and other species of the *Datura* group; the Mescal Bean or Frijolillo in the north; Pipiltzintzintli of the Aztecs; the diviner's sage now known as Hierba de la Pastora; Genista among the Yaqui Indians; Piule, Sinicuichi, Zacatechichi, the puffballs

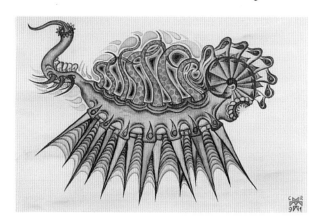

known by the Mixtecs as Gi'-i-Wa; and many others.

South America ranks a close second to Mexico in the number, variety, and deep magico-religious significance of hallucinogens. The Andean cultures had half a dozen species of *Brugmansias*, known as Borrachero, Campanilla, Floripondio, Huanto, Haucacachu, Maicoa, Toé, Tongo, etc. In Peru and Bolivia a columnar cactus called San Pedro or Aguacolla is the basis of the drink *cimora*, used in a vision-seeking ceremony. Mapuche Indian witch doctors (who are mostly female) of Chile formerly employed a hallucinogenic tree of the Nightshade family—Latué or Arbol de los Brujos. Research has indicated the use in various parts of the Andes of the rare shrub Taique *(Desfontainia)*, the mysterious Shanshi, and the fruits of Hierba Loca and Taglli, both of the Heath family. Most recently, a type of Petunia has been reported as an intoxicant used in Ecuador. In the Orinoco and parts of the Amazon, a powerful snuff called Yopo or Niopo is made from the toasted seeds of a tree of the legume

NATIVE USE OF MAJOR HALLUCINOGENS

Notwithstanding the greater age of cultures and the widespread use of hallucinogens in the Eastern Hemisphere, the number of species so used is far greater in the Western Hemisphere. Anthropologists have explained this disparity on cultural grounds. There does not, however, seem to be a significant difference between the two hemispheres in the number of plants possessing hallucinogenic principles.

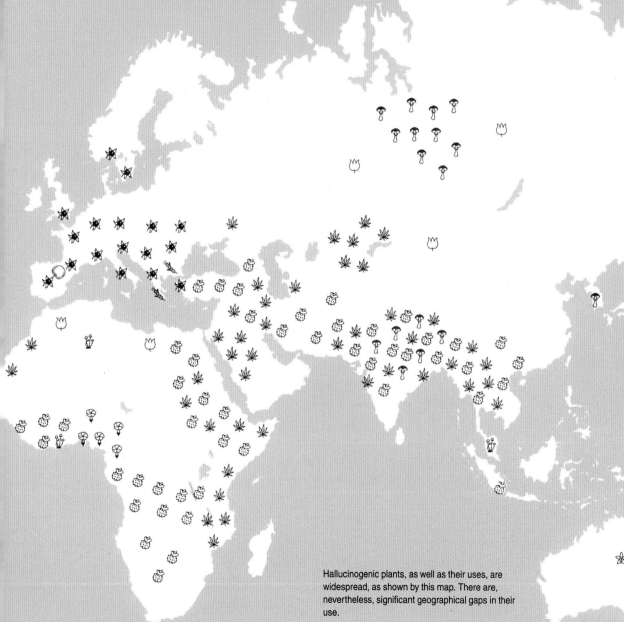

Hallucinogenic plants, as well as their uses, are widespread, as shown by this map. There are, nevertheless, significant geographical gaps in their use.

There are few cultures in the Western Hemisphere that did not value at least one hallucinogenic plant in magico-religious ceremonies. Many cultures had several. In addition to hallucinogens, a number of otherwise psychoactive plants shared the honors: Tobacco, Coca, Guayusa, Yoco, Guarancá. Some of these—especially Tobacco and Coca—rose to exalted positions in the sacred native pharmacopoeias. These major hallucinogens are culturally significant in the areas indicated by the symbols.

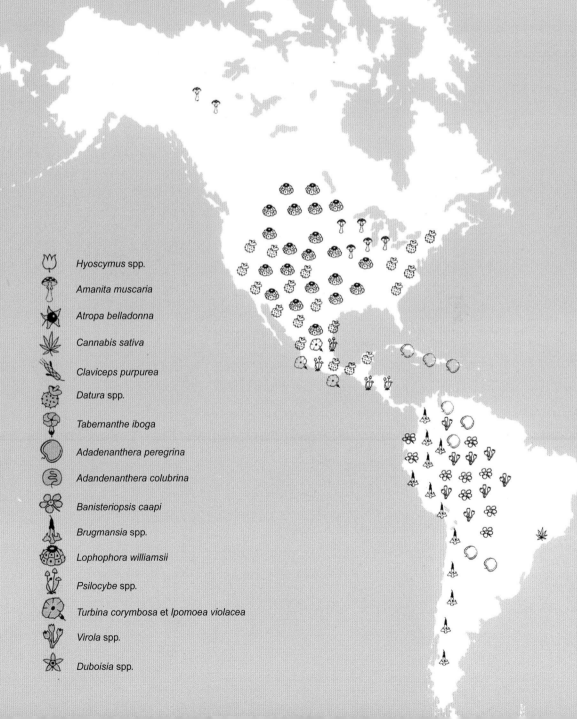

Hyoscymus spp.

Amanita muscaria

Atropa belladonna

Cannabis sativa

Claviceps purpurea

Datura spp.

Tabernanthe iboga

Adadenanthera peregrina

Adandenanthera colubrina

Banisteriopsis caapi

Brugmansia spp.

Lophophora williamsii

Psilocybe spp.

Turbina corymbosa et *Ipomoea violacea*

Virola spp.

Duboisia spp.

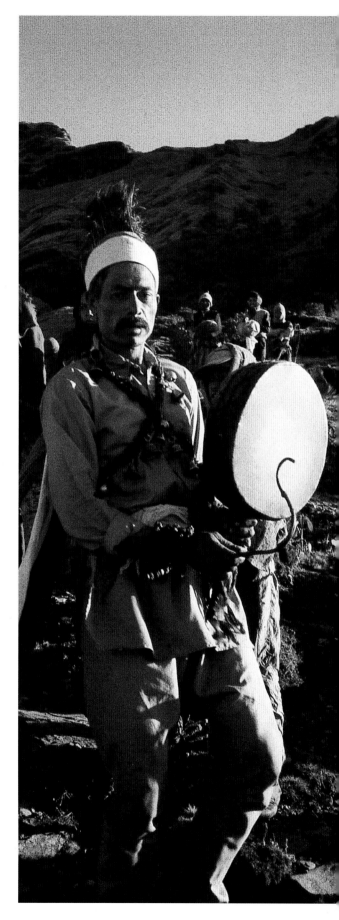

family. The Indians of northern Argentina take a snuff—Cebíl or Villca—prepared from seeds of a species closely related to Yopo. Perhaps the most important lowland hallucinogen in South America is Ayahuasca, Caapi, Natema, Pindé, or Yajé. Employed ceremonially in the western Amazon and in several localities on the Pacific coastal areas of Colombia and Ecuador, it is made basically from several species of lianas of the Malpighia family. *Brunfelsia,* a member of the Nightshade family, known widely in the westernmost Amazon as Chiricaspi, is taken for hallucinatory purposes.

There are more plants utilized as hallucinogens in the New World than in the Old. Nearly 130 species are known to be used in the Western Hemisphere, whereas in the Eastern Hemisphere the number reaches roughly 50. Botanists have no reason to presume that the flora of the New World is richer or poorer than that of the Old in plants with hallucinogenic properties.

PLANT LEXICON

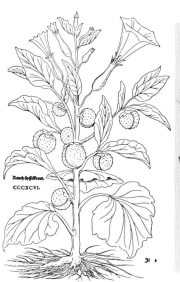

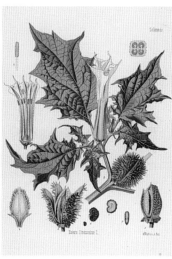

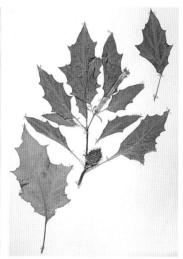

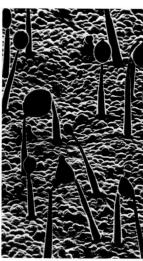

The plant lexicon includes basic descriptions, primarily botanical in nature, of ninety-seven plants that are known to have a hallucinogenic or psychoactive effect.

Emphasis is given to plants that are known from the literature, field experience, and/or laboratory evidence to have definite psychoactive effects. Some species that are reported to have "narcotic" or "intoxicating" uses are included as well.

The plants are arranged alphabetically according to the Latin name of the genus. This order has been followed in view of the many different vernacular names in the great variety of native languages. If a particular name is not listed, it may be sought in the index of vernacular names on pages 32–33 or at the end of the book where these epithets are cross-referenced.

Inasmuch as this volume is written for the general reader, the botanical descriptions are intentionally brief, stressing the obvious and most easily visible characteristics of the plant. Whenever space permits, additional information of historical, ethnological, phytochemical, and, very occasionally, psychopharmacological interest is added. In this way, an attempt has been made in this introductory lexicon to give as broad an interdisciplinary view as possible. The illustrations in the lexicon are of two kinds: some of them are watercolors made whenever possible from living plant material or herbarium specimens. Most are direct reproductions of color photographs. A number of the plants depicted here are illustrated for the first time.

The purpose of the lexicon is manifestly to help guide the reader more easily into the admittedly complex array of facts and stories that comprise only a small fraction of the extensive knowledge from many fields concerning these plants that native peoples around the world have considered plants of the gods.

The botanical investigation of medicinal plants has, over the years, become more and more exact and sophisticated. In 1543, the writer of one of the most beautifully illustrated herbals, Leonard Fuchs, presented this accurate sketch of *Datura stramonium,* the Thorn Apple *(left).* Some three hundred years later, Köhler, in his *Medizinal Pflanzen,* published a more detailed pharmacognostic rendering of this very important therapeutic plant *(center).* In the 125 years since the establishment of Linnaeus's herbarium and the binomial system of nomenclature, our herbaria have greatly enhanced the understanding of the morphological variation of vegetal species through the collection of dried specimens around the world. The third illustration depicts a typical herbarium specimen of the Thorn Apple representing the kind of material that now authenticates botanical identification. Modern technology (for example, the electron-scanning microscope) is making available morphological details, such as the leaf surface hairs of the Thorn Apple, which provide greater accuracy in the work of plant identification.

Index and Key
to the Plant Lexicon

Ninety-seven hallucinogenic plants are illustrated and described on the following pages (34–60).

The lexicon is in alphabetical order by genus name. Each text in the lexicon includes the following information in its heading:

- Genus, author, and, in brackets, the number of species known to exist in the genus.
- Botanical name of the species shown. The species known to contain hallucinogenic properties or to be used as hallucinogens will be found in the reference section "Overview of Plant Use," pages 65–80, which is organized by common name. This reference section/ chart provides the botanical names of the plants and describes the history, ethnography, context, purpose of usage, and preparation, as well as chemical components and effects.
- Plant family.
- Reference number.
- Geographical distribution of the genus.

Common names are listed here below with the number designating each plant's location in the lexicon.

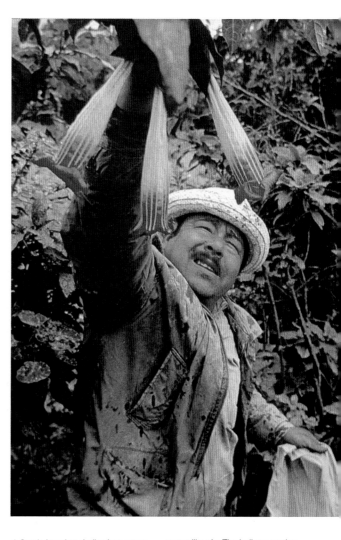

A South American Indian harvests a plant of the gods, a Blood-Red Angel's Trumpet *(Brugmansia sanguinea)*. This alkaloid-rich plant has been cultivated and used for psychoactive purposes for centuries or even millennia. The Indians caution against the thoughtless use of this plant, which causes such strong hallucinations and delirium that only experienced shamans can use it for divination and healing.

ACACIA Mill. (750–800)	ACORUS L. (2)	AMANITA L. (50–60)	ANADENANTHERA Speg. (2)
Acacia maidenii F von Muell. Maiden's Acacia	*Acorus calamus* L. Sweet Flag	*Amanita muscaria* (L. ex Fr.) Pers. Fly Agaric	*Anadenanthera colubruna* (Vellozo) Brennan Cebíl, Villca
Leguminosae (Pea Family)	Araceae (Arum Family)	Amanitaceae	Leguminosae (Pea Family)
1 Australia	**2** Temperate and warm zones of both hemispheres	**3** Europe, Africa, Asia, Americas	**4** Northwest Argentina

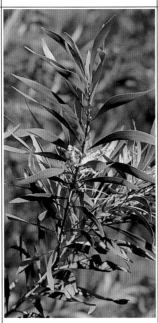

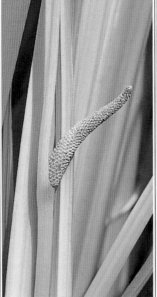

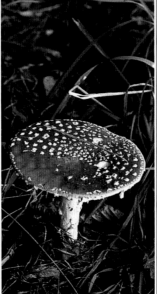

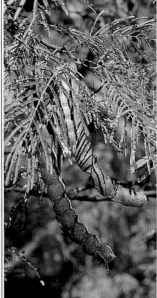

The genus *Acacia* is widely distributed throughout the tropical and subtropical regions of the world. It encompasses for the most part medium-sized trees with pinnate, occasionally smooth leaves. The flowers grow in clusters and the fruit is pea-like. Many acacias are a traditional additive to psychoactive products, such as betel, beer, balché, pituri, and pulque. Some of the species are suited for the preparation of Ayahuasca analogs. Numerous Australian species *(A. maidenii, A. phlebophylla, A. simplicifolia)* contain higher concentrations of DMT in their bark and leaves.

Acacia maidenii, a beautiful erect tree with a silvery splendor, contains different tryptamines. The bark contains 0.36 % DMT. The leaves are usable as a DMT-delivering component of Ayahuasca analogs. These acacias are easy to cultivate in temperate climates such as in California and southern Europe.

Some evidence, although weak and indirect, suggests that the Cree Indians of northwestern Canada may occasionally chew the rootstalk of Sweet Flag for its psychoactive effects.

Sweet Flag is a semiaquatic herb with a long, aromatic, creeping rootstock producing shoots of erect, linear, swordlike leaves up to 6 ft (2 m) in length. The tiny flowers are borne on a solid, lateral, greenish yellow spadix. The rootstalk or rhizome contains an essential oil responsible for the plant's medicinal value.

It has been suggested that the active principles are α-asarone and β-asarone. There is a structural resemblance between asarone and mescaline, a psychoactive alkaloid. No evidence has ever been produced, however, that asarone can be associated with psychotomimetic activity.

Amanita muscaria is a beautiful mushroom growing in thin forests usually under birches, firs, and young pines. It may attain a height of 8–9 in. (20–23 cm). The somewhat viscid, ovate, hemispheric, and finally almost flat cap measures 3–8 in. (8–20 cm) when mature. There are three varieties: one with a blood-red cap with white warts found in the Old World and northwestern North America; a yellow or orange type with yellowish warts common in eastern and central North America; and a white variety that is found in Idaho. The cylindrical stem, which has a bulbous base, is white, ½–1 in (1–3 cm) thick, with a conspicuous cream-white ring covered basically with encircling scales. The white valve adheres to the base of the stem. The gills vary from white to cream color or even lemon yellow.

This mushroom, perhaps man's oldest hallucinogen, has been identified with Soma of ancient India.

This tree grows 9–50 ft (3–18 m) and has an almost black bark often adorned with conical thorns. The leaves are finely locular and reach up to 1 ft (30 cm) long. The yellowish white flowers are round. The leathery dark brown fruit pods grow to 1 ft (35 cm) long and contain very flat red-brown seeds ½ to 1 in. (1–2 cm) wide, with rounded to right angles.

The seeds have been used as a hallucinogen by the Indians of the southern region of the Andes for approximately 4,500 years. They are either worked into a snuff powder, smoked, or used as an additive for beer. Primarily they are used in shamanism.

The seeds of the Cebíl or Villca contain tryptamines, especially bufotenine.

ANADENANTHERA Speg. (2)	ARGYREIA Lour. (90)	ARIOCARPUS Scheidw. (6)

Anadenanthera peregrina (L.) Speg.
Yopo

Leguminosae (Pea Family)

5 Tropical zones of South America, West Indies

Argyreia nervosa (Burman f.) Bojer,
Hawaiian Wood Rose
Convovulaceae
(Morning Glory Family)

6 India, Southeast Asia, Hawaii

Ariocarpus retusus Scheidw.
False Peyote

Cactaceae (Cactus Family)

7 Mexico, Texas

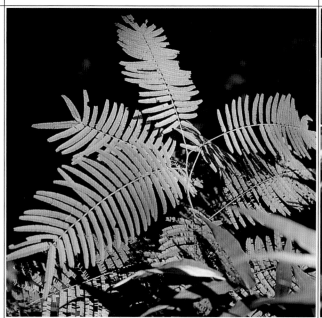

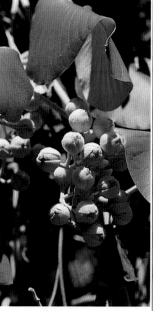

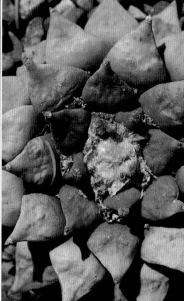

Anadenanthera peregrina is a mimosa-like tree, mainly of open grasslands, attaining a height of 65 ft (20 m) and with a trunk 2 ft (60 cm) in diameter. The blackish bark is coarsely armed with conical mucronate projections. The leaves have from 15 to 30 pairs of pinnae with many very small hairy leaflets. Many minute white flowers in spherical heads arranged in terminal or axillary clusters comprise the inflorescence. Flat, thin, glossy black, roundish seeds occur in rough, woody pods, from 3 to 10 in a pod.

A potent hallucinogenic snuff is made from the beans of *Anadenanthera peregrina* in the Orinoco basin, where it is called Yopo. Its former shamanic and ritual use in the West Indies, under the name Cohoba, was reported as early as 1496. Sadly, this use has disappeared due to the exploitation of the native people.

The tree native to the edges of the large forested areas of Guyana is still used by different tribes, primarily the Yanomano and Waika, for the production of Epená. The shamanic snuff is made from cultivated trees in addition to other substances and plant ashes. The seeds contain mostly *N,N*-Dimethyltryptamine (DMT) as well as 5-MeO-DMT and other tryptamines. The shaman of the rain forest people of the Orinoco region (for example, the Piaroa) cultivate this tree which is not native to that area. That way they secure their snuff supplies.

The mature stems of this vigorously growing twining bindweed climb up to 30 ft (10 m) high and carry a latexlike milk. The stemmed, heart-shaped leaves are finely haired and have a silvery appearance due to a dense white down that covers the young stems and the leaf undersides. The funnel-shaped flowers are violet or lavender and are carried in the leaf axis. Their sepals are finely haired. The round fruit are berrylike and contain smooth brown seeds. In each seed capsule there are 1–4 seeds.

The plant originates in India, where it has been used medicinally since ancient times. A traditional use as an entheogen has not yet been discovered. Phytochemical research is to thank for the awareness of its potent psychedelic constitution. The seeds contain 0.3 % Ergot alkaloids (ergine and lysergic-acid-amides). Most psychonauts describe LSD-like effects after taking 4–8 seeds.

These plants are small, grayish green to purplish gray or brownish cactuses, 4–6 in. (10–15 cm) in diameter. They hardly appear above the ground. Often called Living Rocks, they can easily be mistaken for rocks in the stony desert where they grow. Their horny or fleshy, umbricated, three-angled tubercles are characteristic of the genus. Dense masses of hair often fill the areoles. The flowers vary from white to pink and purplish and measure approximately 2¼ in. (6 cm) long and up to 1½ in. (4 cm) wide when fully open.

Indians in northern and central Mexico consider *A. fissuratus* and *A. retusus* as "false Peyotes."

These species of cactus, related to *Lophophora,* are typical desert plants, growing preferentially in the open sun in sandy or rocky stretches.

Several psychoactive phenylethylamine alkaloids have been isolated from *A. fissuratus* and *A. retusus.*

ATROPA L.   (4)

Atropa belladonna L.
Deadly Nightshade

Solanaceae
(Nightshade Family)

8   Europe, North Africa, Asia

BANISTERIOPSIS   (20–30)
C.B. Robinson et Small

Banisteriopsis caapi (Spruce ex Griseb.) Morton, Ayahuasca

Malpighiaceae
(Malpighia Family)

9   Tropical zones of northern South America, West Indies

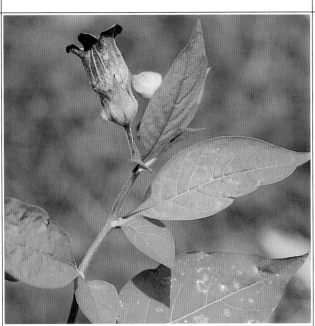

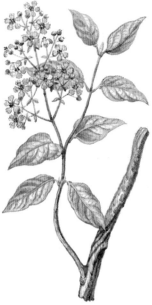

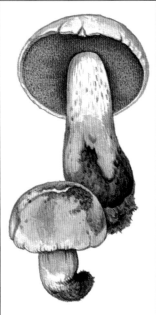

This much-branched perennial herb up to 3 ft (90 cm) tall may be glabrous or pubescent-glandular. The ovate leaves attain a length of 8 in. (20 cm). The solitary, drooping, bell-shaped, brown-purple flowers, approximately 1⅛ in. (3 cm) long, produce shiny black berries 1⅛–1½ in. (3–4 cm) in diameter. All parts of the plant contain potent alkaloids. It grows in thickets and woods on lime soils and is naturalized especially near old buildings and hedges.

It is believed that Belladonna figured as an important ingredient in many of the witches' brews of antiquity. There are, of course, numerous records of accidental and purposeful poisoning associated with the Deadly Nightshade.

This plant played a major role in the war of the Scots under Duncan I against the Norwegian king Sven Canute about A. D. 1035. The Scots destroyed the Scandinavian army by sending them food and beer to which "Sleepy Nightshade" had been added.

The main psychoactive constituent is atropine but lesser amounts of scopolamine and trace amounts of minor tropane alkaloids are also present. The total alkaloid content in the leaves is 0.4 %, in the roots 0.5 %, and in the seeds 0.8 %.

In addition to the usual Belladonna there is a rare, yellow blooming variety (var. *lutea*) as well as little known related kinds. The Indian Belladonna (*Atropa acuminata* Royle ex Lindl.) is cultivated for pharmaceutical purposes because of its high content of scopolamine. In Asia the Caucasian Belladonna (*Atropa caucasia* Kreyer) and the Turkmenish Belladonna (*Atropa komarovii* Blin. et Shal) are found. Belladonna is still cultivated for the pharmaceutical production of atropine.

These giant forest lianas are the basis of an important hallucinogenic drink (Ayahuasca) ritually consumed in the western half of the Amazon Valley and by isolated tribes on the Pacific slopes of the Colombian and Ecuadorean Andes. The bark of *Banisteriopsis caapi* and *B. inebrians,* prepared in cold water or after long boiling, may be taken alone, but various plant additives—especially the leaves of *Diplopteris cabrerana,* known as Oco-Yajé, and of *Psychotria viridis*—are often used to alter the effects of the hallucinogenic drink.

Both species are lianas with smooth, brown bark and dark green, chartaceous, ovate-lanceolate leaves up to about 7 in. (18 cm) in length, 2–3 in. (5–8 cm) wide. The inflorescence is many-flowered. The small flowers are pink or rose-colored. The fruit is a samara with wings about 1⅜ in. (3.5 cm) long. *B. inebrians* differs from *B. caapi* in its thicker ovate, more attenuate leaves and in the shape of the samara wings. The liana contains MAO inhibitors.

Several species of *Boletus* are involved in the curious "mushroom madness" of the Kuma of New Guinea. *Boletus reayi,* one of these, is characterized by a hemispherical, strong brownish red cap that is cream-yellow at the periphery; it measures from ¾ to 1½ in. (2 to 4 cm) in diameter. The flesh of the cap is lemon-colored. The stipe varies from orange at the top, to a marbled green and gray-rose in the middle, to a green at the base. The spores, which are elongated ellipsoidal, have a yellow membrane but are olive-colored within.

B. manicus is a well-known species that, as its name implies, has somewhat toxic properties, (*mania* = insanity). Hallucinogenic properties have not yet been proven.

BRUGMANSIA Pers.   (7–8)

Brugmansia aurea Lagerh.
Golden Angel's Trumpet

Solanaceae
(Nightshade Family)

11   Western South America

BRUGMANSIA Pers.   (9–10)

Brugmansia sanguinea
(Ruíz et Pavón) D. Don
Blood-Red Angel's Trumpet

Solanaceae
(Nightshade Family)

12   South America,
Colombia to Chile

BRUNFELSIA L.   (40)

Brunfelsia grandiflora D. Don
Brunfelsia

Solanaceae
(Nightshade Family)

13   Tropical zones of northern
South America, West Indies

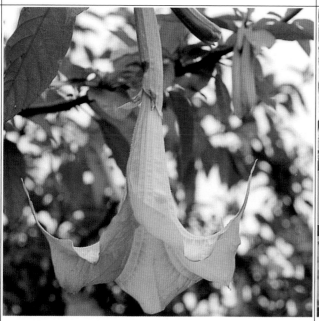

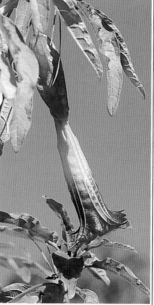

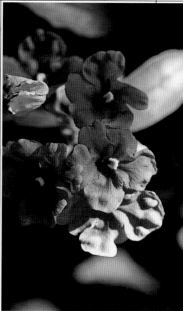

Closely related to *Datura,* the species of *Brugmansia* are arborescent, and it is suspected that they are all cultigens unknown in the wild. Biologically very complex, all species appear to have been used as hallucinogens for millennia. *Brugmansia suaveolens* and *B. insignis* occur in warmer parts of South America, especially in the western Amazonia, where they are employed alone or mixed with other plants, usually under the name Toé. Most of the species, however, prefer the cool, wet highlands above 6,000 ft. (1,830 m). The most widespread species in the Andes is *Brugmansia aurea,* with both yellow and, more commonly, white flower forms. In the horticultural literature it has frequently been misidentified as *Brugmansia* (or *Datura*) *arborea,* which is in reality a much less common plant. *Brugmansia aurea* is a shrub or small tree up to 30 ft (9 m) tall with oblong-elliptic, often minutely hairy leaves, the blade measuring 4–16 in. (10–40 cm) long, 2–6½ in.

(5–16 cm) wide, borne on a petiole up to 5 in. (13 cm) long. The flowers are nodding, not wholly pendulous, usually 7–9 in. (18–23 cm) long and very fragrant, especially in the evening. The trumpet-shaped corolla flaring broadly at the mouth is white or golden yellow, its slender basal part completely enclosed by the calyx, its teeth 1½–2½ in. (4–6 cm) long, recurving. The elongate-ovoid, smooth, green fruit, which is variable in size, remains fleshy, never becoming hard or woolly. The angular, blackish or brownish seeds are relatively large, measuring about ½ by ⅜ in. (12 by 9 mm). In addition to their use as hallucinogens, all species have played major roles as medicines for a large spectrum of ills, especially in the treatment of rheumatic pains. They contain potent hallucinogenic tropane alkaloids.

This perennial *Brugmansia* is heavily branched and reaches 6–16 ft (2–5 m), developing a very woody trunk. The gray-green leaves are furry and roughly serrated at the edge. The Blood-Red Angel's Trumpet does not emit scents in the night. Usually the flowers are green at the base, yellow in the middle, and have a red edge around the top. There are also green-red, pure yellow, yellow-red, and almost completely red varieties. The smooth oval fruits are bulbous in the center and pointed at the ends and are usually partially protected by the dried calyx. In Colombia this powerful shaman plant was ritually used in the cult of the sun of pre-Columbian times. The plant is still used as a hallucinogen by the shamans and Curanderos of Ecuador and Peru.

The entire plant contains tropane alkaloids. The flowers contain essentially atropine and only traces of scopolamine (hyoscine). In the seeds approximately 0.17% total alkaloids are present; of those, 78% are scopolamine.

Several species of *Brunfelsia* have medicinal and psychoactive roles in the Colombian, Ecuadorean, and Peruvian Amazon as well as in Guyana. Scopoletine has been found in *Brunfelsia,* but this compound is not known to be psychoactive.

B. chiricaspi and *B. grandiflora* are shrubs or small trees reaching a height of about 10 ft (3 m). The oblong or lanceolate leaves, measuring 2½–12 in. long (6–30 cm), are scattered along the branchlets. The flowers have a tubular corolla, longer than the bell-shaped calyx and measuring about 4–4¾ in. (10–12 cm) across, blue to violet, fading with age to white. *B. chiricaspi* differs from *B. grandiflora* in having much larger leaves, longer leaf stalks, a few-flowered inflorescence, and deflexed corolla lobes. *B. chiricaspi* occurs in the west Amazonia of Colombia, Ecuador, and Peru. *B. grandiflora* is wide-ranging in western South America from Venezuela to Bolivia. *Brunfelsias* serve as Ayahuasca additives.

CACALIA L. (50)	CAESALPINIA L. (100)	CALEA L. (95)	CANNABIS L. (3)
Cacalia cordifolia L. fil. Matwú	*Caesalpinia sepiaria* Roxb. Yün-Shih	*Calea zacatechichi* Schlecht. Dog Grass	*Cannabis sativa* L. Hemp
Compositae (Sunflower Family)	Leguminosae (Pea Family)	Compositae (Sunflower Family)	Cannabaceae (Hemp Family)
14 East Asia, North America, Mexico	**15** Tropical and warm zones of both hemispheres	**16** Tropical zones of northern South America, Mexico	**17** Warm-temperate zones, worldwide

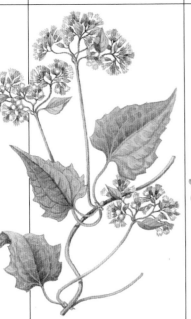

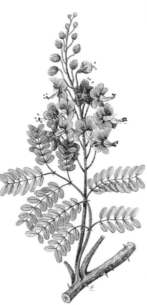

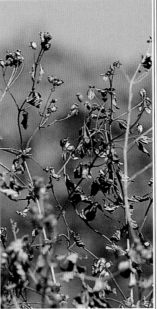

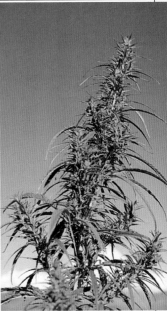

A small shrubby climber, *Cacalia cordifolia* has dusty-puberulent, six-angled stems. The leaves are thin, ovate, and basally cordate, 1½–3⅓ in. (4–9 cm) long. The flowering head is subsessile or pedicellate, about ⅜ in. (1 cm) long.

This and several other species of *Cacalia* have been referred to in parts of northern Mexico as Peyote and may possibly have once been employed for hallucinatory purposes. In Mexico *Cacalia cordifolia* is a presumed aphrodisiac and cure for sterility. An alkaloid has been reported from the plant, but there is no evidence of a chemical constituent with psychoactive properties.

This little researched plant is apparently often confused with *Calea zacatechichi*.

Caesalpinia sepiaria or Yün-Shih, a shrubby vine with retrorsely hooked spines, is reputedly used as a hallucinogen in China. The roots, flowers, and seeds also have value in folk medicine.

The earliest Chinese herbal—*Pen-ts'-ao-ching*—stated that the "flowers could enable one to see spirits and, when taken in excess, cause one to stagger madly." If consumed over a long period, they produce levitation and "communication with the spirits."

This plant is an extensive climber with pinnate leaves 9–15 in. (23–38 cm) long and linear-oblong leaflets in 8–12 pairs. The large, erect, unbranched showy racemes, 21 in. (53 cm) long, bear canary yellow flowers. The smooth, elongate-ovoid, pointed fruit has 4 to 8 ovoid, brown- and black-mottled seeds, ⅖ in. (1 cm) long. An alkaloid of unknown structure has been reported from *Caesalpinia sepiaria*.

Known in Mexico as Zacatechichi ("bitter grass"), this inconspicuous shrub, occurring from Mexico to Costa Rica, has been important in folk medicine. It has also been valued as an insecticide.

Recent reports suggest that the Chontal Indians of Oaxaca take a tea of the crushed, dried leaves as a hallucinogen. Believing in visions seen in dreams, Chontal medicine men, who assert that Zacatechichi clarifies the senses, call the plant Thle-pelakano, or "leaf of god."

Calea zacatechichi is a heavily branching shrub with triangular-ovate, coarsely toothed leaves ¾–2½ in. (2–6.5 cm) long. The inflorescence is densely many-flowered (usually about 12).

No constituent with hallucinatory properties has as yet been isolated from *C. zacatechichi*.

The plant contains germacranolides. The subtle psychoactive effect can be described as dreamlike.

Cannabis sativa has become very polymorphic, but it is usually a rank, robust, erect, loosely branched annual herb, sometimes attaining a height of 18 ft (5.4 m). The sexes are normally on separate plants, the staminate weaker and dying after shedding pollen, the pistillate stockier and more foliose. The membranaceous leaves are digitate, with 3 to 15 (usually 7 to 9) linear-lanceolate, serrated segments commonly 2¼–4 in. (6–10 cm) wide. The flowers are borne in axillary or terminal branches, dark green, yellow-green, or brownish purple. The fruit is an ovoid, slightly compressed, often brownish akene covered by a persistent calyx, enveloped by an enlarged bract, usually lacking a strong marbled pattern; it is firmly attached to the stalk without a definite articulation. The seed is ovoid, mostly ⅛ by ⅙ in. (4 by 2 mm).

Cannabis indica is pyramidal or conical in form and under 4–5 ft (120–150 cm) in height.

Cannabis ruderalis is small and is never cultivated.

CARNEGIEA Britt. et Rose (1)	CESTRUM L. (160)	CLAVICEPS Tulasne (6)	COLEUS Lour. (150)
Carnegiea gigantea (Engelm.) Britt. et Rose Saguaro Cactaceae (Cactus Family) **18** Southwestern North America, northern Mexico	*Cestrum parqui* L'Hérit. Lady of the Night Solanaceae (Nightshade Family) **19** Chile	*Claviceps purpurea* (Fr.) Tulasne Ergot Clavicipitaceae **20** Temperate zones of Europe, northern Africa, Asia, North America	*Coleus blumei* Benth. Painted Nettle Labiatae (Mint Family) **21** Tropical and warm zones of Europe, Africa, Asia

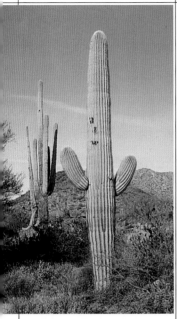 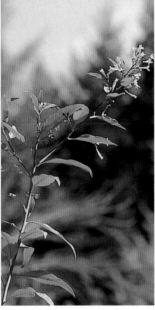 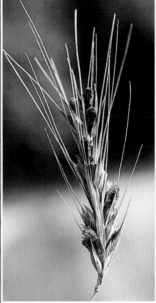 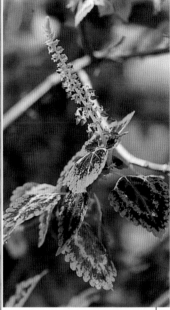

This largest of the columnar cactus plants, Saguaro, reaching a height of some 40 ft (12 m), is a candelabra-branched "tree." The many-ribbed stems and branches attain a diameter of 1–2½ ft (30–75 cm). The spines near the top of the plant are yellow-brown. Measuring 4–5 in. (10–13 cm) in length, the white, funnel-shaped flowers open during the day. The fruit, red or purple, is an ovoid or ellipsoid berry splitting down the side into two or three sections and measuring 2½–3½ in. (6–9 cm) long. The numerous small seeds are black and shining.

Although there are no reports of the Saguaro as a hallucinogen, the plant does contain pharmacologically active alkaloids capable of psychoactivity.

Carnegine, 5-hydroxycarnegine, and norcarnegine, plus trace amounts of 3-methoxytyramine and arizonine (a tetrahydroquinoline base), have been isolated from Saguaro.

The native people make a wine from the pressed fruit.

Cestrum parqui has been used medicinally and ritually for shamanic healing since pre-Columbian times by the Mapuche in southern Chile. The plant has the power to withstand attacks of sorcery or black magic. The dried leaves of *Cestrum parqui* are smoked.

The shrub grows to 5 ft (1.5 m) and has small, lanceolate matte green leaves. The bell-shaped yellow flowers have five pointy petals. They hang from the stem in clusters. The flowers bloom in Chile between October and November and release a powerful, heady aroma. The plant has small oval berries that are a shiny black color.

Cestrum parqui contains solasonine, a glycoside steroid-alkaloid, as well as solasonidine and a bitter alkaloid (Parquin's formula $C_{21}H_{39}NO_8$), which has a similar action to strychnine or atropine.

Ergot is a fungal disease of certain grasses and sedges, primarily of rye. Meaning "spur," Ergot refers to the sclerotium or fruiting body of an ascomycete or sac fungus. The spur is a purplish or black, curved, club-shaped growth ½–2½ in. (1–6 cm) long, which parasitically replaces the endosperm of the kernel. The fungus produces psychoactive and toxic alkaloids.

There are two distinct periods in the life cycle of this fungus: an active and a dormant stage. The Ergot or spur represents the dormant stage. When the spur falls to the ground, the Ergot sprouts globular heads called ascocarps from which grow asci, each with threadlike ascospores that are disseminated when the asci rupture.

In the Middle Ages and earlier in Europe, especially where rye was used in bread-making, whole areas frequently were poisoned, suffering plagues of ergotism, when fungus-infected rye kernels were milled into flour.

Two species of *Coleus* have significance in Mexico. Related to *Salvia divinorum* is La Hembra ("the woman"); *C. pumilus* is El Macho ("the man"); and two forms of *C. blumei* are El Nene ("the child") and El Ahijado ("the godson"). *C. blumei* attains a height of 3 ft (1 m) and has ovate, marginally toothed leaves up to 6 in. (15 cm) in length; the bottom surface is finely hairy, the upper surface usually with large dark red blotches. The more or less bell-shaped blue or purplish flowers, measuring about ½ in. (1 cm) long, are borne in long lax, whorled racemes up to 12 in. (30 cm) in length.

Recently, salvinorine-like substances (diterpene) were discovered. The chemical structure has not yet been determined. It is possible that by drying or burning the diterpene, its chemical structure is modified into potent material. The chemistry and pharmacology must be researched further.

CONOCYBE (40)	CORIARIA L. (15)	CORYPHANTHA (64) (Engelm.) Lem.	CYMBOPOGON Sprengel (60)
Conocybe siligineoides Heim Conocybe	*Coriara thymifolia* HBK ex Willd. Shanshi	*Coryphantha compacta* (Engelm.) Britt. et Rose Pincushion Cactus	*Cymbopogon densiflorus* Stapf Lemongrass
Agaricaceae (Bolbitiaceae) (Agaric Family)	Coriariaceae (Coriaria Family)	Cactaceae (Cactus Family)	Gramineae (Grass Family)
22 Cosmopolitan	**23** Southern Europe, northern Africa, Asia; New Zealand; Mexico to Chile	**24** Southwestern North America, Mexico, Cuba	**25** Warm zones of Africa and Asia

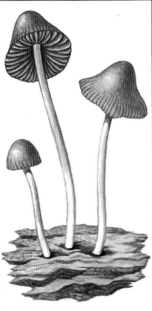

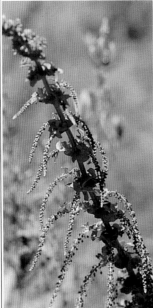

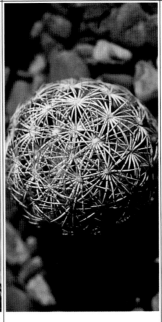

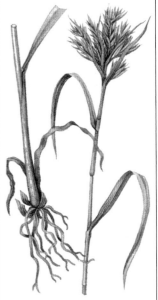

Conocybe siligineoides has been reported as one of the sacred intoxicating mushrooms of Mexico. Psilocybine has not as yet been isolated from this species, but *Conocybe cyanopus* of the United States has been shown to contain this psychoactive alkaloid.

This beautiful mushroom, up to about 3 in. (8 cm) tall, living on rotting wood, has a cap up to 1 in. (2.5 cm) in diameter that is fawn-orange-red, with a deeper orange at the center. The gills are saffron-colored or brownish orange with chrome yellow spores.

Many species of the genus *Conocybe* contain psilocybine, are psychoactive, and are used ritually. Recently a rudimentary cult around Tamu (a *Conocybe* species, "Mushroom of Awareness") has been discovered.

Conocybe siligeneoides is an obscure mushroom which has not been found or analyzed again since its first description.

In the highest Andes from Colombia to Chile, *Coriaria thymifolia* adorns the highways with its frondlike leaves. It has been feared in the Andean countries as a plant toxic to browsing animals. Human deaths have supposedly followed ingestion of the fruit. Reports from Ecuador, nevertheless, suggest that the fruit (shanshi) may be eaten to induce an intoxication characterized by sensations of soaring through the air.

Coriaria thymifolia is a shrub usually up to 6 ft (1.8 m) tall. The leaves are oblong-ovate, ½–¾ in. (1–2 cm) in length, borne on slender, arching lateral branches. The small, dark purple flowers occur densely on long drooping racemes. The round purplish black fruit is composed of five to eight compressed fleshy parts, or carpels. The whole shrub has a fernlike appearance.

No psychoactive properties have been isolated yet.

A small, solitary, globular but somewhat flattened, spiny cactus up to 3¼ in. (8 cm) in diameter, *Coryphantha compacta* grows in dry hilly and mountainous regions. It is hardly visible in the sandy soil where it occurs. The radial spines are whitish, ½–¾ in. (1–2 cm) in length; the central spines are usually absent. The crowded tubercles are arranged in 13 rows. Arising from the center of the crown either singly or in pairs, the yellow flowers measure up to 1 in. (2.5 cm) in length. The Tarahumara of northern Mexico consider *Coryphantha compacta* a kind of Peyote. The plant, called Bakana, is taken by shamans and is respected and feared. It is used as a substitute for Peyote.

Coryphantha palmerii has likewise been reported as a hallucinogen in Mexico. Various alkaloids, including the psychoactive phenylethylamines, have been isolated from several species of *Coryphantha*: hordenine, calipamine, and macromerine.

Native medicine men in Tanzania smoke the flowers of *Cymbopogon densiflorus* alone or with tobacco to cause dreams that they believe foretell the future. The leaves and rhizomes, pleasantly aromatic of citron, are locally used as a tonic and styptic.

This perennial grass has stout, erect culms with linear to linear-lanceolate leaves, basally wide and rounded and tapering to a fine point, 1 ft. (30 cm) in length and ½–1 in. (1–2 .5 cm) in width. The flowering spikes are slender, olive green to brownish. This species grows in Gabon, the Congo, and Malawi.

Little is known about the psychoactive properties of the grass. The genus *Cymbopogon* is rich in essential oils, and steroidal substances have been found in some species.

CYTISUS L. (30)	DATURA L. (14–16)	DATURA L. (14–16)	DATURA L. (14–16)

Cytisus canariensis (L.) O. Kuntze
Genista

Leguminosae (Pea Family)

26 Southern Europe, northern Africa, western Asia; Canary Islands, Mexico

Datura innoxia Mill. *(D. meteloides)*
Toloache

Solanaceae
(Nightshade Family)

27 Tropical and warm-temperature zones of both hemispheres

Datura metel L.
Datura

Solanaceae
(Nightshade Family)

28 Tropical and warm-temperate zones of Asia and Africa

Datura stramonium L.
Thorn Apple

Solanaceae
(Nightshade Family)

29 Tropical and moderate zones of both hemispheres

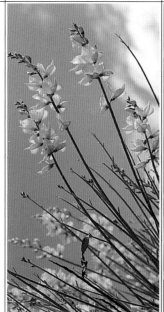 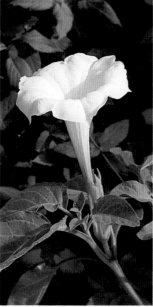 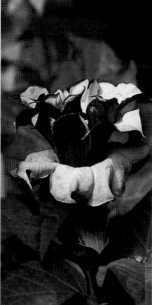 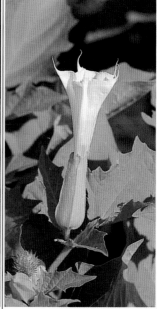

Rarely are foreign plants incorporated in ceremonial use in aboriginal American societies. Native to the Canary Islands, Genista was introduced into Mexico from the Old World, where it has no record of use as a hallucinogen. It apparently has acquired magical use among the Yaquí Indians of northern Mexico, where medicine men value the seed as a hallucinogen.

A coarse, evergreen, much-branched shrub up to 6 ft (1.8 m) tall, *Cytisus canariensis* bears leaves with obovate or oblong, hairy leaflets ¼–½ in. (.5–1 cm) long. The fragrant, bright yellow flowers, in terminal, many-flowered, dense racemes, measure about ½ in. (1 cm) in length. The pods are hairy, ½–¾ in. (1–2 cm) long.

Cytisus is rich in the lupine alkaloid cytisine, which is common in the Leguminosae. Cystine has similar properties as nicotine. For this reason, plants that contain cystine are often smoked as a substitute for Tobacco.

The most extensive use of *Datura* centers in Mexico and the American Southwest, where the most important psychoactive species seems to be *Datura innoxia*. This is the famous Toloache of Mexico, one of the plants of the gods among the Aztecs and other Indians. The modern Tarahumara of Mexico add the roots, seeds, and leaves of *D. innoxia* to tesquino, a ceremonial drink prepared from maize. Mexican Indians believe that, unlike Peyote, Toloache is inhabited by a malevolent spirit.

Datura innoxia is a herbaceous perennial up to 3 ft (1 m) tall, grayish because of fine hairs on the foliage; the leaves, unequally ovate, repand or subentire, measure up to 2 or 2¼ in. (5 cm) in length. The erect, sweet-scented flowers, 5½–9 in. (14–23 cm) long, are white with a 10-pointed corolla. The pendant fruit is nearly globose, 2 in. (5 cm) in diameter, covered with sharp spines.

In the Old World, the most culturally important species of *Datura* for medicinal and hallucinogenic use is *D. metel*.

Datura metel, native probably to the mountainous regions of Pakistan or Afghanistan westward, is a spreading herb, sometimes becoming shrubby, 3–6 ft (1–2 m) tall. The triangular-ovate, sinuate, and deeply toothed leaves measure 5½–8½ in. (14–22 cm) long, 3–4¼ in. (8–11 cm) wide. The solitary flowers, which may be purple, yellowish, or white, are tubular, funnel- or trumpet-shaped, almost circular when expanded, may attain a length of 6½ in. (17 cm). The drooping, round fruit, up to 2¼ in. (6 cm) in diameter, is conspicuously tuberculate or muricate, opening to expose flat, light brown seeds. The flowers are primarily violet and grow at an angle or upright to the sky.

All types of *Datura* contain the hallucinogenic tropane alkaloids scopolamine, hyosyamine and someatropine.

This annual herb grows to about 4 ft (1.2 m) and has many-forked branches and branched, leafless stems. The rich green leaves are coarsely serrated. The funnel-shaped flowers are 5-pointed, stand erect, and open upward. The common variety carries white flowers that at 2–3 in. (6–9 cm) long are among the smallest of the *Datura* species. The *tatula* variety has smaller violet flowers. The green egg-shaped fruit is covered with thorns and stands erect. The flat, liver-shaped seeds are black.

The origins of this powerful hallucinogenic species of Thorn Apple is uncertain and its botanical history ardently argued over. Some authors suggest that *Datura stramonium* is an ancient species that originates in the region of the Caspian Sea. Others believe that Mexico or North America is the original habitat. Today the herb is found throughout North, Central, and South America; North Africa; Central and Southern Europe; in the near East; and in the Himalayas.

DESFONTAINIA R. et P. (1–3)	DUBOISIA R. Br. (3)	ECHINOCEREUS Engelm. (75)	EPITHELANTHA Weber (3) ex Britt. et Rose
Desfontainia spinosa R. et P. Taique	*Duboisia hopwoodii* F. v. Muell. Pituri Bush	*Echinocereus triglochidiatus* Engelm. Pitallito Cactus	*Epithelantha micromeris* (Engelm.) Weber ex Britt. et Rose Hikuli Mulato
Desfontainiaceae	Solanaceae (Nightshade Family)	Cactaceae (Cactus Family)	Cactaceae (Cactus Family)
30 Highlands of Central America and South America	**31** Central Australia	**32** Southwestern North America, Mexico	**33** Southwestern North America, Mexico

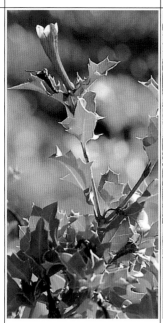 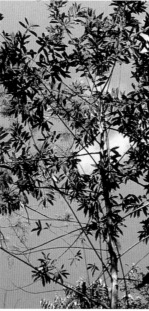 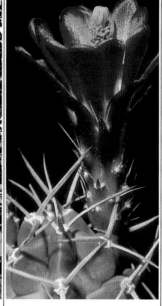 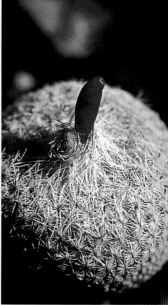

One of the least-known Andean plants, *Desfontainia spinosa* is sometimes assigned to a different family: Loganiaceae or Potaliaceae. Botanists are not in agreement as to the number of species in the genus.

Desfontainia spinosa, a beautiful shrub 1–6 ft (30 cm-1.8 m) in height, has glossy green leaves, resembling those of Christmas holly, and tubular red flowers with a yellow tip. The berry is white or greenish yellow, globose, with many lustrous seeds. It has been reported as a hallucinogen from Chile and southern Colombia. In Chile it is known as Taique, in Colombia as Borrachero ("intoxicator").

Colombian shamans of the Kamsá tribe take a tea of the leaves to diagnose disease or "to dream." Some medicine men assert that they "go crazy" under its influence. Nothing is as yet known of the chemical constituents of *Desfontainia*.

In southern Chile *Desfontainia* is used for shamanic purposes similar to *Latua pubiflora*.

The branched evergreen shrub with woody stems grows to approximately 6–9 ft (2.5–3 m). Its wood has a yellow color and a distinct scent of vanilla. The green leaves are lanceolate, with a continuous margin tapered at the petiole and are 4–5 in. long (12–15 cm). The flowers are white, occasionally with rose speckles, and bell-shaped (to 7 mm long) and hang in clusters off the tips of the branches. The fruit is a black berry with numerous tiny seeds.

The psychoactive Pituri has been hedonistically and ritually used by the Aborigines since their settlement of Australia. The leaves are gathered in August when the plants are in flower. They are hung up to dry or roasted over a fire. They are either chewed as Pituri or smoked in cigarettes rolled with alkaline substances.

Duboisia hopwoodii contains a variety of powerful and stimulating but toxic alkaloids: piturine, dubosine, D-nor-nicotine, and nicotine. The hallucinogenic tropane alkaloids hyoscyamine and scopolamine have been discovered in the roots.

The Tarahumara Indians of Chihuahua consider two species as false Peyotes or Hikuri of the mountainous areas. They are not so strong as *Ariocarpus, Coryphantha, Epithelantha, Mammillaria,* or *Lophophora. Echinocereus salmdyckianus* is a low, caespitose cactus with decumbent, yellow-green stems ¾–1½ in. (2–4 cm) in diameter. The ribs number 7 to 9. The 8 or 9 radial spines are yellow, ½ in. (1 cm) long, central spine solitary and longer than radials. The orange-colored flowers measure 3¼–4 in. (8–10 cm) long and have oblanceolate to spathulate perianth segments. This species is native to Chihuahua and Durango in Mexico. *Echinocereus triglochidiatus* differs in having deep green stems, fewer radial spines, which turn grayish with age, and scarlet flowers 2–2¾ in. (5–7 cm) long.

A tryptamine derivative has been reported from *Echinocereus triglochidiatus* (3-hydroxy-4-methoxyphenethylamine).

This spiny cactus, one of the so-called false Peyotes of the Tarahumara Indians of Chihuahua, has acidic, edible fruit called Chilitos. Medicine men take Hikuli Mulato to make their sight clearer and to permit them to commune with sorcerers. It is taken by runners as a stimulant and "protector," and the Indians believe that it prolongs life. It is reportedly able to drive evil people to insanity or throw them from cliffs.

Alkaloids and triterpenes have been reported from *Epithelantha micromeris*. This very small, globular cactus grows to a diameter of 2½ in. (6 cm). The low tubercles, 1/16 in. (2 mm) long, are arranged in many spirals. The numerous white spines almost hide the tubercles. The lower radial spines measure 1/16 in. (2 mm) long, the upper about 3/8 in. (1 cm). The small flowers, which arise from the center of the plant in a tuft of wool and spines, are whitish to pink, ¼ in. (5 mm) broad. The clavate fruit, 3/8–½ in. (9–13 mm) long, bears rather large, shining black seeds, 1/16 in. (2 mm) across.

ERYTHRINA L. (110)	GALBULIMIMA F. M. Bailey (3)	HEIMIA Link et Otto (3)	HELICHRYSUM Mill (500)
Erythrina americana Mill. Coral Tree	*Galbulimima belgraveana* (F. v. Muell.) Sprague Agara	*Heimia salicifolia* (H.B.K.) Link et Otto Sinicuichi	*Helichrysum* (L.) Moench. Straw Flower
Leguminosae (Pea Family)	Himantandraceae	Lythraceae (Loosestrife Family)	Compositae (Sunflower Family)
34 Tropical and warm zones of both hemispheres	**35** Northeast Australia, Malaysia	**36** Southern North America to Argentina, West Indies	**37** Europe, Africa, Asia, Australia

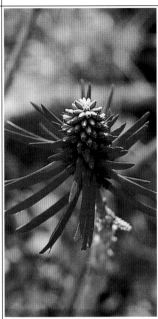

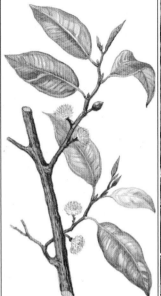

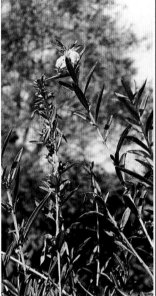

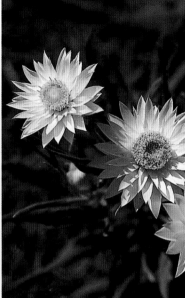

Tzompanquahuitl of the ancient Aztecs may have been from the many species in the genus *Erythrina*, the seeds of which are believed to have been employed as a medicine and hallucinogen. In Guatemala the beans are employed in divination.

The beans of *Erythrina flabelliformis* constitute a Tarahumara Indian medicinal plant of many varied uses, which may have been utilized as a hallucinogen.

Erythrina flabelliformis is a shrub or small tree with spiny branches. The leaflets are 2½– 3½ in. (3–6 cm) long, usually broader than long. The densely many-flowered racemes bear red flowers 1⅕–2½ in. (3–6 cm) long. Sometimes attaining a length of 1 ft (30 cm), the pods, shallowly constricted between the seeds, contain from two to many dark red beans. This species is common in the hot, dry regions of northern and central Mexico and the American Southwest.

Natives in Papua boil the bark and leaves of this tree with a species of *Homalomena* to prepare a tea that causes an intoxication leading to a deep slumber, during which visions are experienced.

This tree of northeastern Australia, Papua, and Molucca is unbuttressed, attaining a height of 90 ft (27 m). The highly aromatic, gray brownish, scaly bark measures ½ in. (1 cm) in thickness. The elliptic, entire leaves are a glossy, metallic green above, brown beneath, and are normally 4½–6 in. (11– 15 cm) long and 2–2¾ in. (5– 7 cm) wide. Lacking sepals and petals but with many conspicuous stamens, the flowers have a pale yellow or brownish yellow hue with a rusty brown calyx. The ellipsoidal or globose fruit is fleshy-fibrous, reddish, ¾ in. (2 cm) in diameter.

Although 28 alkaloids have been isolated from *Galbulimima belgraveana*, a psychoactive principle has not yet been found in the plant.

This genus has three very similar species, and all play important roles in folk medicine. Several vernacular names reported from Brazil seem to indicate knowledge of psychoactivity, e. g., Abre-o-sol ("sun-opener") and Herva da Vida ("herb of life").

Sinicuichi *(Heimia salicifolia)* is 2–6 ft (60 cm-1.8 m) tall with lanceolate leaves ¾–3½ in. (2– 9 cm) long. The yellow flowers are borne singly in the leaf axils; the persistent bell-shaped calyx develops long hornlike appendages. The shrub grows abundantly in moist places and along streams in the highlands.

In the Mexican highlands, the leaves of *H. salicifolia* are slightly wilted, crushed in water, and the preparation is then allowed to ferment into an intoxicating drink. Although it is believed that excessive use of Sinicuichi may be physically harmful, there are usually no uncomfortable aftereffects. This plant contains quinolizidine alkaloids (lythrine, cryogenine, lyfoline, nesidine).

Two species are used by witch doctors in Zululand "for inhaling to induce trances." It is presumed that the plants are smoked for these effects.

Helichrysum foetidum is a tall, erect, branching herb 10–12 in. (25–30 cm) in height. It is slightly woody near the base and is very strongly scented. The lanceolate or lanceolate-ovate, basally lobed, entire leaves, measuring up to 3½ in. (9 cm) long and ¾ in. (2 cm) wide, basally enclasp the stem; they are graywoolly beneath and glandular above. The flowers occur in loose, terminal, corymbose clusters of several stalked heads ¾–1½ in. (2–4 cm) in diameter, subtended by cream-colored or golden yellow bracts. These species of *Helichrysum* are some of the plants known in English as Everlasting.

Coumarine and diterpenes have been reported from the genus, but no constituents with hallucinogenic properties have been isolated.

HELICOSTYLIS Trécul (12)	HOMALOMENA Schott (142)	HYOSCYAMUS L. (10–20)	HYOSCYAMUS L. (20)

Helicostylis pedunculata
Benoist
Takini

Moraceae (Mulberry Family)

38 Central America, tropical zones of South America

Homalomena lauterbachii Engl.
Ereriba

Araceae (Arum Family)

39 South America, tropical zones of Asia

Hyoscyamus albus L.
Yellow Henbane

Solanaceae
(Nightshade Family)

40 Mediterranean, Near East

Hyoscyamus niger L.
Black Henbane

Solanaceae
(Nightshade Family)

41 Europe, northern Africa, southwestern and central Asia

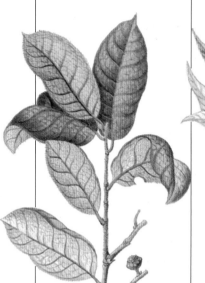

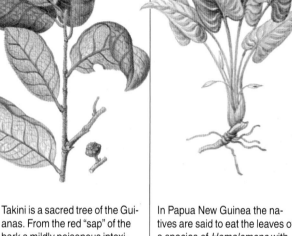

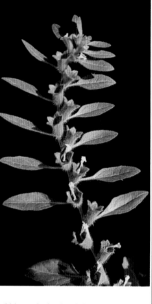

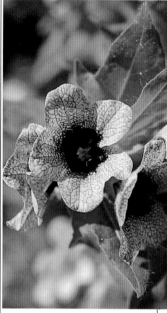

Takini is a sacred tree of the Guianas. From the red "sap" of the bark a mildly poisonous intoxicant is prepared. Extracts from the inner bark of two trees elicit central nervous system depressant effects similar to those produced by *Cannabis sativa*. The two species responsible for this hallucinogen are *H. pedunculata* and *H. tomentosa*.

These two species of trees are similar. Both are cylindrical or very slightly buttressed forest giants 75 ft (23 m) tall with grayish brown bark; the latex is pale yellow or cream-colored. The leathery lanceolate-elliptic leaves attain a length of 7 in. (18 cm) and a width of 3 in. (8 cm). The fleshy, pistillate flowers are borne in globose cauliflorous heads.

Very little is known about these trees and they are rarely studied. The hallucinogen could theoretically originate from either of the related genera *Brosimum* or *Piratinera*. Extracts from the inner bark of both trees have been pharmacologically studied; they have a softening or dampening effect, similar to *Cannabis sativa*.

In Papua New Guinea the natives are said to eat the leaves of a species of *Homalomena* with the leaves and bark of *Galbulimima belgraveana* to induce a violent condition ending in slumber, during which visions are experienced. The rhizomes have a number of uses in folk medicine, especially for the treatment of skin problems. In Malaya an unspecified part of a species was an ingredient of an arrow poison.

The species of *Homalomena* are small or large herbs with pleasantly aromatic rhizomes. The leaves are oblong-lanceolate or cordate-ovate, borne on very short stems, rarely exceeding 6 in. (15 cm) in length. The spathe usually persists in fruit. The male and female portions of the spadix are proximate. The small berries are few or many-seeded.

The chemistry of this group of plants has not yet disclosed any hallucinogenic principle.

Although the herb has erect stems, it often appears bushy. It grows to approximately 8–12 in. (40–50 cm) high. The light green stems and serrated leaves, as well as the funnel-shaped flowers and fruits, are all pileous. The herb blooms from January to July. The color of the flowers is light yellow with deep violet on the interior. The seeds have a whitish or ocher color, occasionally a gray color.

This henbane was the most widely used magical herb and medicinal plant. The hallucinogen was an important medium in antiquity, used to promote a trance and taken by oracles and divinitory women. In the ancient earth oracle of Gaia, it is the "dragon's herb." The goddess of the witches, Hecate, uses "crazy-maker" in the Kolch oracle. Late antiquity gives us "Zeus's Beans" in the oracle of Zeus-Ammon and the Roman god Jupiter. In the Delphi oracles of Apollo, who is the God of "prophetic insanity," it is known as "Apollo's Plant."

The entire plant contains the tropane alkaloids hyoscyamine and scopolamine.

Henbane is a coarse annual or biennial, viscid, hairy, strong-smelling herb up to about 30 in. (76 cm) tall. The leaves are entire or occasionally have a few large teeth, ovate, 6–8 in. (15–20 cm) long, the lower cauline amplexicaul leaves being oblong and smaller. The flowers, yellow or greenish yellow veined with purple, attain a length of about 1½ in. (4 cm) and are borne in two ranks in a scorpioid cyme. The fruit is a many-seeded capsule enclosed in the persistent calyx with its five triangular points becoming rigid. The seeds release a powerful and distinctive odor when squeezed.

In antiquity and the Middle Ages, *Hyoscyamus niger* was employed in Europe as an important ingredient of the witches' brews and ointments. It not only reduced pain but also induced oblivion.

The active principles in this solanaceous genus are tropane alkaloids, especially scopolamine. Scopolamine is a potent hallucinogenic agent.

44

IOCHROMA Benth. (24)	IPOMOEA L. (500)	JUSTICIA L. (350)
Iochroma fuchsioides (Benth.) Miers Paguando	*Ipomoea violacea* L. Morning Glory	*Justicia pectoralis* Jacq. var. *stenophylla* Leonard Mashihiri
Solanaceae (Nightshade Family)	Convolvulaceae (Morning Glory Family)	Acanthaceae (Acanthus Family)
42 Tropical and subtropical zones of South America	**43** Mexico to South America	**44** Tropical and warm zones of Central and South America

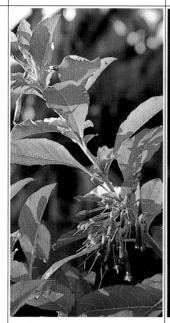

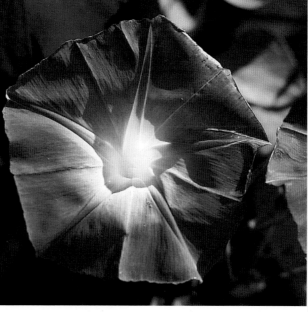

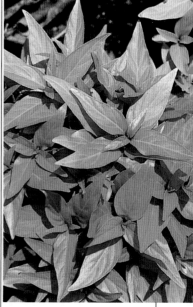

Among the Kamsá Indians of the Colombian Andes, *I. fuchsioides* is taken by shamans for difficult diagnoses.

The intoxication is not pleasant, leaving aftereffects for several days. The shrub is valued also as a medicine for treating difficulties with digestion or bowel function, and to aid in cases of difficult childbirth.

Iochroma fuchsioides, a shrub or small tree 10–15 ft (3–4.5 m) tall, but sometimes larger, occurs in the Colombian and Ecuadorean Andes at about 7,000 ft (2,200 m) altitude. The branches are reddish brown, and the leaves, obovate-oblong, measure 4–6 in. (10–15 cm) in length. The clustered tubular or bell-shaped flowers are red, 1–1½ in. (2.5–4 cm) long. The red fruit is an ovoid or pyriform berry about ¾ in. (2 cm) in diameter, partially enclosed in a persistent calyx.

The plant contains withanolide.

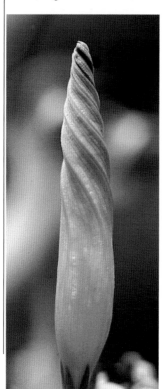

In Oaxaca, in southern Mexico, the seeds of this vine are esteemed as one of the principal hallucinogens for use in divination as well as magico-religious and curing rituals. The Chinan-tec and Mazatec Indians call the seeds Piule; the Zapotecs, Ba-doh Negro. In pre-Conquest days, the Aztecs knew them as Tlililtzin and employed them in the same way as Ololiuqui, the seeds of another Morning Glory, *Turbina corymbosa*.

Ipomoea violacea, known also as *I. rubrocaerulea,* is an annual vine with entire, ovate, deeply cordate leaves 2½–4 in. (6–10 cm) long, ¾–3 in. (2–8 cm) wide. The inflorescence is three- or four-flowered. The flowers vary from white to red, purple, blue or violet-blue, and measure 2–2¾ in. (5–7 cm) wide at the mouth of the trumpet-shaped, corolla tube, 2–2¾ in. (5–7 cm) long. The ovoid fruit, about ½ in. (1 cm) in length, bears elongate, angular black seeds.

This variable species ranges through western and southern Mexico and Guatemala and in the West Indies. It can be found as well in tropical South America. It is well known in horticulture.

Justicia pectoralis var. *stenophylla* differs from the widespread *J. pectoralis* mainly in its smaller stature and its very narrowly lanceolate leaves and shorter inflorescence. It is an herb up to 1 ft (30 cm) tall, with erect or ascending stems, sometimes rooting at the lower nodes. The internodes are short, usually less than ¾ in. (2 cm) long. The numerous leaves measure normally ¾–2¼ in. (2–5 cm) long, ⅜–1 in. (1–2 cm) wide. The dense inflorescence, covered with glandular hairs, may reach a length of 4 in. (10 cm) but is usually much shorter. The inconspicuous flowers, about ¼ in. (5 mm) long, are white or violet, frequently purple-spotted. The fruit, ¼ in. (5 mm) long, bears flat, reddish brown seeds.

Chemical examination of *Justicia* has been inconclusive. Preliminary indications that the leaves of *J. pectoralis* var. *stenophylla* contain tryptamines (DMT) need confirmation. The dried herb contains coumarin.

45

KAEMPFERIA L. (70)	LAGOCHILUS Bunge (35)	LATUA Phil. (1)	LEONOTIS (pers.) R. Br. (3–4)
Kaempferia galanga L. Galanga	*Lagochilus inebrians* Bunge Turkestan Mint	*Latua pubiflora* (Griseb.) Baill. Latúe	*Leonotis leonurus* (L.) R. Br. Lion's Tail
Zingiberaceae (Ginger Family)	Labiatae (Mint Family)	Solanaceae (Nightshade Family)	Labiatae (Mint Family)
45 Tropical zones of Africa, southeastern Asia	**46** Central Asia	**47** Chile	**48** South Africa

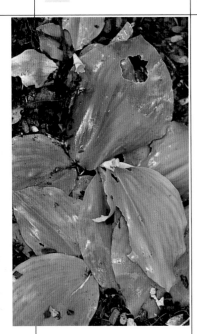

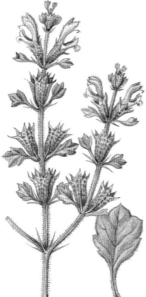

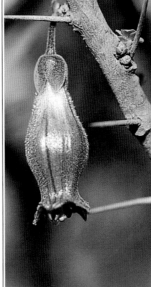

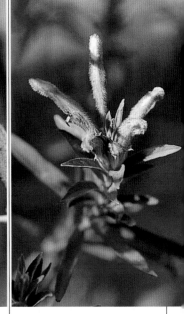

Kaempferia galanga is used as a hallucinogen in New Guinea. Throughout the range of this species, the highly aromatic rhizome is valued as a spice to flavor rice, and also in folk medicine as an expectorant and carminative as well as an aphrodisiac. A tea of the leaves is employed for sore throat, swellings, rheumatism, and eye infections. In Malaysia, the plant was added to the arrow poison prepared from *Antiaris toxicaria*.

This short-stemmed herb has flat-spreading, green, round leaves measuring 3–6 in. (8–15 cm) across. The white flowers (with a purple spot on the lip), which are fugacious, appear singly in the center of the plant and attain approximately 1 in. (2.5 cm) in breadth.

Beyond the high content of essential oil in the rhizome, little is known of the chemistry of the plant. Psychoactive activity might possibly be due to constituents of the essential oils.

On the dry steppes of Turkestan, the Tajik, Tatar, Turkoman, and Uzbek tribesmen have used a tea made from the toasted leaves of the mint *Lagochilus inebrians* as an intoxicant. The leaves are frequently mixed with stems, fruiting tops, and flowers, and honey and sugar may occasionally be added to lessen the intense bitterness of the drink.

This plant has been well studied from the pharmacological point of view in Russia. It is recommended for its antihemorrhagic and hemostatic effects to reduce permeability of blood vessels and as an aid in blood coagulation. It has also been considered helpful in treating certain allergies and skin problems. It has sedative properties.

Phytochemical studies have shown the presence of a crystalline compound called lagochiline—a diterpene of the grindelian type.
This compound is not known to be hallucinogenic.

Latua, 6–30 ft (2–9 m) tall, has one or more main trunks. The bark is reddish to grayish brown. The spiny branches, rigid and 1 in. (2.5 cm) long, arise in the leaf axils. The narrow elliptic leaves, dark to light green above, paler beneath, are marginally entire or serrate and measure 1⅜–1¾ in. (3½–4½ cm) by ⅝–1½ in. (1.5–4 cm). The flowers have a persistent, bell-shaped, green to purplish calyx and a larger, magenta to red-violet, urceolate corolla 1⅜–1½ in. (3.5–4 cm) long, ½ in. (1 cm) wide at the mouth. The fruit is a globose berry about 1 in. (2.5 cm) in diameter, with numerous kidney-shaped seeds.

The leaves and fruit of *L. pubiflora* contain 0.18 % hyoscyamine and atropine and 0.08 % scopolamine

This South African shrub has orange-colored flowers and is reported to be "hallucinogenic." In Africa it is called Dacha, Daggha, or Wild Dagga, which means "wild hemp." The Hottentots and the Bush people smoke the buds and the leaves as a narcotic. It is possible that this plant is one of the narcotic plants called Kanna (compare to *Sceletium tortuosum*). The resinous leaves, or the resin extracted from the leaves, are smoked alone or mixed with tobacco. Chemical studies are lacking.

In California the plant has been grown and tested, revealing a bitter-tasting smoke and a lightly psychoactive effect that is reminiscent of both *Cannabis* and *Datura*. In eastern South Africa, the closely related *Leonotis ovata* is reportedly used for the same purpose.

LEONURUS L. (5–6)	LOBELIA L. (250)	LOPHOPHORA Coult. (2)
Leonurus sibiricus L. Siberian Motherwort	*Lobelia tupa* L. Tabaco del Diablo	*Lophophora williamsii* (Lem.) Coult. Peyote
Labiatae (Mint Family)	Campanulaceae (Lobeliaceae) (Harebell Family)	Cactaceae (Cactus Family)
49 Siberia to East Asia, Central and South America (naturalized)	**50** Tropical and warm zones	**51** Mexico, Texas

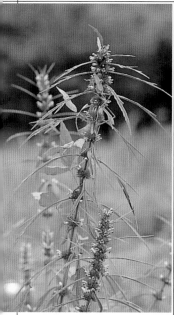

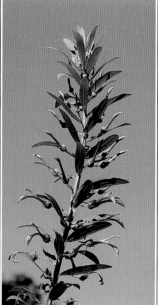

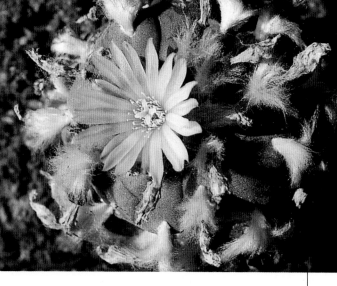

This herb grows erect and tall, reaching over 6 ft (2 m) often on a single stem. It has maxilliform branches and finely serrated, dark green leaves. The violet flowers appear on the ends of each stem and the inflorescence can be long and attractive.

The Siberian Motherwort is mentioned in the ancient Chinese *Shih Ching* (the Book of Songs, written approximately 1000–500 B.C.), where it is called *t'uei*. Later it was occasionally praised as a medicinal plant in old Chinese herbals.

The dried leaves, harvested from the flowering plant, are smoked as marijuana substitute in Central and South America (1–2 g per cigarette).
In the plant, 0.1 % of the flavonoid glycoside rutin has been ascertained. Of particular interest with regard to the psychoactive properties was the discovery of three new diterpenes: leosibiricine, leosibirine, and the isomers isoleosibiricine in essential oil.

This beautiful, red- or red-purple-flowered, 6–9 ft (2–3 m) high polymorphic *Lobelia* is well recognized as toxic in the Andes of southern Peru and northern Chile, where it is called Tupa or Tabaco del Diablo ("devil's tobacco"). It flourishes in dry soil, and its stems and roots have a white latex that irritates the skin.

The luxuriant foliage clothes nearly the whole length of the plant with grayish green, elliptic, often minutely hairy leaves 4–9 in. (10–23 cm) long. 1¼–3¼ in. (3–8 cm) wide. Carmine red or purple, the flowers, 1½ in. (4 cm) in length, are borne densely on a stalk 14 in. (36 cm) long. The corolla is decurved, sometimes recurved with the lobes united at the apex.

Tupa leaves contain the piperidine alkaloid lobeline, a respiratory stimulant, as well as the diketo- and dihydroxy-derivatives lobelamidine and nor-lobedamidine. These constituents are not known to possess hallucinogenic properties. Nevertheless, the smoked leaves have a psychoactive effect.

Two species of *Lophophora* are recognized: they differ morphologically and chemically.

Both species of *Lophophora* are small, spineless gray-green or bluish green top-shaped plants. The succulent chlorophyll-bearing head or crown measures up to 3¾ in. (8 cm) in diameter and is radially divided in from 5 to 13 rounded ribs. Each tubercle bears a small, flat areole from the top of which arises a tuft of hairs ¾ in. (2 cm) long. The whitish or pinkish campanulate, usually solitary, ⅝–1 in. (1.5–2.5 cm) long flowers are borne in the umbilicate center of the crown.

The Indians cut off the crown and dry it for ingestion as a hallucinogen. This dry, disklike head is known as the Mescal Button or Peyote Button.
Lophophora williamsii is usually blue-green with from 5 to 13 ribs and normally straight furrows. It has up to 30 alkaloids—primarily Mescaline—as well as further psychoactive phenylethylamines and isoquinolines. *L. diffusa* has a gray-green, sometimes even a rather yellowish green crown with indefinite ribs and sinuate furrows. The flowers are usually much larger than in *L. williamsii*. The chemical constitution is much simpler.

Both species of *Lophophora* inhabit the driest and stoniest of desert regions, usually on calcareous soil. When the crown is removed, the plant will often grow new crowns and thus Peyotes with multiple heads are commonly seen. The hallucinogenic effects of Peyote are strong, with kaleidoscopic, richly colored visions. The other senses—hearing, feeling, taste—can also be affected. There are reportedly two stages in the intoxication. At first, a period of contentment and sensitivity occurs. The second phase brings great calm and muscular sluggishness, with a shift in attention from external stimuli to introspection and meditation.

LYCOPERDON L. (50–100)	MAMMILLARIA Haw. (150–200)	MANDRAGORA L. (6)
Lycoperdon mixtecorum Heim *Lycoperdon marginatum* Vitt. Bovista	*Mammillaria* spp. Pincushion Cactus	*Mandragora officinarum* L. Mandrake
Lycoperdaceae (Club Moss Family)	Cactaceae (Cactus Family)	Solanaceae (Nightshade Family)
52 Temperate zones of Mexico	**53** Southwestern North America, Central America	**54** Southern Europe, northern Africa, western Asia to Himalayas

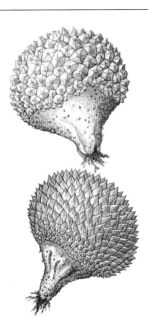

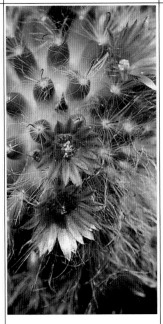

Probably no plant has had a more fantastic history than the Mandrake. As a magical plant and hallucinogen, its extraordinary place in European folklore can nowhere be equaled. Known for its toxic and real and presumed medicinal properties, Mandrake commanded the fear and respect of Europeans throughout the Middle Ages and earlier. Its folk uses and attributes were inextricably bound up with the Doctrine of Signatures, because of its anthropomorphic root.

While there are six species of *Mandragora,* it is *M. officinarum* of Europe and the Near East that has played the most important role as a hallucinogen in magic and witchcraft. It is a stemless perennial herb up to 1 ft (30 cm) high, with a thick, usually forking root and large, stalked, wrinkled, ovate leaves, marginally entire or toothed and measuring up to 11 in. (28 cm) in length. The whitish green, purplish, or bluish bell-shaped flowers, 1¼ in. (3 cm) in length, are borne in clusters among the tufted leaves. The globose or ovoid, succulent yellow berry has a delightful fragrance.

The total content of tropane alkaloids in the root is 0.4 %. The principal alkaloids are hyoscyamine and scopolamine, but atropine, cuscohygrine, or mandragorine is also present.

In northern Mexico, among the Tarahumara of Chihuahua, a species of *Lycoperdon,* known as Kalamoto, is taken by sorcerers to enable them to approach people without being detected and to make people sick. In southern Mexico, the Mixtecs of Oaxaca employ two species to induce a condition of half-sleep, during which it is said that voices and echoes can be heard.

Lycoperdon mixtecorum, known only from Oaxaca, is small, attaining a diameter of no more than 1¼ in. (3 cm). It is subglobose, somewhat flattened, abruptly constricted into a peduncle scarcely ⅛ in. (3 mm) long. The exterior surface is densely cobbled-pustuliform and light tan in color. The interior substance is straw colored.

The spherical spores, brownish tawny with a subtle tinge of violet, measure up to 10 μ. This terrestrial species grows in light forest and in pastures.

Psychoactive constituents have not yet been isolated.

Among the most important "false Peyotes" of the Tarahumara Indians are several species of *Mammillaria,* all of them round and stout-spined plants.

N-methyl-3,4-dimethoxy-phenylethylamine has been isolated from *M. heyderii,* a species closely related to *M. craigii.* Hordenine is present in many species.

Mammillaria craigii is globose but apically somewhat flattened with conical, angled tubercles about ½ in. (1 cm) long and axils and areoles at first woolly; the central spines are about ¼ in. (5 mm) long. The rose-colored flower attains a length of ⅝ in. (1.5 cm). *M. grahamii* may be globose or cylindric, 2½ in. (6 cm) in diameter with small tubercles and naked axils; the central spines are ¾ in. (2 cm) or less in length. The flowers, which attain a length of 1 in. (2.5 cm), have violet or purplish segments, sometimes with white margins.

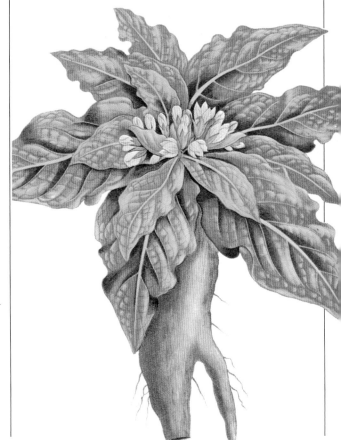

MAQUIRA Aubl. (2)	MIMOSA L. (500)	MITRAGYNA Korth. (20–30)

Maquira sclerophylla (Ducke) C. C. Berg Rapé dos Indios	*Mimosa hostilis* (Mart.) Benth. *(Mimosa tenuiflora)* Jurema Tree	*Mitragyna speciosa* Korthals Kratom
Moraceae (Mulberry Family)	Leguminosae (Pea Family)	Rubiaceae (Madder Family)
55 Tropical zones of South America	**56** Mexico and Brazil	**57** Southeast Asia (Thailand, northern Malay Peninsula to Borneo, New Guinea)

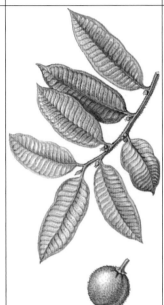
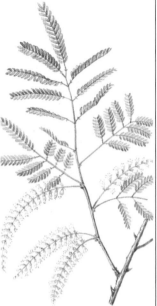
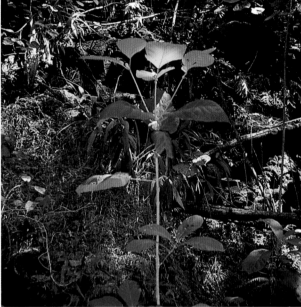

In the Pariana region of the Brazilian Amazon, the Indians formerly prepared a potent hallucinogenic snuff that, although no longer prepared and used, is known as Rapé dos Indios ("Indian snuff"). It is believed to have been made from the fruit of an enormous forest tree, *Maquira sclerophylla* (known also as *Olmedioperebea sclerophylla*).

Maquira sclerophylla attains a height of 75–100 ft (23–30 m). The latex is white. Very thick and heavy, the ovate or oblong-ovate, marginally inrolled leaves are 8–12 in. (20–30 cm) long, 3–6½ in. (8–16 cm) wide. The male flowering heads are globose, up to about ½ in. (1 cm) in diameter; the female inflorescences are borne in the leaf axils and have one or rarely two flowers. The drupe or fruit, cinnamon-colored and fragrant, is globose, ¾–1 in. (2–2.5 cm) in diameter. The tree contains cardiac glycosides.

In the dry *caatingas* of eastern Brazil, this busy, sparsely spiny treelet flourishes abundantly. The spines are basally swollen, ⅛ in. (3 mm) long. Its finely pinnate leaves are 1¼–1¾ in. (3–5 cm) long. The flowers, which occur in loosely cylindrical spikes, are white and fragrant. The legume or pod, about 1–1¼ in. (2.5–3 cm) long, breaks into 4–6 sections. An alkaloid was isolated from the root of this treelet and called nigerine. It was later shown to be identical with the hallucinogenic N,N-dimethyltryptamine.

Several species of *Mimosa* are called Jurema in eastern Brazil. *M. hostilis* is often known as Jurema Prêta ("black jurema"). It is identical to the Mexican Tepescohuite *(M. tenuiflora)*. The related *M. verrucosa*, from the bark of which a stupefacient is said to be derived, is frequently called Jurema Branca ("white jurema").

The tropical tree or shrub grows in marshy areas. Often it grows only to 6–9 ft (3–4 m) high, occasionally to 36–42 ft (12–16 m). It has an erect stem with forked branches that grow obliquely upward. The green oval leaves (8–12 cm) are very broad and become narrower toward the tip, which is pointed. The flowers are deep yellow and hang in globular clusters. The seeds are winged.

The dried leaves are smoked, chewed, or worked into an extract called Kratom or Mambog.

The psychoactive properties of kratom are paradoxical. Personal research, the descriptions of it in the literature, as well as the pharmacological characteristics of the material have revealed kratom to be simultaneously stimulating like cocaine and soothing like morphine. The stimulating effects begin within 5 to 10 minutes of chewing the fresh leaves.

As early as the 19th century the use of Kratom as an opium substitute and a curative for opium addiction was reported. There are numerous indole alkaloids present in the plant. The primary constituent is mitragynine, which is apparently easily tolerated and shows barely any toxicity even in high doses.

MUCUNA Adans. (120)	MYRISTICA Gronov. (120)	NYMPHAEA L. (50)	ONCIDIUM Sw. (350)

Mucuna pruriens (L.) DC.
Cowhage

Leguminosae (Pea Family)

58 Tropical and warm zones of both hemispheres

Myristica fragrans Houtt.
Nutmeg

Myristicaceae (Nutmeg Family)

59 Tropical and warm zones of Europe, Africa, Asia

Nymphaea ampla (Salisb.) DC.
Water Lily
Nymphaeaceae
(Water Lily Family)

60 Temperate and warm zones of both hemispheres

Oncidium cebolleta (Jacq.) Sw.
Hikuri Orchid

Orchidaceae (Orchid Family)

61 Central America, South America, Florida

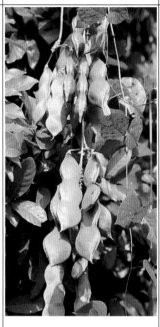
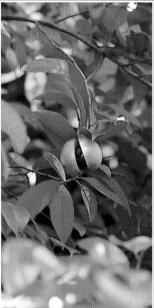
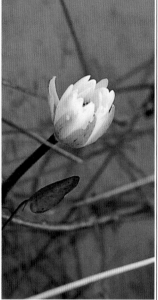
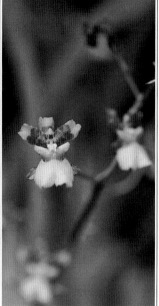

Mucuna pruriens has not been reported as a hallucinogen, but the plant has been chemically shown to be rich in psychoactive constituents (DMT, 5-MeO-DMT).

This stout, scandent herb, with acute angulate stems, has three-foliolate leaves. The leaflets, oblong or ovate, are densely hairy on both surfaces. The dark purple or bluish flowers, ¾–1¼ in. (2–3 cm) long, are borne in short hanging racemes. The pods, with long, stiff, stinging hairs, measure about 1½–3½ in. (4–9 cm) long, ½ in. (1 cm) thick.

The total indole alkylamine content was studied from the point of view of its hallucinogenic activity. It was found that marked behavioral changes occurred that could be equated with hallucinogenic activity. It is possible that Indian peoples may have discovered and utilized some of these psychoactive properties of *M. pruriens*. The powdered seeds are considered aphrodisiac in India. The seeds contain DMT and are used as an Ayahuasca analog today.

Nutmeg and mace can, in large doses, induce an intoxication characterized by space and time distortion, a feeling of detachment from reality, and visual and auditory hallucinations. Frequently with unpleasant effects such as severe headache, dizziness, nausea, tachycardia, nutmeg intoxication is variable.

Myristica fragrans is a handsome tree, unknown in a truly wild state, but widely cultivated for nutmeg, from the seed, and for mace, from the red aril surrounding the seed. The two spices have different tastes because of differing concentrations of components of their essential oils. The aromatic fraction of oil of nutmeg is made up of nine components belonging to the groups terpenes and aromatic ethers. The major component—myristicine—is a terpene, but its biological activity is believed to be that of an irritant.

The psychotropic activity is thought to be due primarily to aromatic ethers (myristicine and others).

There is evidence that *Nymphaea* may have been employed as a hallucinogen in both the Old and New Worlds. The isolation of the psychoactive apomorphine has offered chemical support to this speculation. Nuciferine and nornuciferine are also isolated from *N. ampla*.

Nymphaea ampla has thickish dentate leaves, purple beneath, measuring 5½–11 in. (14–28 cm) across. The beautiful, showy white flowers, with 30–190 yellow stamens, become 3–5¼ in. (7–13 cm) across at maturity. The Egyptian native *N. caerulea*'s oval, peltate leaves, irregularly dentate, measure 5–6 in. (12–15 cm) in diameter and are green-purple blotched beneath. The light blue flowers, dull white in the center, open three days in the midmorning; they measure 3–6 in. (7.5–15 cm) across; the petals, acute-lanceolate, number 14 to 20, while the stamens number 50 or more.

Oncidium cebolleta is an epiphytic orchid that grows on steep, stone cliffs and trees in the Tarahumara Indian country of Mexico. It is employed as a temporary surrogate of Peyote or Hikuri *(Lophophora williamsii)*. Little is known, however, of its use.

The tropical orchid is widely distributed in the New World. The pseudo-bulbs appear as little more than a swelling at the base of the fleshy, erect, round leaves, grayish green, often spotted with purple. The flowering spike, often arching, has a green stalk with purplish or purple-brown spots. The flowers have brownish yellow sepals and petals spotted with dark brown blotches. The three-lobed lip, ¾ in. (2 cm) long by 1⅛ in. (3 cm) across the mid-lobe, is bright yellow with reddish brown marks.

An alkaloid has been reported from *Oncidium cebolleta*.

PACHYCEREUS (A. Berger) (5) Britt. et Rose	PANAEOLUS (Fr.) (20–60) Quélet	PANAEOLUS (Fr.) (20–60) Quélet
Pachycereus pecten-aboriginum (Engelm.) Britt. et Rose Cawe	*Panaeolus cyanescens* Berk. et Br. Blue Meanies	*Panaeolus sphinctrinus* (Fr.) Quélet Hoop-petticoat
Cactaceae (Cactus Family) **62** Mexico	Coprinaceae **63** Warm zones of both hemispheres	Coprinaceae **64** Cosmopolitan

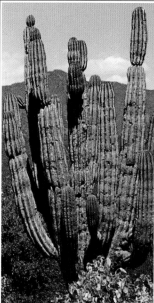 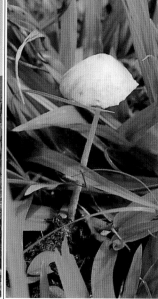 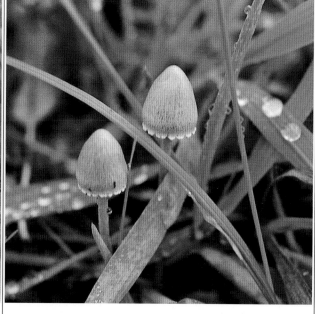

A plant of many uses among the Indians, this tall, treelike columnar cactus, arising from a 6 ft (1.8 m) trunk, attains a height of 35 ft (10.5 m). The short spines are characteristically gray with black tips. The 2–3 in. (5–8 cm) flowers are purplish in the outermost petals, white in the inner parts. The fruit, globose and measuring 2½–3 in. (6–8 cm) in diameter, is densely covered with yellow wool and long yellow bristles.

The Tarahumara, who know the plant as Cawe and Wichowaka, take a drink made from the juice of the young branches as a narcotic. It causes dizziness and visual hallucinations. The term *Wichowaka* also means "insanity" in the Tarahumara language. There are a number of purely medicinal uses of this cactus. Recent studies have isolated 4-hydroxy-3-methoxyphenylethylamine and 4-tetrahydroisoquinoline alkaloids from this plant.

Panaeolus cyanescens is a small, fleshy or nearly membranaceous, campanulate mushroom. The slender stipe is fragile and the lamellae are variegated, with metuloid colored, pointed cystidia on the sides. The spores are black. The fruiting bodies take on bluish flecks with age or after bruising.

The islanders of Bali pick *Panaeolus cyanescens* from cow and water buffalo dung and ingest them for celebrations and artistic inspiration. The mushroom is also sold as a hallucinogen to strangers as they pass through on their travels.

Although this mushroom is primarily tropical, the discovery that it contains psilocybine was made with material collected in a garden in France. Up to 1.2% of psilocine and 0.6% of psilocybine has been found in this species.

One of the sacred hallucinogenic mushrooms employed in divination and other magic ceremonies in northeastern Oaxaca, Mexico, among the Mazatec and Chinantec Indians is this member of the small genus *Panaeolus*. It is known in Mazatec as T-ha-na-sa, She-to, and To-shka. *She-to* means "pasture mushroom" and *To-shka,* "intoxicating mushroom." While not so important as the several species of *Psilocybe* and *Stropharia, P. sphinctrinus* is on occasion used by certain shamans. This and other species of *Panaeolus* have been reported to contain the hallucinogenic alkaloid psilocybine.

Growing on cow dung in forests, open fields, and along roads, *P. sphinctrinus* is a delicate yellowish brown mushroom up to 4 in. (10 cm) in height. It has an ovoid-campanulate, obtusely pointed, tan-gray cap up to 1¼ in. (3 cm) in diameter. The stipe is dark grayish. The dark brownish black gills bear black, lemon-shaped spores that vary in size; they can measure 12 to 15 by 7.5 to 8.3 µ.

The flesh is thin, in color similar to the surface, with scarcely any odor. Several investigators have at times argued that *P. sphinctrinus* is not among the hallucinogenic mushrooms used by shamans in Indian communities of Oaxaca, but this view is contradicted by ample evidence. Its use by Oaxacan Indians along with so many other mushroom species demonstrates the tendency among shamans to use a surprisingly wide range of different mushrooms, depending on season, weather variation, and specific usage. Investigators now believe that there may be more species and genera of mushrooms in use among Mexican Indian populations than those now known.

In European *Panaeolus sphinctrinus* no psilocybine has been detected. Neither have psychoactive effects been determined in human pharmacological experiments. It is possible that chemically different types exist.

PANAEOLUS (Fr.) (20–60) Quélet	PANCRATIUM L. (15)	PANDANUS L. fil. (600)	PEGANUM L. (6)
Panaeolus subbalteatus Berk. et Broome Dark-rimmed Mottlegill	*Pancratium trianthum* Herbert Kwashi	*Pandanus* sp. Screw Pine	*Peganum harmala* L. Syrian Rue
Coprinaceae	Amaryllidaceae (Amaryllis Family)	Pandanaceae (Screwpine Family)	Zygophyllaceae (Caltrop Family)
65 Eurasia, North and Central America	**66** Tropical and warm zones of Africa and Asia	**67** Tropical and warm zones of Europe, Africa, Asia	**68** Western Asia to northern India; Mongolia, Manchuria

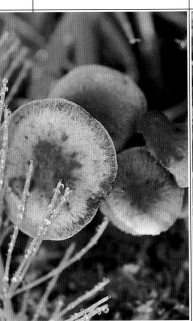

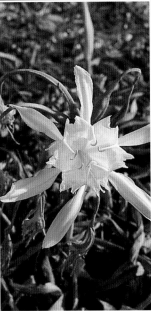

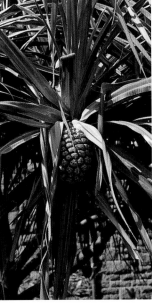

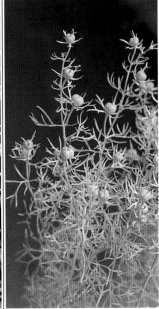

The Dark-rimmed Mottlegill is widely distributed throughout Europe. It grows in dung-fertilized, grassy earth, in particular in horse pastures and in conjunction with horse manure. The cap is ¾–2⅜ in. (2–6 cm) wide and somewhat smooth. This mushroom spreads rapidly. It is at first damp brown and grows drier toward the middle, so that the edge often appears markedly darker. The red-brown lamellae are curved and eventually become black due to the spores.

There is no information passed on about a traditional use of this mushroom. It is possible that it was an ingredient in the mead or beer of the Germans. Nevertheless, this mushroom has a symbiotic relationship with the horse, the sacred animal of the German god of ecstasy, Wodan.

The fruiting body contains 0.7% psilocybine as well as 0.46% baeocystine, a fair amount of serotonine and also 5-hydroxy-tryptophane, but no psilocine. Activity is experienced with 1.5 g dried mushroom; 2.7 g are visionary.

Many of the 15 species of this plant are potent cardiac poisons; others are emetics; one is said to cause death by paralysis of the central nervous system. *P. trianthum* is reputedly one of the most toxic species.

Little is known of the use of *Pancratium trianthum*. In Dobe, Botswana, the Bushmen reportedly value the plant as a hallucinogen, rubbing the sliced bulb over cuts made in the scalp. In tropical west Africa, *P. trianthum* seems to be religiously important.

The species of *Pancratium* have tunicated bulbs and linear leaves, mostly appearing with the flowers. The white or greenish white flowers, borne in an umbel terminating in an erect, solid, stout scape, have a funnel-shaped perianth with a long tube and narrow segments. The stamens, located at the throat of the perianth, are joined together at the base into a kind of cup. The seeds are angled and black.

In the bulb of *P. trianthum* the alkaloids lycorine and hordenine have been detected.

Natives of New Guinea employ the fruit of a species of *Pandanus* for hallucinogenic purposes, but little is known of this use.

Dimethyltryptamine has been isolated and identified in *Pandanus* nuts. *Pandanus* is a very large genus of the Old World tropics. It is dioecious, treelike, sometimes climbing, with prominent flying-buttress- or stiltlike roots. The leaves of some species attain a length of 15 ft (4.5 m) and are used for matting: they are commonly long, stiff, swordlike, armed with prickles, hooked forward and backward. The naked flowers occur in large heads enclosed in spathes. The aggregate fruit or syncarpium, is a large, heavy, hard, composite ball-like, orconelike mass comprising the union of the angled, easily detachable carpels. Most species of *Pandanus* occur along the seacoast or in salt marshes. The fruits of some species are used as food in Southeast Asia.

The Syrian Rue is an herb native to desert areas. It is a bushy shrub attaining a height of 3 ft (1 m). The leaves are cut into narrowly linear segments, and the small white flowers occur in the axils of branches. The globose, deeply lobed fruit contains many flat, angled seeds of a brown color, bitter taste, and narcotic odor. The plant possesses psychoactive principles: β-carboline alkaloids—harmine, harmaline, tetrahydroharmine—and related bases known to occur in at least eight families of higher plants. These constituents are found in *Peganum harmala* in the seeds.

The high esteem that *P. harmala* enjoys in folk medicine wherever the plant occurs may indicate a former semisacred use as a hallucinogen in native religion and magic. It has recently been postulated that *P. harmala* may have been the source of Soma or Huoma of the ancient peoples of Persia and India.

PELECYPHORA Ehrenb. (2)	PERNETTYA (20) Gaud.-Beaup.	PETUNIA Juss. (40)	PEUCEDANUM L. (125)
Pelecyphora aselliformis Ehrenb. Peyotillo	*Pernettya furens* (Hook. ex DC.) Klotzch Hierba Loca	*Petunia violacea* Lindl. Shanin	*Peucedanum japonicum* Thunb. Fang-K'uei
Cactaceae (Cactus Family)	Ericaceae (Heath Family)	Solanaceae (Nightshade Family)	Umbelliferae (Parsley Family)
69 Mexico	**70** Mexico to the Andes; Galápagos and Falkland Islands; New Zealand	**71** Warm zones of North America, South America	**72** Temperate zones of Europe, southern Africa, Asia

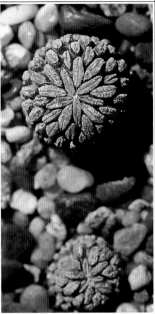

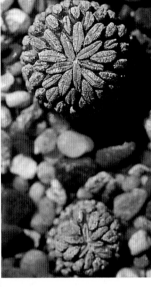

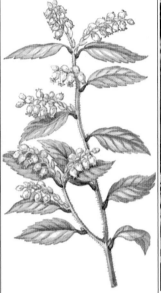

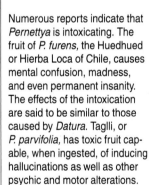

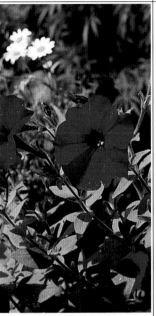

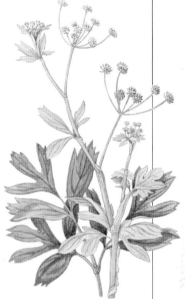

There are suspicions that this round cactus may be valued in Mexico as a "false Peyote." It is locally known as Peyote and Peyotillo.

A beautiful cactus, *P. aselliformis* is a solitary, gray-green, tufted, cylindric-conical plant 1–2½ in. (2.5–6.5 cm), although rarely up to 4 in. (10 cm) in diameter. The laterally flattened tubercles are spiraled, not arranged on ribs, and bear very small, scalelike, pectinate spines. The apical bell-shaped flowers measure up to 1¼ in. (3 cm) in width; the outer segments are white, the inner red-violet.

Recent investigations have indicated the presence of alkaloids, mescaline among others. When consumed, the cactus has a similar effect to Peyote.

Numerous reports indicate that *Pernettya* is intoxicating. The fruit of *P. furens,* the Huedhued or Hierba Loca of Chile, causes mental confusion, madness, and even permanent insanity. The effects of the intoxication are said to be similar to those caused by *Datura*. Taglli, or *P. parvifolia,* has toxic fruit capable, when ingested, of inducing hallucinations as well as other psychic and motor alterations.

It has been suggested that *Pernettya* was employed by aboriginal peoples as a magico-religious hallucinogen.

These two species of *Pernettya* are small, sprawling to suberect shrubs with densely leafy branches. The flowers are white to rose-tinted. The berrylike fruit is white to purple.

A recent report from highland Ecuador has indicated that a species of *Petunia* is valued as a hallucinogen. It is called Shanin in Ecuador. Which group of Indians employs it, what species, and how it is prepared for use are not known. It is said to induce a feeling of levitation or of soaring through the air, a typical characteristic of many kinds of hallucinogenic intoxications.

Most of the cultivated types of *Petunia* are hybrids derived from the purple-flowered *Petunia violacea* and the white *Petunia axillaris*. These species are native to southern South America.

Phytochemical studies of the horticulturally important genus *Petunia* are lacking, but as a solanaceous group allied to *Nicotiana*—the tobaccos—it may well contain biologically active principles.

Peucedanum japonicum is a stout perennial, blue-green herb with thick roots and short rhizomes. The solid, fibrous stems attain a length of 20–40 in. (0.5–1 m). The thick leaves are 8–24 in. (20–61 cm) long, twice or thrice ternate with obovate-cuneate leaflets 1¼–2½ in. (3–6 cm) long. The flowers are borne in umbellate clusters. The 10 to 20 rays are ¾–1¼ in. (2–3 cm) long. The ellipsoid fruit is minutely hairy, 1½–2 in. (3.5–5 cm) long. This plant is common on sandy places near seashores.

The root of Fang-K'uei is employed medicinally in China as an eliminative, diuretic, tussic, and sedative. Although thought to be rather deleterious, it may, with prolonged use, have tonic effects.

Alkaloidal constituents have been reported from *Peucedanum*. Coumarin and furocoumarin are widespread in the genus and occur in *P. japonicum*.

PHALARIS L. (10)	PHRAGMITES Adans. (1)	PHYTOLACCA L. (36)	PSILOCYBE (Fr.) Quélet (180)

Phalaris arundinacea L. Red Canary Grass	*Phragmites australis* (Cav.) Trin. ex Steud. Common Reed	*Phytolacca acinosa* Roxb. Pokeberry	*Psilocybe cubensis* (Earle) Sing. San Isidro
Graminaea (Grass Family)	Gramineae (Grass Family)	Phytolaccaceae	Strophariaceae
73 Cosmopolitan	**74** Cosmopolitan	**75** Tropical and warm zones of both hemispheres	**76** Nearly cosmopolitan in the tropics

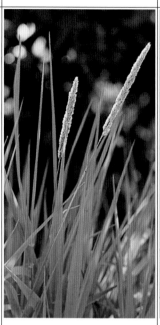

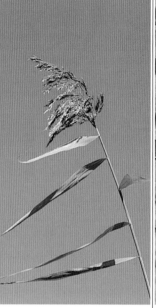

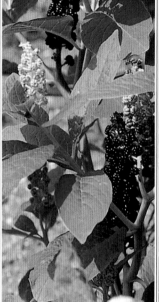

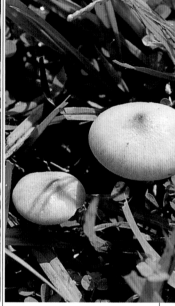

This perennial grass has grayish green stalks that grow to 6 ft (2 m) and can be split lengthwise. The long, broad leaves have rough edges. The panicle can take on a light green or red-violet coloration. The calyx holds one flower.

The Red Canary Grass was known already in antiquity. Thus far, no traditional use of *Phalaris arundinacea* as a psychoactive substance is known.

The psychoactive constituents of *Phalaris* were first noticed by a phytochemical study on grasses done for agricultural purposes. It is possible that in the past few years "cellar shamans" might have been experimenting with a possible psychoactive use for the grass in Ayahuasca analogs and DMT extracts.

The entire grass contains indole alkaloids, which are highly variable according to their species, tribe, position, and harvest. In most, DMT, MMT, and 5-MeO-DMT are to be found. The grass can also contain high concentrations of gramine, an extremely toxic alkaloid.

The Common Reed, the largest grass in Central Europe, often grows in harbors. It has a thick, many-branched rhizome. The stalks are 3–9 ft (1–3 m) high; the leaves have rough edges and grow up to 16–20 in. (40–50 cm) long and ¼–¾ in. (1–2 cm) wide. The very long panicle, 6–16 in. (15–40 cm) long, has many dark purple flowers. It flowers from July to September. Seeds mature in winter, at which point the leaves drop and the panicle turns white.

The Common Reed had many uses in ancient Egypt, particularly as fibrous material. Traditional use for psychoactive purposes has been documented, only as a fermented ingredient in a beerlike drink.

The rootstalk contains DMT, 5-MeO-DMT, bufotenine, and gramine. Reports concerning psychoactive properties are primarily from experiences with an Ayahuasca analog made from an extract of the roots, lemon juice, and the seeds of *Peganum harmala*. Unpleasant side effects such as nausea, vomiting, and diarrhea have been described.

Phytolacca acinosa is a glabrous perennial with robust, branching green stems up to 3 ft (91 cm) in length. The elliptic leaves average about 4¾ in. (12 cm) long. The white flowers, about ⅜ in. (1 cm) in diameter, are borne on densely flowered racemes 4 in. (10 cm) in length. The purple-black, berrylike fruit bears small black kidney-shaped seeds ⅛ in. (3 mm) long.

A well-known *Phytolacca* in China, Shang-lu exists in two forms: one with white flowers and a white root and one with red flowers and a purplish root. The latter type is considered to be highly toxic, although the former is cultivated as a food. The flowers—Ch'ang-hau'—are esteemed for treating apoplexy. The root is so poisonous that it is normally used only externally.

Phytolacca acinosa is high in saponines and the sap of the fresh leaves has been reported to have antiviral properties.

This mushroom, known in Oaxaca as Hongo de San Isidro, is an important hallucinogen, although it should be noted that not all shamans will use it. The Mazatec name is Di-shi-tjo-le-rra-ja ("divine mushroom of manure").

The mushroom may attain a height of 1¾–3 in. (4–8 cm), very rarely up to 5¾ in. (15 cm). The cap, usually ¾–2 in. (2–5 cm) in diameter (rarely larger), is conic-campanulate, at first especially papillose, then becoming convex to plane. It is golden yellow, pale tan to whitish near the margin; in age or upon injury, it may become cyanaceous. The stipe is hollow, usually thickened at the base, white but yellowing or becoming ashy red, and strongly lined. The gills vary from whitish to deep gray-violet or purple-brown. The ellipsoid spores are purple-brown.

The active principle in *Psilocybe cubensis* is psilocybine.

54

PSILOCYBE (Fr.) Quélet (180)	PSILOCYBE (Fr.) Quélet (180)	PSILOCYBE (Fr.) Quélet (180)	PSYCHOTRIA L. (1200–1400)

Psilocybe cyanescens Wakefield emend. Kriegelsteiner
Wavy Cap
Strophariaceae

77 North America, Central Europe

Psilocybe mexicana Heim
Teonanácatl
Strophariaceae

78 Nearly cosmopolitan

Psilocybe semilanceata (Fr.) Quélet
Liberty Cap
Strophariaceae

79 Cosmopolitan, except Mexico

Psychotria viridis Ruíz et Pavón
Chacruna
Rubiaceae (Madder Family)

80 Amazonia—from Colombia to Bolivia and eastern Brazil

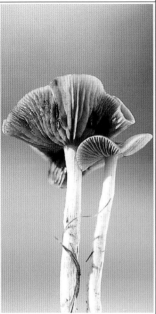
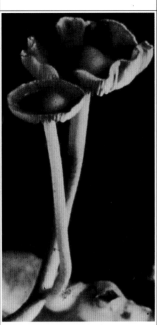
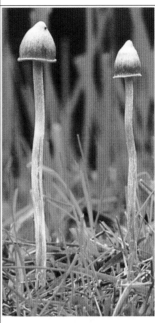
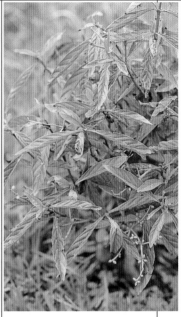

Psilocybe cyanescens is relatively easy to identify by its wavy brown cap ¾–1⅝ in. (2–4 cm) wide. It doesn't live on dung, but on decaying plants, coniferous mulch, and humus-rich earth. In older mushroom guides it is often called *Hyphaloma cyanescens*. It is very closely related to the species *Psilocybe azurescens* and *Psilocybe bohemica*, both also very powerful hallucinogens.

A traditional or shamanic use of this highly potent *Psilocybe* has not yet been documented.

Today, *Psilocybe cyanescens* is used in Central Europe and North America in neo-pagan rituals. In addition, cultivated mushrooms that have a very high concentration of psilocybine are eaten. Visionary doses are 1 g of the dried mushroom, which contains approximately 1 % tryptamine (psilocybine, psilocine, and baeocystine).

Many species of *Psilocybe* are employed in southern Mexico as sacred mushrooms, *P. mexicana* being one of the most widely used.

P. mexicana grows at altitudes of 4,500–5,500 ft (1,375–1,675 m), especially in limestone regions, isolated or very sparsely in moss along trails, in wet meadows and fields, and in oak and pine forests. One of the smallest of the hallucinogenic species, it attains a height of 1– (rarely) 4 in. (2.5–10 cm). The conic campanulate or frequently hemispherical cap, ¼–1⅓ in. (1–3 cm) in diameter, is a weak straw color or greenish straw color (sometimes even brownish red) when living, drying to a greenish tan or deep yellow; it has brown striations, and the terminal nipple is often reddish. The flesh of the cap turns bluish on bruising. The hollow stipe is yellow to yellowish pink, red-brown near the base. The spores are deep sepia to dark purple-brown.

Psilocybe semilanceata is the most common and widespread mushroom in the *Psilocybe* genus. The Liberty Cap prefers to grow in fields with old manure piles and on grassy, fertile meadows. Its cap, ⅜–1 in. (1–2.5 cm) wide, is conical and often peaked. It usually feels damp and slimy. The "head skin" is easy to peel off. The small lamels are olive to red-brown; the spores are dark brown or purple-brown.

P. semilanceata contains high concentrations of psilocybine (0.97 % up to 1.34 %), some psilocine, and less baeocystine (0.33 %). This species is one of the most potent *Psilocybe* mushrooms.

Toward the end of the Middle Ages in Spain, *P. semilanceata* was probably used as a hallucinogen by women who were accused of being witches. Allegedly the nomads of the Alps named *P. semilanceata* the "dream mushroom" and traditionally used it as a psychoactive substance. Today this mushroom is ritually taken in certain circles.

The evergreen shrub can grow into a small tree with a woody trunk, but usually remains at a height of 6–9 ft (2–3 m). Its whorled leaves are long and narrow with a color ranging from light green to dark green and a shiny top side. The flowers have greenish white petals on long stalks. The red fruit is a berry that contains numerous small long oval seeds, about 1 in. (4 mm) long.

The leaves must be gathered in the morning. They are used either fresh or dried in the production of Ayahuasca. Today they are also used as an Ayahuasca analog.

The leaves contain 0.1–0.61 % DMT, as well as traces of similar alkaloids (MMT, MTHC); most of the leaves contain around 0.3 % DMT.

RHYNCHOSIA Lour. (300)	SALVIA L. (700)	SCELETIUM (1000)	SCIRPUS L. (300)
Rhynchosia phaseoloides DC. Piule	*Salvia divinorum* Epl. et Játiva-M. Diviner's Sage	*Sceletium tortuosum* L. Kougued	*Scirpus atrovirens* Willd. Bakana
Leguminosae (Pea Family)	Labiatae (Mint Family)	Aizoaceae (Carpetweed Family)	Cyperaceae (Sedge Family)
81 Tropical and warm zones of both hemispheres	**82** Oaxaca, Mexico	**83** South Africa	**84** Cosmopolitan

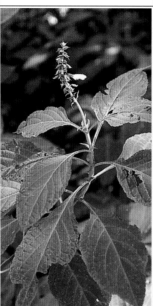

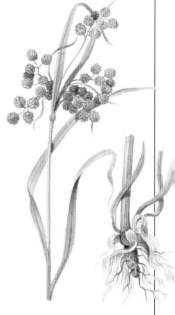

The beautiful red and black beans of several species of *Rhynchosia* may have been employed in ancient Mexico as a hallucinogenic. Paintings of these seeds on frescoes dated A.D. 300–400 at Tepantitla suggest former use as a sacred plant.

These two species are similar—scandent vines with flowers in long racemes. The flowers of *R. longeracemosa* are yellow; the seeds are mottled light and dark brown. *R. pyramidalis* has greenish flowers and handsome half-red, half-black seeds.

Chemical studies of *Rhynchosia* are still preliminary and indecisive. An alkaloid with curare-like activity has been reported from one species. Early pharmacological experiments with an extract of *R. phaseoloides* produced a kind of semi-narcosis in frogs.

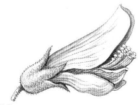

In Oaxaca, Mexico, the Mazatec Indians cultivate *Salvia divinorum* for the leaves, which are crushed on a metate, diluted in water, and drunk or chewed fresh for their hallucinogenic properties in divinatory rituals. The plant, known as Hierba de la Pastora ("herb of the shepherdess") or Hierba de la Virgen ("herb of the Virgin"), is cultivated in plots hidden away in forests far from homes and roads.

Salvia divinorum is a perennial herb 3 ft (1 m) tall or more, with ovate leaves up to 6 in. (15 cm) and finely dentate along the margin. The bluish flowers, borne in panicles up to 16 in. (41 cm) in length, are approximately ⅝ in. (15 mm) long.

It has been suggested that the narcotic Pipiltzintzintli of the ancient Aztecs was *Salvia divinorum,* but at present the plant seems to be used only by the Mazatecs. The plant contains the potent compound salvinorin A.

Over two centuries ago, Dutch explorers reported that the Hottentots of South Africa chewed the root of a plant known as Kanna or Channa as a vision-inducing hallucinogen. This common name is today applied to several species of *Sceletium* that have alkaloids—mesembrine and mesembrenine—with sedative, cocainelike activities capable of inducing torpor.

Sceletium expansum is a shrub up to 12 in. (30 cm) tall with fleshy, smooth stems and prostrate, spreading branches. The lanceolate-oblong entire, smooth, unequal leaves, measuring 1½ in. (4 cm) long, ½ in. (1 cm) wide, are of a fresh green color and very glossy. Borne on solitary branches in groups of one to five, the white or dull yellow flowers are 1½–2 in. (4–5 cm) across. The fruit is angular.

Both *S. expansum* and *S. tortuosum* were formerly *Mesembryanthemum.*

One of the most powerful herbs of the Tarahumara of Mexico is apparently a species of *Scirpus.* Tarahumara Indians fear to cultivate Bakana lest they become insane. Some medicine men carry Bakana to relieve pain. The tuberous underground part is believed to cure insanity, and the whole plant is a protector of those suffering from mental ills. The intoxication that it induces enables Indians to travel far and wide, talk with dead ancestors, and see brilliantly colored visions.

Alkaloids have been reported from *Scirpus* as well as from the related genus *Cyperus.*

The species of *Scirpus* may be annuals or perennials and are usually grasslike herbs with few- to many-flowered spikelets that are solitary or in terminal clusters. The fruit is a three-angled akene with or without a beak. They grow in many habitats but seem to prefer wet soil or bogs.

56

SCOPOLIA (3–5)	SIDA L. (200)	SOLANDRA Sw. (10–12)	SOPHORA L. (50)
Jacq. Corr. Link			
Scopolia carniolica Jacques	*Sida acuta* Burm.	*Solandra grandiflora* Sw.	*Sophora secundiflora* (Ort.) Lag. ex DC.
Scopolia	Axocatzín	Chalice Vine	Mescal Bean
Solanaceae		Solanaceae	
(Nightshade Family)	Malvaceae (Mallow Family)	(Nightshade Family)	Leguminosae (Pea Family)
85 Alps, Carpathian Mountains, Caucasus Mountains, Lithuania, Latvia, and Ukraine	**86** Warm zones of both hemispheres	**87** Tropical zones of South America, Mexico	**88** Southwestern North America, Mexico

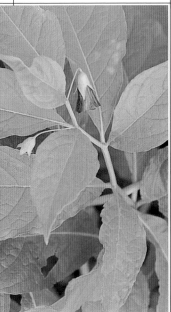 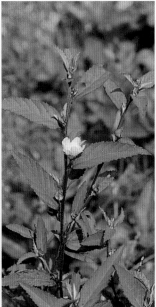 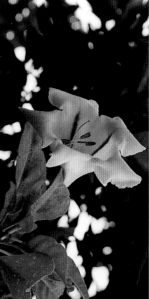 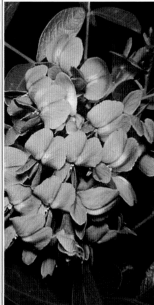

This herbaceous annual often grows 1–3 ft (30–80 cm). The dull green leaves are longish, pointed, and slightly pileous. The fleshy root is tapered. The small, bell-shaped flowers are violet to light yellow and hang down individually from the rachis and look similar to the flowers of henbane (*Hyoscyamus albus*). It flowers April to June. The fruit develops a capsule with doubled dividing wall and many small seeds.

In Slovenia, Scopolia was possibly used for the preparation of witches' salves. In East Prussia, the root was used as a native narcotic, beer additive, and aphrodisiac. Women allegedly used it to seduce young men into being willing lovers.

The whole plant contains coumarins (scopoline, scopoletine) as well as hallucinogenic alkaloids (hyoscyamine, scopolamine) and chlorogenic acid. Today the plant is grown for the industrial harvest of *L*-hyoscyamine and atropine.

These two species are herbs or shrubs often up to 9 ft (2.7 m) in height, found in hot lowlands. The stiff branches are employed in making rough brooms. The leaves, lanceolate to obovoid and measuring about 1 in. (2.5 cm) wide and up to 4 in. (10 cm) long, are beaten in water to produce a soothing lather for making skin tender. The flowers vary from yellow to white.

Sida acuta and *S. rhombifolia* are said to be smoked as a stimulant and substitute for Marijuana along the Gulf coastal regions of Mexico. Ephedrine is found in the roots of these species of *Sida*. The dried herb smells distinctly like coumarine.

A luxuriant climbing bush with showy flowers resembling those of *Brugmansia*, *Solandra* is valued for its hallucinogenic purposes in Mexico. A tea made from the juice of the branches of *S. brevicalyx* and of *S. guerrerensis* is known to have strong intoxicant properties. Mentioned by Hernández as Tecomaxochitl or Hueipatl of the Aztecs, *S. guerrerensis* is used as an intoxicant in Guerrero.

These two species of *Solandra* are showy, erect, or rather scandent shrubs with thick elliptic leaves up to about 7 in. (18 cm) in length and with large, cream-colored or yellow, fragrant, funnel-form flowers, up to 10 in. (25 cm) in length and opening wide at maturity.

The genus *Solandra*, as would be expected in view of its close relationship to *Datura*, contains tropane alkaloids: hyoscyamine, scopolamine, nortropine, tropine, cuscohygrine, and other bases have been reported.

The beautiful red beans of this shrub were once used as a hallucinogen in North America.

Sophora secundiflora seeds contain the highly toxic alkaloid cytisine, belonging pharmacologically to the same group as nicotine. It causes nausea, convulsions, and eventually, in high doses, death through respiratory failure. Truly hallucinogenic activity is unknown for cytisine, but it is probable that the powerful intoxication causes, through a kind of delirium, conditions that can induce a visionary trance.

Sophora secundiflora is a shrub or small tree up to 35 ft (10.5 m) in height. The evergreen leaves have 7 to 11 glossy leaflets. The fragrant, violet-blue flowers, borne in drooping racemes about 4 in. (10 cm) long, measure up to 1¼ in. (3 cm) in length. The hard, woody pod, constricted between each seed, bears two to eight bright red beans.

TABERNAEMONTANA L. (120)	TABERNANTHE Baill. (2–7)	TAGETES L. (50)

Tabernaemontana spp.
Sanango

Apocynaceae (Dogbane Family)

89 Tropical zones of both hemispheres

Tabernanthe iboga Baill.
Iboga

Apocynaceae (Dogbane Family)

90 Tropical zones of western Africa

Tagetes lucida Cav.
Yauhtli

Compositae (Sunflower Family)

91 Warm zones of the Americas mostly Mexico

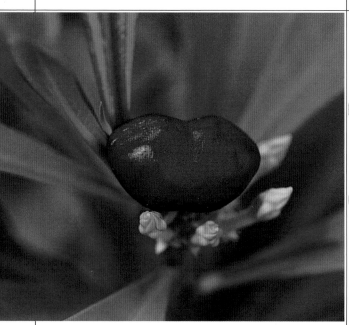

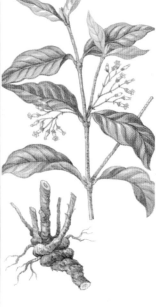

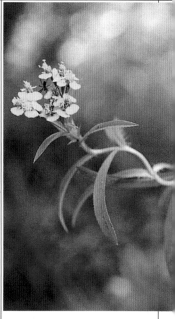

Most species of *Tabernaemontana* are bushy shrubs, climbers, or small trees. The leaves are evergreen, lanceolate, often with a leathery top side. The flowers consist of five pointed petals that mostly grow in clusters out of the calyx. The two symmetrical fruits are divided and marked with fairly visible veins. Because of this, they are easily confused with the testes of a mammal.

In the Amazon, the Sanango (*Tabernaemontana sananho* R. et P.) is considered a panacea. The leaves, roots, and the latex-rich bark are used in folk medicine. The tree grows as tall as 15 ft (5 m). The leaves are used as a psychoactive additive to Ayahuasca. It is used in combination with *Virola* in the production of an orally effective hallucinogen. In the Amazon, Sanango is also considered a "memory plant." Ayahuasca is enhanced with it in order that the visions can be better recalled.

Phytochemical research has recently been done on the genus. Indole alkaloids are the primary constituent, in some even ibogaine and voacangine have been ascertained. For this reason, this species is of particular interest for the discovery of new psychoactive plants. A few of the species (*Tabernaemontana coffeoides* Bojer ex DC., *Tabernaemontana crassa* Benth.) have already revealed psychoactive properties and uses.

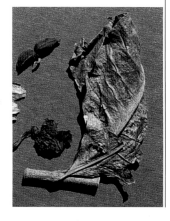

Tabernanthe iboga is a shrub 3–4½ ft (1–1.5 m) tall, found in the undergrowth of tropical forests but often cultivated in native dooryards. The shrub has copious white, vile-smelling latex. The ovate leaves, usually 3½–4 in. (9–10 cm) long, about 1¼ in. (3 cm) wide (but occasionally up to 8½ by 2¾ in. or 22 by 7 cm), are yellowish green beneath. The tiny yellowish, pinkish, or white- and pink-spotted flowers, which grow in groups of 5 to 12, have a crateriform corolla (a long, slender tube abruptly flaring at the mouth) with twisted lobes ¼ in. (1 cm) long. The ovoid, pointed yellow-orange fruits occur in pairs and become as large as olives.

Chemical studies on *Tabernanthe iboga* have shown at least a dozen indole alkaloids, the most active being ibogaine, the effects of which, in toxic doses, lead to extraordinary visions; an overdose, to paralysis and death.

The Huichol of Mexico induce visions by smoking a mixture of *Nicotiana rustica* and *Tagetes lucida*. They frequently drink a fermented beer from maize along with the smoking in order "to produce clearer visions." *Tagetes lucida* is occasionally smoked alone.

Tagetes lucida is a strongly scented perennial herb up to 1½ ft (46 cm) tall. The opposite leaves are ovate-lanceolate, toothed, and punctated with oil glands. The flowering heads are produced in dense terminal clusters ½ in. (1 cm) in diameter, usually yellow to yellow-orange. This species is native to Mexico, where it is very abundant in the states of Nayarit and Jalisco. No alkaloids have been isolated from *Tagetes,* but the genus is rich in essential oils and thiophene derivatives; *l*-inositol, saponines, tannins, coumarine derivatives, and cyanogenic glycosides have been reported.

TANAECIUM Sw. (7)	TETRAPTERIS Cav. (80)	TRICHOCEREUS (A. Berger) Riccob.
Tanaecium nocturnum (Barb.-Rodr.) Bur. et K. Schum. Koribo	*Tetrapteris methystica* R. E. Schult. Caapi-pinima	*Trichocereus pachanoi* Britt. et Rose San Pedro Cactus
Bignoniaceae (Bignonia Family)	Malpighiaceae (Malpighia Family)	Cactaceae (Cactus Family)
92 Tropical zones of Central America and South America, West Indies	**93** Tropical zones of South America, Mexico, West Indies	**94** Temperate and warm zones of South America

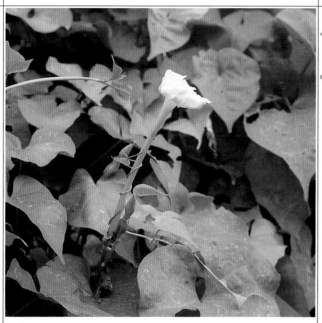

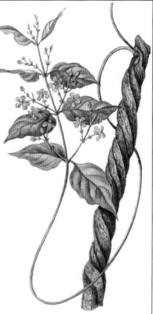

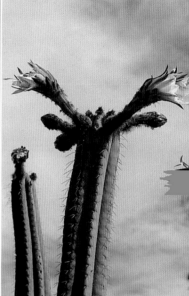

Tanaecium nocturnum is a much-branched climber with broadly elliptic leaves 5⅓ in. (13.5 cm) long, 4 in. (10 cm) wide. The white flowers, 6½ in. (16.5 cm) long, are tubular, borne in five- to eight-flowered racemes 3 in. (8 cm) long, arising from the stem. The stem, when cut, emits an odor of almond oil.

The Paumari, who live on the Rio Purus, create a ritual snuff that they call *koribo-nafuni* out of the leaves. The shamans sniff it when they are dealing with difficult cases—for example, in order to extract a magical object out of the body of the sick person. They also sniff it during a ritual for protection of children, during which they fall into a trance. The snuff is used only by the men. This species is said to be prized as an aphrodisiac by Indians of the Colombian Chocó.

Saponines and tannins have been found in *Tanaecium*. The leaves contain prussic acid and cyanoglycosides, which disintegrate when roasted.

It is uncertain as to whether the toxin's waste products contribute to the psychoactive effect of *T. nocturnum*. It is not yet known if there are other active compounds in the leaves or other parts of the plant. It is possible that this plant contains substances of unknown chemical structure and pharmacological effect.

The nomadic Makú Indians of the Rio Tikié in the northwestern most Amazonas of Brazil prepare a hallucinogenic drink, a sort of Ayahuasca or Caapi, from the bark of *Tetrapteris methystica*. Reports of the effects of the drug would suggest that β-carboline alkaloids are present.

Tetrapteris methystica (T. mucronata) is a scandent bush with black bark. The leaves are characeous, ovate, 2¼–3⅜ in. (6–8.5 cm) long, 1–2 in. (2.5–5 cm) wide, bright green above, ashy green beneath. The inflorescence is few-flowered, shorter than the leaves. The sepals are thick, hairy without, ovate-lanceolate, with eight black oval-shaped glands; the petals, spreading, membranaceous, yellow with red or brown in the center, elongate-orbicular, ½ in. (1 cm) long, ¹⁄₁₆ in. (2 mm) wide. The fruit, or samara, is ovoid, ⅛ by ⅛ by ¹⁄₁₆ in. (4 by 4 by 2 mm), with brownish wings about ½ by ¹⁄₁₆ in. (10 by 2 mm).

This cactus is a branched, often spineless, columnar plant 9–20 ft (2.75–6 m) in height. The branches, which have 6 to 8 ribs, are glaucous when young, dark green in age. The pointed buds open at night to produce very large, 7½–9¼ in. (19–24 cm), funnel-shaped, fragrant flowers with the inner segments white, the outer segments brownish red, and long, greenish stamen filaments. The fruit, as well as the scales on the floral tube, have long black hairs.

Trichocereus pachanoi is rich in mescaline: 2 % of the dried material or 0.12 % of the fresh material. Other alkaloids have been reported from the plant: 3,4-dimethoxyphenylethylamine, 3-methoxy-tyramine, and traces of other bases.

Trichocereus pachanoi (Echinopsis pachanoi) occurs in the central Andes between 6,000 and 9,000 ft (1,830–2,750 m), particularly in Ecuador and northern Peru.

Turbina corymbosa (L.) Raf.
Ololiuqui

Convolvulaceae
(Morning Glory Family)

95 Tropical zones of the Americas, mostly Mexico and Cuba

Virola theiodora (Spr.) Warb.
Cumala Tree

Myristicaceae (Nutmeg Family)

96 Tropical zones of Central America and South America

Voacanga spp.
Voacanga

Apocynaceae (Dogbane Family)

97 Tropical Africa

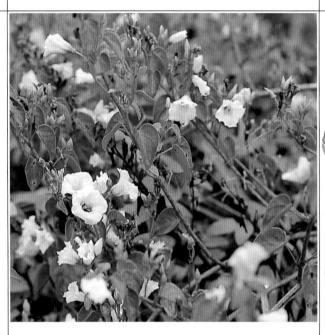

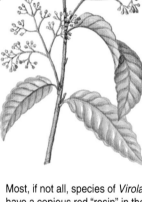

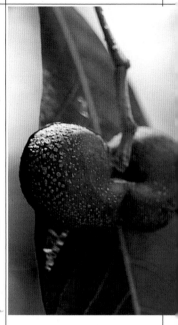

The seeds of *Turbina corymbosa,* better known as *Rivea corymbosa,* are valued as one of the major sacred hallucinogens of numerous Indian groups in southern Mexico. Their use goes back to early periods. Known as Ololiuqui, they were important in Aztec ceremonies as an intoxicant with reputedly analgesic properties.

Turbina corymbosa is a large woody vine with heart-shaped leaves 2–3½ in. (5–9 cm) long and 1–1¾ in. (2 .5–4.5 cm) wide. The cymes are many-flowered. The bell-shaped corollas, ¾–1½ in. (2–4 cm) long, are white with greenish stripes. The fruit is dry, indehiscent, ellipsoidal with persistent, enlarged sepals, and bears a single hard, roundish, brown, minutely hairy seed about ⅛ in. (3 mm) in diameter. The seeds contain lysergic acid amide, analogous to LSD.

Classification of genera in the Morning Glory family or Convolvulaceae has always been difficult. This species has at one time or another been assigned to the genera *Convolvulus, Ipomoea, Legendrea, Rivea,* and *Turbina.* Most chemical and ethnobotanical studies have been reported under the name *Rivea corymbosa,* but recent critical evaluation indicates that the most appropriate binomial is *Turbina corymbosa.*

Most, if not all, species of *Virola* have a copious red "resin" in the inner bark. The resin from a number of species is prepared as a hallucinogenic snuff or small pellets.

Probably the most important species is *Virola theiodora,* a slender tree 25–75 ft (7.5–23 m) in height, native to the forests of the western Amazon basin. The cylindrical trunk, 1½ ft (46 cm) in diameter, has a characteristic smooth bark that is brown mottled with gray patches. The leaves (with a tea-like fragrance when dried) are oblong or broadly ovate, 3½–13 in. (9–33 cm) long, 1½–4½ in. (4–11 cm) wide. The male inflorescences are many-flowered, usually brown- or gold-hairy, shorter than the leaves; the very small flowers, borne singly or in clusters of 2 to 10, are strongly pungent. The fruit is subglobose, ⅜–¾ in. (1–2 cm) by ¼–⅝ in. (.5–1.5 cm); the seed is covered for half its length by a membranaceous, orange-red aril.

The resin of the *Virola* contains DMT and 5-MeO-DMT.

The *Voacanga* genus has received little research. The species are similar to one another. They are multiple-branched, evergreen shrubs or small trees. The flowers are mostly yellow or white with five united petals. There are two symmetrical fruits. Latex runs in the bark.

The bark and seeds of the African *Voacanga africana* Stapf. contain up to 10% indole alkaloids of the iboga type (voacamine is the primary alkaloid, ibogaine) and should be simulating and hallucinogenic. In West Africa the bark is used as a hunting poison, stimulant, and potent aphrodisiac. Supposedly the seeds are used by African magicians in order to produce visions.

The seeds of the *Voacanga grandiflora* (Miq.) Rolfe are used by magicians in West Africa for visionary purposes. Unfortunately the details are not yet uncovered, as the knowledge of the magicians is a closely guarded secret.

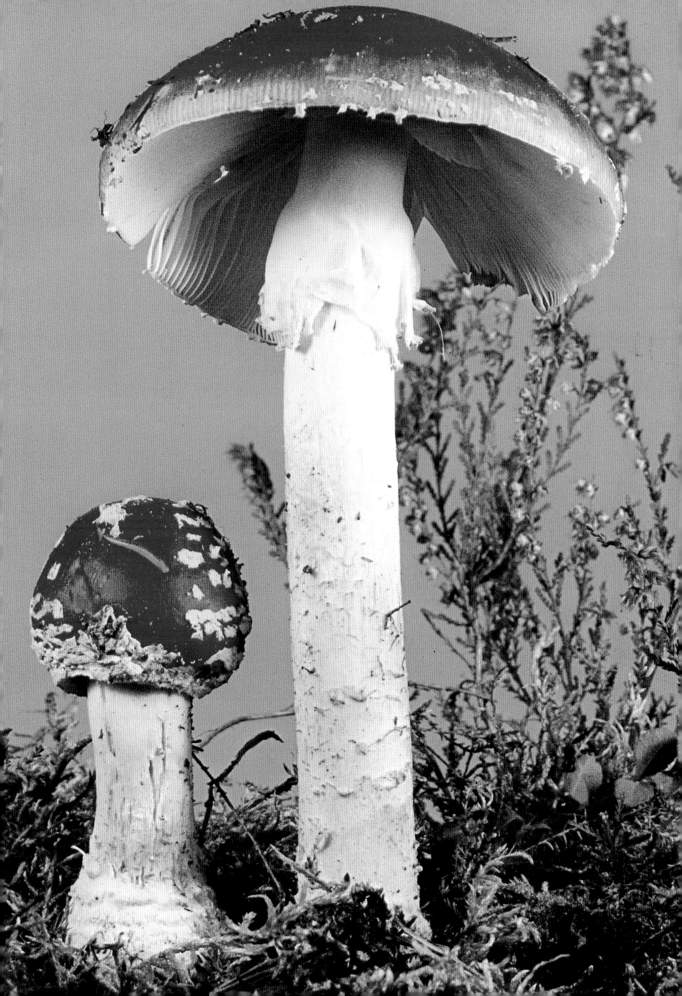

WHO USES HALLUCINOGENIC PLANTS?

Page 61: The Fly Agaric is used for shamanic purposes worldwide. It has even been linked to the ancient Indian Soma.

Notwithstanding the recent upsurge in the use of psychoactive plants in modern Western societies, the thrust of this book emphasizes almost exclusively the employment of hallucinogens among aboriginal peoples who have restricted the use of these plants mostly to magic, medical, or religious purposes. The outstanding difference between the use of hallucinogens in our culture and their use in preindustrial societies is precisely the difference in the belief concerning their purpose and origin: all aboriginal societies have considered—and still do—that these plants are the gifts of the gods, if not the gods themselves. It is obvious that our culture does not view hallucinogenic plants in this light.

There are many examples—and more will be discussed in the following pages—of plants that are sacred and even revered as gods. Soma, the ancient god-narcotic of India, may be the most outstanding example. Most hallucinogens are holy mediators between man and the supernatural, but Soma was deified. So holy was Soma that it has

South America, Ayahuasca reveals the real world, while daily living is an illusion. *Ayahuasca* means "tendril of the soul" in Kechwa and comes from the frequent experience that the soul separates from the body during the intoxication, communing with the ancestors and forces of the spirit world. The drinking of Caapi is a return "to the maternal womb, to the source and origin of all things," and participants see "all the tribal divinities, the creation of the universe, the first human beings and animals and even the establishment of the social order" (Reichel-Dolmatoff).

It is not always the shaman or medicine man who administers these sacred plants. The general population—usually the adult male portion—often shares in the use of hallucinogens. Under

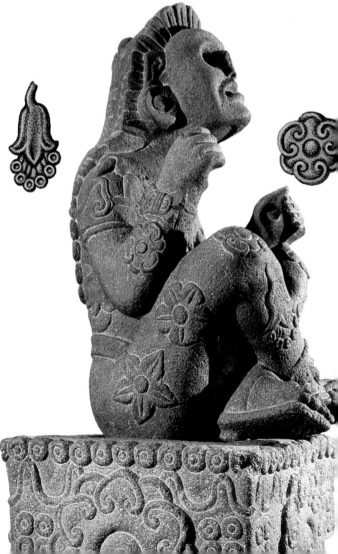

been suggested that even the idea of deity may have arisen from experiences with its unearthly effects. The sacred Mexican mushrooms have a long history that is closely linked to shamanism and religion. The Aztecs called them Teonanácatl ("divine flesh"), and they were ceremonially ingested. Highland Maya cultures in Guatemala apparently had, more than three thousand years ago, a sophisticated religion utilizing mushrooms. Probably the most famous sacred hallucinogen of the New World, however, is Peyote, which, among the Huichol of Mexico, is identified with the deer (their sacred animal) and maize (their sacred vegetal staff of life). The first Peyote-collecting expedition was led by Tatewari, the original shaman, and subsequent annual trips to collect the plant are holy pilgrimages to Wirikuta, original paradisiacal home of the ancestors. In

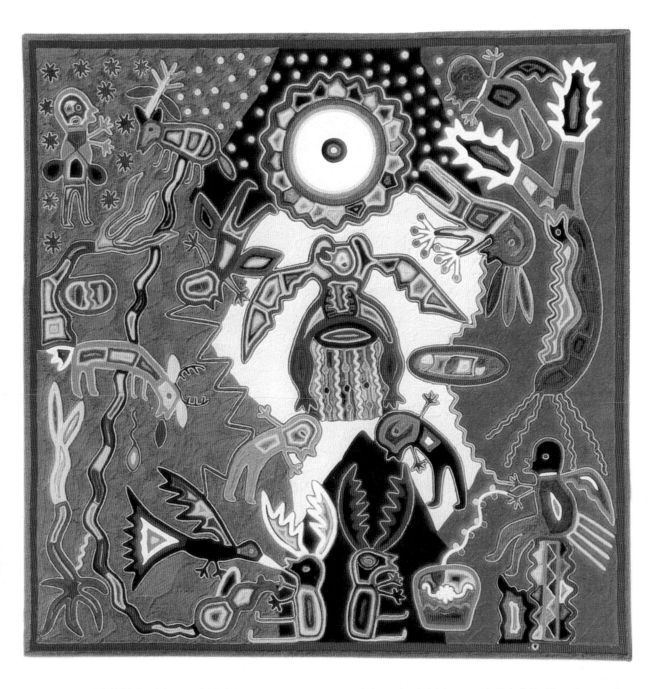

Above: The symbols in Huichol mythology are vividly depicted in their popular sacred art. The beauty of the forms has as a basis the ceremonial use of Peyote. The yarn painting above, like an Aztec Codex, is a chronicle of the creation of the world. The gods emerged from the Underworld to Mother Earth. This was possible because Kauyumari, Our Elder Brother Deer, found the *nierika,* or portway. The *nierika* of Kauyumari *(top center)* unifies the spirit of all things and all worlds. Through it all life came into being.

Below Kauyumari's *nierika,* Our Mother Eagle *(center)* lowers her head to listen to Kauyumari, who sits on a rock, bottom right. His sacred words travel down a thread to a prayer bowl and are transformed into life energy, depicted as a white blossom.

Above Kauyumari, the Spirit of Rain, a serpent, gives life to the gods. Tatewari, first shaman and Spirit of Fire *(top center right)*, is bending down toward Kauyumari listening to his chant. Both are connected to a medicine basket *(center right)*, which binds them together as shamanic allies. Our Father Sun, seen opposite Tatewari on the left, is connected with the Spirit of Dawn, the orange figure below. The Sun and Spirit of Dawn are both found in Wirikuta, the Sacred Land of Peyote. Also in Wirikuta is Kauyumari's *nierika* and the temple of Elder Brother Deer Tail. The temple is the black field, lower center. Deer Tail, with red antlers, is seen with his human manifestation above him. Behind Deer Tail is Our Mother the Sea. A crane brings her a prayer gourd containing the words of Kauyumari. Blue Deer *(left center)* enlivens all sacred offerings. A stream of energy goes from him to our Mother Sea's prayer gourd; he also offers his blood to the growing corn, the staff of life germinating below him. Above Blue Deer is the First Man, who invented cultivation. First Man faces a sacrificed sheep.

Page 62: This early-sixteenth-century Aztec statue of Xochipilli, the ecstatic Prince of Flowers, was unearthed in Tlamanalco on the slopes of the volcano Popocatepetl. The stylized glyphs depict various hallucinogenic plants. From left to right, the glyphs represent: mushroom cap; tendril of the Morning Glory; flower of Tobacco; flower of the sacred Morning Glory; bud of Sinicuiche; and, on the pedestal, stylized caps of *Psilocybe aztecorum.*

these circumstances, however, use is often strictly controlled by taboos or ceremonial circumscriptions. In almost all instances, in both the Old and the New World, the use of hallucinogenic drugs is restricted to adult males. There are, however, striking exceptions. Among the Koryak of Siberia, *Amanita* may be used by both sexes. In southern Mexico, the sacred mushrooms can be taken by both men and women; in fact, the shaman is usually a woman. Similarly, in the Old World, Iboga may be taken by any adult, male or female. While purely speculative, there may be a basic reason for the exclusion of women from ingesting narcotic preparations. Many hallucinogens are possibly sufficiently toxic to have abortifacient effects. Since women in aboriginal societies are frequently pregnant during most of their childbearing years, the fundamental reason may be purely an insur-

ance against abortions—even though this reason has been forgotten.

Sometimes hallucinogens are administered to children. Among the Jívaro, *Brugmansia* may be given to boys, who are then admonished by the ancestors during the intoxication. Frequently, the first use of a hallucinogen occurs in puberty rituals.

There is hardly an aboriginal culture without at least one psychoactive plant: even Tobacco and Coca may, in large doses, be employed for the induction of visions. An example is the smoking of Tobacco among the Warao of Venezuela, who use it to induce a trancelike state accompanied by what, for all practical purposes, are visions.

Although the New World has many more species of plants purposefully employed as hallucinogens than does the Old World, both hemispheres have very limited areas where at least one hallucinogen is not known or used. So far as we know, the Inuit have only one psychoactive plant; the Polynesian Islanders of the Pacific had Kava-kava *(Piper methysticum),* but they seem never to have had a true hallucinogen in use: Kava-kava is classed as a hypnotic.

Africa has been poorly studied from the point of view of drug plants, and may have hallucinogenic species that have not yet been introduced to the scientific world. It is, however, possible to assert that there are few parts of the continent where at least one such plant is not now utilized or was not employed at some time in the past.

Asia, a vast continent, has produced relatively few major hallucinogenic varieties but their use has been widespread and extremely significant from a cultural point of view; furthermore, the use of them is extremely ancient. Numerous sources describe the use of hallucinogenic and other intoxicating plants in ancient Europe. Many researchers see the roots of culture, shamanism, and religion in the use of psychoactive or hallucinogenic plants.

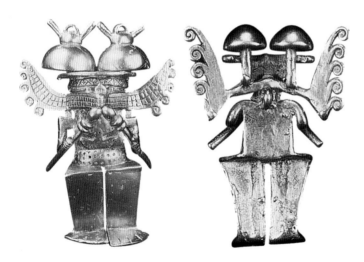

"Whether shaman alone,
or shaman and communicants,
or communicants alone
imbibe or ingest *Ilex* drinks,
Datura infusions, Tobacco, . . .
Peyote cactus, Ololiuqui seeds, mushrooms,
narcotic Mint leaves or Ayahuasca
. . . the ethnographic principle is the same.
These plants contain spirit power."
—Weston La Barre

OVERVIEW OF PLANT USE

Two points stand out in clear relief in this tabular summary of material set forth in greater detail in other sections of the book. It is obvious that: (1) the sources of information are interdisciplinary in nature; and (2) there is urgent need for deeper studies in view of the sparsity or vagueness of knowledge in so many cases.

That progress in future studies will be made only when they are based on integration of data from sundry fields—anthropology, botany, chemistry, history,

NOTES OF A BOTANIST

ON THE

AMAZON · & ANDES

BEING RECORDS OF TRAVEL ON THE AMAZON AND
ITS TRIBUTARIES, THE TROMBETAS, RIO NEGRO,
UAUPÉS, CASIQUIARI, PACIMONI, HUALLAGA,
AND PASTASA; AS ALSO TO THE CATAR-
ACTS OF THE ORINOCO, ALONG THE
EASTERN SIDE OF THE ANDES OF
PERU AND ECUADOR, AND THE
SHORES OF THE PACIFIC,
DURING THE YEARS
1849-1864

BY RICHARD SPRUCE, Ph.D.

EDITED AND CONDENSED BY
ALFRED RUSSEL WALLACE, O.M., F.R.S.
WITH A
BIOGRAPHICAL INTRODUCTION
PORTRAIT, SEVENTY ONE ILLUSTRATIONS
AND
SEVEN MAPS

IN TWO VOLUMES—VOL. I

MACMILLAN AND CO., LIMITED
ST. MARTIN'S STREET, LONDON
1908

medicine, mythology, pharmacology, philology, religion, and so on—should be obvious. And wise handling of such a wealth of information calls for patience and breadth of understanding. One of the first steps in this direction must be presentation of such diverse material in easily assimilated outline form—an end that we have tried to accomplish in this overview.

It is man living in so-called archaic so-cieties and intimately familiar with his ambient vegetation who has discovered the hallucinogens and bent them to his use. The relentless march of civilization is ever increasing in speed and intensity, reaching even the most remote and hidden peoples. Acculturation inevitably spells the doom of native lore and leads to the disappearance of knowledge built up through the ages. It is, therefore, urgent that we step up the tempo of research before this knowledge will forever be entombed with the culture that gave it birth.

Accurate botanical identification of the source plant is basic to a sound understanding of hallucinogens. We do not always have this knowledge. Ideally, botanical determination of a product should be made on the basis of a voucher specimen: only in this way can exactness be ensured. It is sometimes necessary to base an identification on a common name or on a description, in which case there always may exist some doubt as to its accuracy. It is equally essential that chemical investigations be founded upon properly vouchered material. Brilliant phytochemical work too often is worthless simply because grave doubts about the identity of the original vegetal material cannot be dispelled.

Similar deficiencies in other aspects of our knowledge of hallucinogens and their use hamper our understanding. The full cultural significance of mind-altering plants may not be appreciated. It is only in very recent years that anthropologists have begun to comprehend the deep and all-encompassing role that hallucinogens play in the history, mythology, and philosophy of aboriginal societies. In time as this understanding is appreciated, anthropology will advance in its explanation of many basic elements of human culture.

The material presented in this book is of necessity concentrated in detail. It may also at times be diffuse. Realizing the desirability occasionally of having a quick means of consultation, we have striven to assemble the essential facts and present them in skeletal form in this Overview of Plant Use.

Key symbols designating plant types in Overview of Plants Use

 XEROPHYTES AND SUCCULENTS

 LIANAS

 VINES AND TWINERS

 GRASSES AND SEDGES

 HERBS

 LILY-LIKE PLANTS

 FUNGI

 ORCHIDS

 SHRUBS

 TREES

 AQUATIC PLANTS

Left: The English botanist Richard Spruce spent fourteen years in field research in South America during the 1800's. An insatiable plant-explorer, he might be called the prototype of ethnobotanists of tropical America. His studies laid the foundation of research on the hallucinogens Yopo and Caapi—research still in progress.

Page 64: The Sinú culture of Colombia (from 1200 to 1600) has yielded many enigmatic gold pectorals with mushroomlike representations. They may imply the existence of a cult using these intoxicating fungi, species of which occur in the area. Many of the pectorals have winglike structures, possibly signifying magic flight, a frequent characteristic of hallucinogenic intoxication.

REF. NUMBER	COMMON NAME	TYPE OF PLANT	BOTANICAL NAME	USAGE: HISTORY AND ETHNOGRAPHY
35	Agara		*Galbulimima belgraveana* (F. Muell.) Sprague	Natives in Papua
11 12	Angel's Trumpets Floripondio Borrachero Huacacachu Huanto Maicoa Toé Tonga (see also pages 140–143)		*Brugmansia arborea* (L.) Lagerh.; *B. aurea* Lagerh.; *B.* x *insignis* (Barb.-Rodr.) Lockwood ex R. E. Schult.; *B. sanguinea* (R. et P.) Don; *B. suaveolens* (H. et B. ex Willd.) Bercht. et Presl.; *B. versicolor* Lagerh.; *B. vulcanicola* (A. S. Barclay) R. E. Schult.	*Brugmansia* are employed in the warmer parts of South America, especially in the western Amazon, under the name of Toé. Also used by the Mapuche Indians of Chile, the Chibcha of Colombia, and known to Peruvian Indians as Huacacachu.
9	Ayahuasca Caapi Yajé (see also pages 124–139)		*Banisteriopsis caapi* (Spruce ex Griseb.) Morton; *B. inebrians* Morton; *B. rusbyana* (Ndz.) Morton; *Diplopterys cabrerana* (Cuatr.) B. Gates	Used in the western half of the Amazon Valley and by isolated tribes on the Pacific slopes of the Colombian and Ecuadorean Andes.
43	Badoh Negro Piule Tlililtzin (see also pages 170–175)		*Ipomoea violacea* L.	Oaxaca, southern Mexico. Known to the Aztecs as Tlililtzin and employed in the same way as Ololiuqui, *Ipomoea* is called Piule by the Chinantec and Mazatec, and Badoh Negro by the Zapotec.
24	Bakana Hikuli Wichuri		*Coryphantha compacta* (Engelm.) Britt. et Rose; *C.* spp.	The Tarahumara Indians of Mexico consider *C. compacta* (Wichuri, also referred to as Bakana or Bakana-wa) a kind of Peyote or Hikuli (see Peyote).
84	Bakana		*Scirpus* sp.	A species of *Scirpus* is apparently one of the most powerful herbs of the Tarahumara Indians of Mexico. The Indians fear the plant because of possible insanity.
60	Blue Water Lily Ninfa Quetzalaxochiacatl		*Nymphaea ampla* (Solisb.) DC.; *N. caerulea* Sav.	Water Lilies enjoyed an exceptionally prominent place in the mythology and art of Minoan and dynastic Egyptian cultures, in India and China, as well as in the Mayan world from the Middle Classical period until the inception of the Mexican period. Among Old and New World similarities is the relation of *N. ampla* to the toad, itself associated with hallucinogenic agents, and the relation of the plant to death.
93	Caapi-Pinima Caapi (see Ayahuasca)		*Tetrapteris methystica* R. E. Schul.; *T. mucronata* Cav.	Caapi-Pinima is employed by the nomadic Makú Indians of the Rio Tikié in the northwestern Amazon of Brazil. They call it Caapi, the same as *Banisteriopsis*. Several writers have mentioned "more than one kind" of Caapi in the Rio Vaupés area of Brazil and adjacent Colombia.
62	Cawe Wichowaka		*Pachycereus pecten-aboriginum* (Engelm.) Britt. et Rose	Employed by the Tarahumara Indians of Mexico, *Wichowaka* means "insanity" in the local language.
4 5	Cebíl Villca Yopo (see also pages 116–119)		*Anadenanthera colubrina* (Vell.) Brenan; *A. colubrina* (Vell.) Brenan var. *Cebil* (Griseb.) Altschul; *A. peregrina* (L.) Speg.; *A. peregrina* (L.) Speg. var. *falcata* (Benth.) Altschul	*A. peregrina* is used today by tribes of the Orinoco basin (Yopo) and was first reported in 1946. No longer used in the West Indies. Indians of Argentina (Villca or Huilca) and southern Peru (Cebíl) are believed to have employed *A. colubrina* in precolonial times.
61	Cebolleta		*Oncidium cebolleta* (Jacq.) Sw.	It is suspected that the Tarahumara of Mexico make use of this orchid.
80	Chacruna Chacruna Bush Cahua		*Psychotria viridis* Ruíz et Pavón	Used for ages in the Amazon region as a significant ingredient of Ayahuasca.

USAGE: CONTEXT AND PURPOSE	PREPARATION	CHEMICAL COMPONENTS AND EFFECTS
Hallucinogenic intoxication	The bark and leaves of this tree are boiled with a species of *Homalomena* to prepare a tea.	Although 28 alkaloids have been isolated, a psychoactive principle has not yet been found. Visions of men and animals to be killed are experienced.
The Indians of Sibundoy use *Brugmansia* for magico-medicinal purposes, the Mapuche as medicine for recalcitrant children. The Chibcha formerly gave fermented Chicha with *Brugmansia* seeds to wives and slaves of dead chieftains to induce a stupor before they were buried alive with their husbands or masters. Indians in Peru still believe that *Brugmansia* permits them to communicate with ancestors and that it can reveal treasures preserved in graves.	The drug is usually taken in the form of powdered seeds added to fermented drinks, or as a tea made of the leaves.	All species of *Brugmansia* are chemically similar, with scopolamine as their principal psychoactive constituent. Content of lesser alkaloids is also similar. A dangerous hallucinogen, *Brugmansia* brings on an intoxication often so violent that physical restraint is necessary before the onset of a deep stupor, during which visions are experienced.
Usually drunk in religious ceremonies. In the famous Tukanoan Yuruparí ceremony in Colombia—an adolescent initiation ritual for boys. The Jívaro believe that Ayahuasca makes possible communication with ancestors and that, under its influence, a man's soul may leave the body and wander free.	The bark, prepared in cold or boiling water, may be taken alone or with additives—especially the leaves of *B. rusbyana (Diplopterys cabrerana)* and of *Psychotria viridis*—which alter the effects. The bark can also be chewed. Recent evidence from the northwestern Amazon suggests that the plants are also used in the form of a snuff.	The hallucinogenic activity is primarily due to harmine, the major β-carboline alkaloid in the plants. Effects of taking the bitter and nauseating drink range from pleasant intoxication with no hangover to violent reactions with sickening aftereffects. Usually, visual hallucinations in color occur. The intoxication ends with a deep sleep and dreams.
In southern Mexico, this vine is respected as one of the principal hallucinogens for use in divination, magico-religious, and curing rituals.	A drink is prepared from about a thimbleful of the crushed seeds.	The alkaloid content is five times that of *Turbina corymbosa*; accordingly natives use fewer seeds. The same alkaloids are found in other Morning Glories but usage is restricted to Mexico. (See Ololiuqui.)
Medicinal purposes. Taken by shamans as a potent medicine and greatly feared and respected by the Indians.	The aboveground Teuile ("meat" of the cactus) is eaten fresh or dried. Eight to twelve cactus "tops" are an adequate dose.	Various alkaloids, including phenylethylamines, have been isolated from *Coryphantha*, a promising genus for future studies.
Scirpus plays an important role in folk medicine and as a hallucinogen; it must be treated with great reverence.	The tuberous roots of *Scirpus* are often collected from faraway places.	Alkaloids have been reported from *Scirpus* and related sedges. The Indians believe that they can travel to distant places, talk with their ancestors, and have colored visions.
There exist numerous interesting parallels between the ritualistic (shamanic) significance of *Nymphaea* in the Old and the New Worlds, suggesting that *Nymphaea* may have been used as a narcotic, possibly a hallucinogen. *N. ampla* has recently been reported to be used in Mexico as a recreational drug with "powerful hallucinatory effects."	Dried flowers and buds of *Nymphaea ampla* are smoked. The rhizomes are eaten raw or cooked. The buds of *N. caerula* are used to make a tea.	The alkaloids apomorphine, nuciferine, and nornuciferine, isolated from the rhizomes of *N. ampla*, may be responsible for the psychotropic activity.
Hallucinogenic intoxication.	A drink is prepared from the bark of *T. methystica* in cold water. The infusion is yellowish, unlike the brownish color of the beverage prepared from *Banisteriopsis*.	It has not been possible as yet to carry out chemical examination of *T. methystica*, but reports of the effects of the drug would suggest that the same or similar β-carboline alkaloids are present as in *Banisteriopsis*.
There are several purely medicinal uses of this cactus.	A hallucinogenic drink is prepared from the juice of the young branches of *P. pecten-aboriginum*.	4-hydroxy-3-methoxyphenylethylamine and four tetrahydroisoquinoline alkaloids have been isolated. It causes dizziness and visual hallucinations.
Now smoked as a hallucinogenic intoxicant by Indians in northern Argentina.	The snuff is prepared from the beans, which are usually moistened, rolled into a paste, and dried by toasting. When pulverized to a gray-green powder, it is mixed with an alkaline plant ash or snail shell lime.	Tryptamine derivatives and β-carbolines. A twitching of the muscles, slight convulsions, and lack of muscular coordination followed by nausea, visual hallucinations, and disturbed sleep. Macropsia.
Reportedly used as a hallucinogen, *O. cebolleta* is employed as a temporary surrogate for Peyote.	Unknown.	An alkaloid has been reported from *O. cebolleta*.
This bush has great cultural significance as a DMT-providing ingredient of the hallucinogen Ayahuasca, which has a central place in the shamanic tradition of the Amazon.	Fresh or dried leaves are mixed with vines or the husk of *Banisteriopsis caapi* and cooked. The preparation is drunk as Ayahuasca *(Caapi, Yagé)*.	The leaves contain 0.1% to 0.61% *N,N,*-DMT, as well as traces of other alkaloids.

REF. NUMBER	COMMON NAME	TYPE OF PLANT	BOTANICAL NAME	USAGE: HISTORY AND ETHNOGRAPHY
13	Chiricaspi Chiric-Sanango Manaka		*Brunfelsia chiricaspi* Plowman; *B. grandiflora* D. Don; *B. grandiflora* D. Don subsp. *schultesii* Plowman	*Brunfelsia* is known as Borrachero ("the intoxicator") t Colombian Indians, and as Chiricaspi ("cold tree") in westernmost Amazonia (Colombia, Ecuador, and Per
34	Colorines Chilicote Tzompanquahuitl		*Erythrina americana* Mill.; *E. coralloides* Moc. et Sesse ex DC.; *E. flabelliformis* Kearney	The beans of various species are frequently sold with those of *Sophora secundiflora* (Mescal Beans) in Mexico. They are used as amulets or charms.
74	Common Reed		*Phragmites australis* (Cav.) Trinius ex Steudel	Used for medicinal purposes since ancient times. Ps choactive use is a recent phenomenon.
63	Copelandia Jambur		*Panaeolus cyanescens* Berk. et Br.; *Copelandia cyanescens* (Berk. et Br.) Singer	Cultivated on cow and buffalo dung in Bali.
58	Cowhage		*Mucuna pruriens* (L.) DC.	India. Used in Ayurvedic medicine. The seeds are us worldwide as charms or amulets.
19	Dama da Noite (Lady of the Night) Palqui Maconha		*Cestrum laevigatum* Schlecht; *Cestrum parqui* L'Herit.	Coastal regions of southern Brazil, southern Chile.
28	Datura Dutra (see also pages 106–111)		*Datura metel* L.	*D. metel* is mentioned as a hallucinogenic plant in ea Sanskrit and Chinese writings. Known as a drug to the Arabian physician Avicenna the eleventh century. Employed today especially in India, Pakistan, and *A* ghanistan. *D. ferox,* a related Old World species, plays a mino role.
8	Deadly Nightshade Belladonna (see also pages 86–91)		*Atropa belladonna* L.	Europe, Near East. Deadly Nightshade figured as an important ingredien many of the witches' brews of the Middle Ages. *Atropa* played a prominent role in the mythology of most European peoples.
21	El Nene El Ahijado El Macho		*Coleus blumei* Benth.; *C. pumilus* Blanco	Native to the Philippine Islands, two species of this pl have acquired significance similar to Salvia in southe Mexico among the Mazatec Indians.
96	Epená Nyakwana Yakee (see also pages 176–181)		*Virola calophylla* Warb.; *V. calophylloidea* Markgr.; *V. elongata* (Spr. ex Benth.) Warb.; *V. theiodora* (Spr.) Warb.	In Brazil, Colombia, Venezuela and Peru a number of species of *Virola* are used, the most important of whi appears to be *V. theiodora.* The hallucinogenic snuff has various names depen ing on the locality or tribe, with the most commonly re cognized terms being Paricá, Epená, and Nyakwana Brazil, Yakee and Yato in Colombia.
39	Ereriba		*Homalomena* sp.	The natives of Papua are reported to use *Homalome*
20	Ergot (see also pages 102–105)		*Claviceps purpurea* (Fr.) Tulasne	It has recently been convincingly argued that Ergot played a role in the Eleusinian mysteries of ancient Greece. When accidentally ground up with rye flour during Middle Ages, Ergot (which grows primarily as a funga disease on rye) poisoned whole districts with ergotis These mass poisonings became known as St. Antho ny's fire.

USAGE: CONTEXT AND PURPOSE	PREPARATION	CHEMICAL COMPONENTS AND EFFECTS
In Amazonian folk medicine, *Brunfelsia* plays a major magico-religious role. Used as an additive to the hallucinogenic drink Yajé (see Ayahuasca).	The Kofán of Colombia and Ecuador and the Jívaro of Ecuador add *Brunfelsia* to Yajé, prepared basically from *Banisteriopsis* (see Ayahuasca). It heightens the hallucinogenic effects.	Scopoletine has been found in *Brunfelsia,* but this compound is not known to be psychoactive. A sensation of chills follows ingestion, an effect that has given rise to the name Chiricaspi ("cold tree").
The plant may once have been used by the Tarahumara, who value the beans medicinally.	The red beans are often mixed with the similar ones of *Sophora secundiflora.*	Some species of *Erythrina* contain alkaloids of the erythran type, producing effects similar to those of curare or cytisine.
Used today as a DMT-delivering agent for Ayahuasca analogs.	Twenty to 50 g of roots are boiled with 3 g of seeds from *Peganum harmala* and the preparation is consumed as a drink.	The roots contain the psychedelic or vision-inducing alkaloid N, N-DMT, 5-MEO-DMT, Bufotenin, and the toxin gramine.
Used in native festivals in Bali and reportedly sold to foreign visitors as a hallucinogen.	The mushrooms are eaten fresh or dried.	Up to 1.2% of psilocine and 0.6% of psilocybine have been found in *C. cyanescens,* which is the highest content of these alkaloids found in hallucinogenic mushrooms.
Indian peoples may have utilized the psychoactive properties. *Mucuna* is considered an aphrodisiac in India.	Powdered seeds. Source of DMT for Ayahuasca analogs.	Although *Mucuna* has not been reported as a hallucinogen, it is rich in psychoactive alkaloids (such as DMT) capable of inducing behavioral changes equitable with hallucinogenic activity.
The Mapuche of southern Chile smoke Palqui.	The leaves are smoked as a substitute for Marijuana.	The unripened fruit, leaves, and flowers contain saponines that are not known to be hallucinogenic.
Used as an aphrodisiac in the East Indies. Valuable drug. Ceremonial intoxication and recreation.	Powdered seeds added to wine. The seeds are added to alcoholic drinks, to *Cannabis* cigarettes or tobacco, and occasionally to the betel chew mixture.	See Toloache.
Witches' brews; the sabbat. Today, *A. belladonna* is an important source for medicinal drugs.	The entire plant contains psychoactive constituents.	The plant contains alkaloids, capable of inducing hallucinations. The main psychoactive constituent is hyoscyamine, but lesser amounts of scopolamine and trace amounts of minor tropane alkaloids are also present.
Having magico-religious significance, *Coleus* is used as a divinatory plant.	The leaves are chewed fresh or the plants are ground, then diluted with water for drinking.	No hallucinogenic principle has yet been discovered in the 150 known *Coleus* species.
Epená or Nyakwana may be snuffed ceremonially by all adult males, occasionally even without any ritual connection. The medicine men use the drug in diagnosis and treatment of illnesses. The use of Yakee or Paricá is restricted to shamans.	Some Indians scrape the inner layer of the bark and dry the shavings over a fire. When pulverized, powdered leaves of *Justicia,* the ashes of Amasita, the bark of *Elizabetha princeps* may be added. Other Indians fell the tree, collect the resin, boil it to a paste, sun-dry the paste, crush and sift it. Ashes of several barks and the leaf powder of *Justicia* may be added. A further method is to knead the inner shavings of freshly stripped bark and to squeeze out the resin and boil it to a paste, which is sun-dried and prepared into snuff with ashes added. A group of Makú Indians in the Colombian Vaupés ingest the unprepared resin as it is collected from the bark.	Tryptamine and β-carboline alkaloids, 5-methoxydimethyltryptamine and dimethyltryptamine (DMT), being the main constituents, are responsible for the hallucinogenic activity. Effects of the intoxication vary. They usually include initial excitability, setting in within several minutes from the first snuffing. Then follows numbness of the limbs, twitching of the facial muscles, inability to coordinate muscular activity, nausea, visual hallucinations, and finally, a deep, disturbed sleep.
Plants are used in traditional medicine and to create hallucinogenic dreams.	The leaves are eaten with the leaves and bark of *Galbulimima belgraveana* (see Agara).	Little is known still of the constituents of this genus. Violent derangement is followed by slumber with visions.
It appears that Ergot has never been utilized purposefully as a hallucinogen in medieval Europe. Employed extensively as a medicine by midwives in cases of difficult childbirth during the Middle Ages, Ergot induced contractions of involuntary muscles and was a strong vasoconstrictor.	Used for psychoactive purposes. Taken as a coldwater infusion. Dosage is difficult to determine and can be dangerous!	Ergoline alkaloids, mainly derivatives of lysergic acid, are the pharmacologically active constituents of Ergot. Ergot alkaloids or derivatives of them are the basis of important medicines used today in obstetrics, internal medicine, and psychiatry. The most potent hallucinogen, lysergic acid diethylamide (LSD), is a synthetic derivative of Ergot.

REF. NUMBER	COMMON NAME	TYPE OF PLANT	BOTANICAL NAME	USAGE: HISTORY AND ETHNOGRAPHY
25	Esakuna		*Cymbopogon densiflorus* Stapf	Used by medicine men in Tanzania.
72	Fang-K'uei		*Peucedanum japonicum* Thunb.	China
3	Fly Agaric (see also pages 82–85)		*Amanita muscaria* (L. ex Fr.) Pers.	Finno-Ugrian peoples in eastern and western Siberia. Several groups of Athabaskan peoples of North America. *A. muscaria* could very well be the mysterio[us] god-narcotic Soma of ancient India, taken by the Arya[n] 3,500 years ago.
45	Galanga Maraba		*Kaempferia galanga* L.	There are vague reports that Galanga is employed as [a] hallucinogen in New Guinea.
26	Genista		*Cytisus canariensis* (L.) O. Kuntze	Although native to the Canary Islands, Genista was in[-] corporated in aboriginal American societies. Genista has apparently acquired an important role among the Yaqui Indians of Mexico.
52	Gi'-i-Wa Gi'-i-Sa-Wa		*Lycoperdon marginatum* Vitt.; *L. mixtecorum* Heim	In southern Mexico, the Mixtec of Oaxaca employ two species to induce a condition of half-sleep. There seem[s] to be no ceremony connected with the use. In northern Mexico, among the Tarahumara of Chihuahua, a species of *Lycoperdon,* known as Kalamot[a], is employed.
40 41	Henbane (see also pages 86–91)		*Hyoscyamus niger* L.; *H. albus* L.	During the Middle Ages, Henbane was an ingredient [of] the witches' brews and ointments. In ancient Greece and Rome, reports of "magic drinks" indicate that Henbane frequently served as an[] ingredient. It has been suggested that the priestesses[] Delphi prophesied under the influence of Henbane.
82	Hierba de la Pastora Hierba de la Virgen Pipiltzintzintli		*Salvia divinorum* Epl. et Jativa-M.	Used by the Mazatec Indians of Mexico as a substitu[te] for psychoactive mushrooms, *S. divinorum* ("of the div[i]ners") is called "herb of the shepherdess." It is commo[nly] believed to be the narcotic Pipiltzintzintli of the Aztec Indians.
33	Hikuli Mulato Hikuli Rosapara		*Epithelantha micromeris* (Engelm.) Weber ex Britt. et Rose	One of the "false Peyotes" of the Tarahumara Indians Chihuahua and the Huichol of northern Mexico.
7	Hikuli Sunamé Chautle Peyote Cimarrón Tsuwiri		*Ariocarpus fissuratus* Schumann; *A. retusus* Scheidw.	The Tarahumara Indians in northern and central Mexi[co] assert that *A. fissuratus* is stronger than Peyote *(Lophophora).* Huichol Indians of Mexico.
90	Iboga (see also pages 112–115)		*Tabernanthe iboga* Baill.	In Gabon and the Congo, the cult surrounding Iboga provides the natives with the strongest single force against the missionary spread of Christianity and Isla[m] in this region.
56	Jurema Ajuca Tepescohuite		*Mimosa hostilis* (Mart.) Benth.; *M. verrucosa* Benth. = *Mimosa tenuiflora* (Willd.) Poir.	Valued in eastern Brazil, where several tribes in Pernan[a]buco use the plant in ceremonials; also employed by va[r]ious now extinct tribes of the same area.
83	Kanna		*Mesembryanthemum expansum* L.; *M. tortuosum* L. = *Sceletium tortuosum* (L.) N.E.Br.	Over two centuries ago, Dutch explorers reported that the Hottentots of South Africa employed the root of a plant known as Channa or Kanna.

USAGE: CONTEXT AND PURPOSE	PREPARATION	CHEMICAL COMPONENTS AND EFFECTS
Employed to cause dreams in order to foretell the future.	Smoking of the flowers, either alone or with tobacco.	It is not known to which compound the alleged hallucinogenic activity has to be attributed.
Folk medicine.	The root of Fang-K'uei is employed medicinally in China.	Alkaloidal constituents have been reported from *Peucedanum,* but whether or not they are of hallucinogenic types is not known. Coumarins and furocoumarins are widespread in the genus; both occur in *P. japonicum.*
Shamanistic inebriation. Religious significance; healing ceremonies. Religious ceremonies.	One or several mushrooms are taken sun-dried or slowly toasted over a fire. They may also be drunk as an extract in water or reindeer milk or with the juice of *Vaccinium oliginorum* or *Epilobium angustifolium.* Ritualistic drinking of the urine of intoxicated individuals in Siberia also occurs.	Ibotenic acid, Muscimole, Muscazone. Euphoria, colored visions, macropsia; on occasion religious fervor and deep sleep may occur.
Hallucinogenic intoxication (?), folk medicine, aphrodisiac.	The highly aromatic rhizome is valued locally as a condiment; a tea from the leaves is employed in folk medicine.	Beyond the high content of essential oil (to which hallucinogenic activity might be due) in the rhizome of this relative of Ginger, little is known of the chemistry.
Ceremonial use in Native American tribes. Employed especially by the medicine men as a hallucinogen in magic ceremonies.	The seeds are valued by Yaqui medicine men.	*Cytisus* is rich in the lupine alkaloid cytisine. Hallucinogenic activity has not been reported from cytisine, but it is known to be toxic.
Used as auditory hallucinogen. Taken by sorcerers to enable them to approach people without being detected and to make people sick.	The fungi are eaten.	There is as yet no phytochemical basis to explain the psychotropic effects.
Witches' brews; magic infusions. Induces a clairvoyant trance.	The dried herb is smoked as a cigarette or smoked in a smokehouse. The seeds are mainly smoked. The seeds are used as a substitute for hops in making beer. Dosage varies from person to person.	The active principles in this solanaceous genus are tropane alkaloids, especially hyoscyamine and scopolamine, the latter being mainly responsible for the hallucinogenic effects.
In Oaxaca, Mexico, the Mazatec Indians cultivate *S. divinorum* for its hallucinogenic properties in divinatory rituals. It is apparently used when Teonanácatl or Ololiuqui seeds are rare.	The leaves are chewed fresh or crushed on a metate, then diluted with water and filtered for a drink.	The main active ingredient, salvinorin A, can bring about extreme hallucinations when inhaled in amounts of 250 to 500 mcg.
Medicine men take Hikuli Mulato to make their sight clearer and permit them to commune with sorcerers. It is taken by runners as a stimulant and "protector" and the Indians believe that it prolongs life.	Cactus flesh is eaten fresh or dried.	Alkaloids and triterpenes have been reported. This cactus is reportedly able to drive evil people to insanity and throw them from cliffs.
Valuing it in witchcraft, the Tarahumara believe that thieves are powerless to steal when this cactus calls its soldiers to its aid. The Huichol consider *Ariocarpus* to be evil, insisting that it may cause permanent insanity.	Consumed either fresh or crushed in water.	Several phenylethylamine alkaloids have been isolated.
Iboga is known to be used as a hallucinogen in magicoreligious context, especially the Bwiti cult, and serves to seek information from ancestors and the spirit world, hence "a coming to terms with death." Moreover, intoxication is practiced in the initiation ceremonies. The drug also has the reputation of a powerful stimulant and aphrodisiac.	Fresh or dried roots are eaten pure, or added to palm wine. Roughly 10 g of dried root powder induces a psychedelic effect.	Iboga contains at least a dozen indole alkaloids, ibogaine being the most important. Ibogaine is a strong psychic stimulant that in high doses produces also hallucinogenic effects.
The hallucinogenic use of *Mimosa hostilis* in ceremonies seems to have nearly disappeared today. Employed in connection with warfare.	The root of *Mimosa hostilis* was the source of a "miraculous drink," known locally as Ajuca or Vinho de Jurema.	One active alkaloid identical with the hallucinogenic *N, N*-dimethyl-tryptamine has been isolated.
Probably once used as a vision-inducing hallucinogen.	In the hinterlands of South Africa, the roots and leaves are still smoked. Apparently, the leaves are sometimes dried after fermentation and chewed as an inebriant.	The common name is today applied to several species of *Sceletium* and *Mesembryanthemum* that have alkaloids – mesembrine and mesembrenine – with sedative activities capable of inducing torpor. Kanna produces a strong intoxication.

71

REF. NUMBER	COMMON NAME	TYPE OF PLANT	BOTANICAL NAME	USAGE: HISTORY AND ETHNOGRAPHY
87	Kieli/Kieri Hueipatl Tecomaxochitl		*Solandra brevicalyx* Standl.; *S. guerrerensis* Martinez	Mentioned by Hernández as Tecomaxochitl or Hueipatl of the Aztec Indians. In the mythology and symbolism of the Mexican Huichol and other tribes, several species of *Solandra* are important.
92	Koribo		*Tanaecium nocturnum* (Barb.-Rodr.) Bur. et K. Schum.	Employed by the Karitiana Indians of the Rio Madeira in Amazonian Brazil.
57	Kratom Biak-Biak		*Mitragyna speciosa* Korthals	In the 19th century, Kratom was known as an opium substitute in Thailand and Malaysia.
66	Kwashi		*Pancratium trianthum* Herbert	Kwashi is employed by the Bushmen in Dobe, Botswana.
47	Latúe Arbol de los Brujos		*Latua pubiflora* (Griseb.) Baill.	Formerly used by the Mapuche Indian shamans of Valdivia, Chile.
79	Liberty Cap		*Psilocybe semilanceata* (Fries) Quélet	It is possible that this fungus has been used for psychoactive purposes in Central Europe for about 12,000 years. Earlier, it was used as a hallucinogen by the Alpen nomads and has also been used in European witchcraft.
48	Lion's Tail Wild Dagga Dacha		*Leonitis leonurus* (L.) R. Br.	This herb has been used as a narcotic in southern Africa since ancient times.
1	Maiden's Acacia		*Acacia maidenii* F. von Muell.; *A. phlebophylla* F. von Muell.; *A. simplicifolia* Druce	Many Acacias are used in traditional medicine. The psychoactive use of Acacia, which contains DMT, is very recent and has been developed especially in Australia and California.
86	Malva Colorada Chichibe Axocatzin		*Sida acuta* Burm.; *S. rhombifolia* L.	*Sida acuta* and *Sida rhombifolia* are said to be smoked along the Gulf Coast of Mexico.
54	Mandrake (see also pages 86–91)		*Mandragora officinarum* L.	Mandrake has a complex history in the Old World. The root of Mandrake can be likened to the human form, hence its magic.
17	Marijuana Bhang Charas Dagga Ganja Hashish Hemp Kif Ta Ma (see also pages 92–101)		*Cannabis sativa* L.; *C. indica* Lam.	In India, use of *Cannabis* has had religious significance. Specimens nearly 4,000 years old have turned up in an Egyptian site. In ancient Thebes, the plant was made into a drink with opium-like effects. The Scythians, who threw Hemp seeds and leaves on hot stones in steam baths to produce an intoxicating smoke, grew the plant along the Volga 3,000 years ago. Chinese tradition puts the use of the plant back 4,800 years. Indian medical writing, compiled before 1000 B. C., reports therapeutic uses of *Cannabis*. The Greek physician Galen wrote, about A. D. 160, that general use of *Cannabis* in cakes produced intoxication. In 13th-century Asia Minor, organized murderers, rewarded with Hashish, were known as *hashishins*, from which may come the term *assassin* in European languages.
44	Mashihiri		*Justicia pectoralis* Jacq. var. *stenophylla* Leonard	The Waiká and other Indians of the uppermost Orinoco and the adjacent parts of northwestern Brazil cultivate *Justicia*.

USAGE: CONTEXT AND PURPOSE	PREPARATION	CHEMICAL COMPONENTS AND EFFECTS
The Huichol worship and fear *Solandra* as a god-narcotic, Kieli, a powerful aid in sorcery. Realizing the close relationship of *Solandra*, *Datura*, and *Brugmansia*, the Huichol sometimes combine their use: they distinguish between *Datura inoxia* or Kielitsa ("bad Kieli") and the real Kieli or *Solandra*. *S. guerrerensis* is known to be employed as an intoxicant in the state of Guerrero.	A tea made from the juice of the branches of both species is known to be employed as an intoxicant.	The genus *Solandra*, closely related to *Datura*, contains hyoscyamine, scopolamine, nortropine, tropine, scopine, cuscohygrine, and other tropane alkaloids with strong hallucinogenic effects.
Folk medicine. This species is said to be praised as an aphrodisiac by Indians of the Colombian Chocó.	A tea is made of the leaves of this liana and those of an unidentified plant as a remedy for diarrhea.	Reports from botanical collectors of the odor of *T. nocturnum* suggest that cyanogenesis occurs in this species. Saponines and tannins have been isolated.
In Southeast Asia, the leaves are chewed or smoked for use as a stimulant or a narcotic.	Fresh leaves are chewed, dried, and smoked, or taken internally as a tea or extract. The leaves are sometimes used together with Betel.	The entire plant contains alkaloids, of which Mitragynine is the main active ingredient. Mitragynine, which is chemically similar to yohimbine and psilocybine, is a very powerful psychoactive substance.
Reportedly used as a hallucinogen and in folk medicine. Religious importance assumed in tropical West Africa.	The bulbs are cut in two and rubbed over incisions on the scalp. This custom most closely approaches the Western habit of injecting medicine.	Many of the 15 species contain very toxic alkaloids. The toxic state may be accompanied by hallucinogenic symptoms.
Latúe is a virulent poison once used to induce delirium, hallucinations, and even permanent insanity.	Dosages were a secret closely guarded. The fresh fruit was preferentially employed.	The leaves and fruit contain 0.15 % hyoscyamine and 0.08 % of scopolamine, responsible for hallucinogenic activity.
This mushroom has been used worldwide for its hallucinogenic and vision-inducing qualities.	Eaten fresh or dried. Thirty fresh mushrooms or roughly 3 g of dried mushrooms is a sufficient psychedelic dose.	Contains high concentrations of psilocybin, and some psilocine and baeocystine (the total alkaloid concentration is roughly 1 % of the dried mass). This is a potent hallucinogen.
The Hottentots and bush people smoke the plant as a narcotic or as a substitute for *Cannabis*.	The dried buds and leaves are smoked either alone or mixed with tobacco.	There have been no chemical studies to date.
Acacia resin is used in conjunction with Pituri by the Australian Aborigines. Today, various varieties of Acacia are used as DMT sources and also in the preparation of Ayahuasca analogs for hallucinogenic experiences.	Extracts from the husk and leaves of *A. maidenii*, the bark of *A. simplicifolia*, or the leaves of *A. phlebophylla* are combined with the seeds from *Peganum harmala*.	Many varieties of Acacia contain the psychedelic substance, DMT. The bark of *A. maidenii* contains 0.36 % DMT; the leaves of *A. phlebophylla* contain 0.3 % DMT. The bark of *A. simplicifolia* can contain up to 3.6 % alkaloids, of which DMT accounts for roughly one third.
Employed as a stimulant and substitute for Marijuana.	Smoking.	Ephedrine, which induces a mild stimulating effect, has been reported from these species of *Sida*.
Used as a panacea, Mandrake played an extraordinary role as a magic plant and hallucinogen in European folklore. An active hallucinogenic ingredient of the witches' brews, Mandrake was probably the most potent admixture.	There existed various precautions in pulling the root from the earth because the plant's unearthly shrieks could drive collectors mad.	Tropane alkaloids with hyoscyamine as the main constituent besides scopolamine, atropine, mandragorine, and others are the psychoactive constituents. The total content of tropane alkaloids in the root is 0.4 %.
Cannabis has a long history of use in folk medicine and as a psychoactive substance. It is the source of fiber, an edible fruit, an industrial oil, a medicine, and an intoxicant. Use of *Cannabis* has grown in popularity in the past 40 years as the plant has spread to nearly all parts of the globe. Increase in the plant's use as an inebriant in Western countries, especially in urban centers, has led to major problems and dilemmas for European and American authorities. There is a sharp division of opinion as to whether the widespread use of *Cannabis* is a vice that must be stamped out or is an innocuous habit that should be permitted legally. The subject is debated hotly, usually with limited knowledge.	Methods of consuming *Cannabis* vary. In the New World, Marijuana (Maconha in Brazil) is smoked—the dried, crushed flowering tips or leaves are often mixed with tobacco or other herbs in cigarettes. Hashish, the resin from the female plant, is eaten or smoked, often in water pipes, by millions in Muslim countries of northern Africa and western Asia. In Afghanistan and Pakistan, the resin is commonly smoked. East Indians regularly employ three preparations: Bhang consists of plants that are gathered green, dried and made into a drink with water or milk or into a candy (majun) with sugar and spices; Charas, normally smoked or eaten with spices, is pure resin; Ganja, usually smoked with tobacco, consists of resin-rich dried tops from the female plant.	The psychoactive principles—cannabinotic compounds—are found in greatest concentration in a resin produced most abundantly in the region of the pistillate inflorescence. A fresh plant yields mainly cannabidiolic acids, precursors of the tetrahydrocannabinols and related constituents, such as cannabinol and cannabidiol. The main effects are attributable to Δ^1–3,4-trans-tetrahydrocannabinol. The principal effect is euphoria. Everything from a mild sense of ease to hallucinations, from feelings of exaltation and inner joy to depression and anxiety have been reported. The drug's activities beyond the central nervous system seem to be secondary. They consist of a rise in pulse rate and blood pressure, tremor, vertigo, difficulty in muscular coordination, increased tactile sensitivity, and dilation of the pupils.
The natives mix *Justicia* leaves with the snuff prepared from *Virola* (see Epená) to "make the snuff smell better."	The leaves are dried and pulverized.	Tryptamines have been suspected from several species of *Justicia*.

REF. NUMBER	COMMON NAME	TYPE OF PLANT	BOTANICAL NAME	USAGE: HISTORY AND ETHNOGRAPHY
14	Matwú Huilca		*Cacalia cordifolia* L. fil.	Mexico
88	Mescal Bean Coral Bean Colorines Frijoles Red Bean		*Sophora secundiflora* (Ort.) Lag. ex DC.	Use of Mescal Bean goes far back into prehistory in the Rio Grande basin, where they have had ritual uses for at least 9,000 years. The Arapaho and Iowa tribes in the United States were using the beans as early as 1820. At least a dozen tribes of Indians in northern Mexico and southern Texas practiced a vision-seeking dance.
85	Nightshade		*Scopolia carniolica* Jacques	Probably used as an ingredient of witches' salves and ointments; used in Eastern Europe as a substitute for Mandrake; also used as an intoxicating ingredient in beer.
10	Nonda		*Boletus kumeus* Heim; *B. manicus* Heim; *B. nigroviolaceus* Heim; *B. reayi* Heim	New Guinea
59	Nutmeg Mace		*Myristica fragrans* Houtt.	Known as "narcotic fruit" in ancient Indian writings. Occasionally used as a surrogate for Hashish in Egypt. Unknown in classical Greece and Rome, Nutmeg was introduced to Europe in the first century A. D. by the Arabs, who employed it as a medicine. Nutmeg poisoning was common in the Middle Ages, and during the 19th century in England and America.
95	Ololiuqui Badoh Xtabentum (see also pages 170–175)		*Turbina corymbosa* (L.) Raf. [= *Rivea corymbosa*]	The seeds of this Morning Glory, formerly known as *Rivea corymbosa,* are valued as one of the major sacred hallucinogens of numerous Indian groups in southern Mexico. Their use goes back to early periods, and they were important in Aztec ceremonies as an intoxicant and as a magic potion with reputedly analgesic properties.
42	Paguando Borrachero Totubjansush Arbol de Campanilla		*Iochroma fuchsioides* Miers	Used by the Indians of the Sibundoy Valley of southern Colombia and the Kamsá of the southern Andes of Colombia.
51	Peyote Hikuli Mescal Button (see also pages 144–155)		*Lophophora diffusa* (Croizat) Bravo; *L. williamsii* (Lem.) Coult.	Spanish chronicles described use of Peyote by the Aztec Indians. *Lophophora* is valued today by the Tarahumara, Huichol, and other Mexican Indians as well as by members of the Native American Church in the United States and western Canada.
69	Peyotillo		*Pelecyphora aselliformis* Ehrenb.	There are suspicions that this round cactus may be valued in Mexico as a "false Peyote."
32	Pitallito Hikuri		*Echinocereus salmdyckianus* Scheer; *E. triglochidiatus* Engelm.	The Tarahumara Indians of Chihuahua consider both species as "false Peyotes."
31	Pituri Pituri Bush Poison Bush		*Duboisia hopwoodii* F. con Muell.	Pituri leaves have been used for at least 40,000 years in Australian rituals and are used for both medicinal and pleasurable purposes.
81	Piule		*Rhynchosia longeracemosa* Mart. et Gal.; *R. phaseoloides; R. pyramidalis* (Lam.) Urb.	The red/black beans of several species of *Rhynchosia* may have been employed in ancient Mexico as a hallucinogen.
55	Rapé dos Indios		*Maquira sclerophylla* (Ducke) C. C. Berg	Indians of the Pariana region of the Brazilian Amazon formerly used *Maquira,* but encroaching civilization has ended this custom.

USAGE: CONTEXT AND PURPOSE	PREPARATION	CHEMICAL COMPONENTS AND EFFECTS
Presumed aphrodisiac and cure for sterility.	The dried herb is smoked.	One alkaloid has been reported. No evidence of hallucinogenic properties.
The arrival of the Peyote cult, centering on *Lophophora,* a safer hallucinogen, led the natives to abandon the Red Bean Dance, which had made use of the beans as an oracular, divinatory, and hallucinogenic medium.	A drink was prepared from the red beans of *S. secundiflora.*	The seeds contain the highly toxic alkaloid cytisine, which pharmacologically belongs to the same group as nicotine. Hallucinogenic activity is unknown from cytisine, but the powerful intoxication may cause a kind of delirium comparable to a visionary trance. In high doses, respiratory failure may lead to death.
Used as an aphrodisiac and psychoactive love potion in Lithuania and Latvia.	The roots are used as an ingredient in beer. The dried herb can be smoked alone or mixed with other herbs.	The whole plant contains strong hallucinogenic tropanalkaloids, especially hyoscyamine and scopolamine. Also contains scopoletine.
Several species of *Boletus* are involved in the reported "mushroom madness" of the Kuma.	The dried, ground fruit is eaten.	Active principles unknown.
The most notable use of Nutmeg is found in Western society, especially among prisoners deprived of other drugs.	At least one teaspoon is used when taken orally or snuffed for narcotic purposes, although usually much more is required to bring on full intoxication. Nutmeg is on occasion added to the betel chew.	The main active ingredient of nutmeg's essential oils is myristicine; safrol and eugenol are also present. In high doses extremely toxic and dangerous, the components of Nutmeg oil so upset normal body functions that they evoke a delirium comparable to hallucinations, usually accompanied by severe headache, dizziness, nausea, etc.
At the present time the small round seeds are utilized in divination and witchcraft by Chinantec, Mazatec, Mixtec, Zapotec, and others and, as has recently been stated, "today in almost all villages of Oaxaca one finds seeds still serving the natives as an ever-present help in time of trouble."	The seeds, which must be collected by the person who is to be treated, are ground by a virgin on a metate, water is added, and then the drink is filtered. The patient drinks it at night in a quiet, secluded place.	Ergoline alkaloids were found to be the psychoactive principles, lysergic acid amide and lysergic acid hydroxyethylamide, closely related to the potent hallucinogen LSD, being the most important constituents.
According to shamans, the aftereffects are so strong that the plant is used for divination, prophecy, and diagnosis of disease only when other "medicines" are unavailable, or for especially difficult cases.	The fresh bark is rasped from the stem and boiled with an equal amount of leaves, usually a handful. The resulting tea, when cooled, is drunk with no admixture. The dose is said to be one to three cupfuls of a strong decoction over a three-hour period.	Although chemical investigation of this genus has not been carried out, it belongs to the Nightshade family, well recognized for its hallucinogenic effects. The intoxication is not pleasant, having after effects of several days.
Mythological and religious significance; healing ceremonies. In the United States, use of Peyote is a vision-quest ritual with a combination of Christian and Native elements and high moral principles.	The cactus may be eaten raw, dried, or made into a mash or a tea. From 4 to 30 tops are consumed during the ceremony.	Contains up to 30 alkaloids of the phenylethylamine and tetrahydroisoquinoline type. The main constituent responsible for the hallucinogenic activity is trimethoxyphenylethylamine, named mescaline. Hallucinations are characterized by colored visions.
The cactus is used in northern Mexico as Peyote (*Lophophora williamsii*).	Cactus flesh is eaten fresh or dried.	Recent investigations have indicated the presence of alkaloids.
The Tarahumara sing to Pitallito during collection and say it has "high mental qualities."	Cactus flesh is eaten fresh or dried.	A tryptamine derivative has been reported from *E. triglochidiatus.*
Pituri has been of central importance in Australian Aboriginal society as a substance for social enjoyment, a shamanic magic drug, and a valuable good for trade. Pituri is chewed for its narcotic effects, as a stimulant to dreams and visions, and simply to be enjoyed.	The fermented leaves are mixed with alkaline plant ashes and other resins (such as Acacia resin) and chewed.	The leaves contain various psychoactive alkaloids (piturine, nicotine, nornicotine, anabasine, and others). The roots also contain nornicotine and scopolamine. The chewed leaves can act as a narcotic, stimulant, or hallucinogen.
Hallucinogenic intoxication (?)	The seeds are referred to by Indians of Oaxaca by the same name used for the hallucinogenic seeds of Morning Glory (*Turbina corymbosa*).	Chemical studies of *Rhynchosia* are still indecisive. An alkaloid with curare-like activity has been reported from one species. Pharmacological experiments with *R. phaseoloides* produced a kind of seminarcosis in frogs.
The snuff was taken during tribal ceremonials.	The method of preparation from the dried fruit is apparently remembered only by the very old.	No chemical studies have been carried out on *M. sclerophylla.*

75

REF. NUMBER	COMMON NAME	TYPE OF PLANT	BOTANICAL NAME	USAGE: HISTORY AND ETHNOGRAPHY
73	Reed Grass		*Phalaris arundinacea* L.	Although Reed Grass was familiar to writers of antiquity, its psychoactive use is very recent.
18	Saguaro		*Carnegiea gigantea* (Engelm.) Britt. et Rose	Southwestern United States and Mexico. Although there are apparently no ethnological reports of Saguaro as a hallucinogen, the plant is an important medicine among the Indians.
89	Sanango Tabernaemontana		*Tabernaemontana coffeoides* Bojer ex DC.; *T. crassa* Bentham; *T. dichotoma* Roxburgh; *T. pandacaqui* Poir. [= *Ervatamia pandacaqui* (Poir.) Pichon]	There are many varieties of the genus *Tabernaemontana* in Africa and South America. Especially in Africa, some varieties seem to have been used for a long time in shamanic or traditional medicine practices.
94	San Pedro Aguacolla Gigantón (see also pages 166–169)		*Trichocereus pachanoi* Britt. et Rose [= *Echinopsis pachanoi*]	Used by the natives of South America, especially in the Andes of Peru, Ecuador, and Bolivia.
67	Screw Pine		*Pandanus* sp.	New Guinea
75	Shang-la		*Phytolacca acinosa* Roxb.	China
71	Shanin Petunia		*Petunia violacea* Lindl.	A recent report from highland Ecuador has indicated that a species of *Petunia* is valued as a hallucinogen.
23	Shanshi		*Coriaria thymifolia* HBK. ex Willd.	Peasants in Ecuador.
49	Siberian Lion's Tail Marijuanillo Siberian Motherwort		*Leonurus sibiricus* L.	The Siberian Motherwort has been used medicinally from the very beginning of Chinese medicine. Since the plant was transplanted to the Americas, it has been used as a substitute for Marijuana.
36	Sinicuichi		*Heimia salicifolia* (HBK) Link et Otto	Although all three species of *Heimia* are important in Mexican folk medicine, mainly *H. salicifolia* has been valued for its hallucinogenic properties.
37	Straw Flower		*Helichrysum foetidum* (L.) Moench; *H. stenopterum* DC.	Zululand, South Africa.
2	Sweet Flag Flag Root Sweet Calomel Calamus		*Acorus calamus* L.	Cree Indians of northwest Canada.
68	Syrian Rue		*Peganum harmala* L.	*P. harmala* is valued today from Asia Minor across to India with extraordinary esteem, suggesting former religious use as a hallucinogen.
70	Taglli Hierba Loca Huedhued		*Pernettya furens* (Hook. ex DC.) Klotzch; *P. parvifolia* Bentham	*P. furens* is called Hierba Loca in Chile ("maddening plant"), while *P. parvifolia* is known as Taglli in Ecuador.
30	Taique Borrachero Latuy		*Desfontainia spinosa* R. et P.	Reported as a hallucinogen from Chile (Taique) and southern Colombia (*Borrachero* = "intoxicant").

USAGE: CONTEXT AND PURPOSE	PREPARATION	CHEMICAL COMPONENTS AND EFFECTS
In connection with research on the so-called Ayahuasca analogs, a species of Reed Grass has been discovered that has a high DMT content and can be used psychoactively.	An extract is made from the leaves. In combination with *Peganum harmala*, it has visionary effects, and can be drunk as a substitute for Ayahuasca.	This grass contains many indole alkaloids, especially *N,N*-DMT, 5-MeO-DMT, MMT and [sometimes] gramine. DMT and 5-MeO-DMT have very strong psychedelic effects, while gramine is very toxic.
The Seri Indians of Sonora consider Saguaro efficacious against rheumatism.	The fruit of *Carnegiea* is valued as food and in wine-making.	The plant contains pharmacologically active alkaloids capable of psychoactivity. Carnegine, 5-hydroxycarnegine, and norcarnegine, plus trace amounts of 3-methoxytyramine and the new alkaloid arizonine (a tetrahydroquinoline base), have been isolated.
Tabernaemontana crassa is used in West Africa as a narcotic in traditional medicine. *T. dichotoma* is used for its psychoactive effects in India and Sri Lanka.	The seeds of *T. dichotoma* are used as a hallucinogen. Unfortunately, very little is known about this interesting genus.	Most varieties contain ibogaine-like alkaloids (such as voacangine), which have very strong hallucinogenic and vision-inducing effects.
Hallucinogenic intoxication. The use of *T. pachanoi* appears to be primarily for divination, diagnosis of disease, and to make oneself owner of another's identity.	Short pieces of the stem are sliced and boiled in water for several hours. Several other plants, *Brugmansia*, *Pernettya*, and *Lycopodium*, for example, are sometimes added.	*T. pachanoi* is rich in mescaline: 2% of dried material (or 0.12% of fresh material).
A species of *Pandanus* is said to be used for hallucinogenic purposes, while others are known to be valued in folk medicine, in magic, and for ceremonial purposes.	It has recently been reported that natives of New Guinea employ the fruit of a species of *Pandanus*.	Dimethyltryptamine (DMT) has been detected in an alkaloid extract. Eating substantial amounts of the nuts is said to cause an "outbreak of irrational behavior" known as Karuka madness among local people.
Shang-la is a well-known medicinal plant in China. It was reportedly used by sorcerers, who valued its hallucinogenic effects.	The flowers and roots enter Chinese medicine: the former for treating apoplexy, the latter for external use only.	*P. acinosa* has a high concentration of saponines. The toxicity and hallucinogenic effects of Shang-la are commonly mentioned in Chinese herbals.
Taken by the Indians of Ecuador to induce a sensation of flight.	The dried herb is smoked.	Phytochemical studies of *Petunia* are lacking. The plant is said to induce a feeling of flying.
Recent reports suggest that the fruit may purposefully be eaten to induce intoxication.	The fruit is eaten.	The chemistry is still poorly known. Levitation or sensations of soaring through the air.
This herb is smoked in Brazil and Chiapas as a substitute for *Cannabis*.	The flowering herb is dried and smoked alone or mixed with other plants. One to 2 g of the dried plant is an effective dose.	Contains alkaloids, flavonglycosides, diterpenes, and an essential oil. The psychoactive effects may be attributable to the diterpenes (leosibiricine, leosibirine, and isoleosibirine).

Mexican natives report that Sinicuichi possesses supernatural virtues, but the plant does not appear to be taken ritually or ceremonially.
    Some natives assert that it helps them clearly to recall happenings of long ago—even prenatal events.
	In the Mexican highlands the leaves of *H. salicifolia* are slightly wilted, crushed in water, and then allowed to ferment into an intoxicating drink.	Alkaloids of the quinolizidine type have been isolated, among them cryogenine (vertine), to which the psychotropic activity may be attributed.
		    The beverage induces giddiness, a darkening of the surroundings, shrinkage of the world around, and a pleasant drowsiness. Auditory hallucinations may occur with voices and distorted sounds that seem to come from far away.

These herbs are used by native doctors "for inhaling to induce trances."	The dried herb is smoked.	Coumarins and diterpenes are reported, but no constituents with hallucinogenic properties have been isolated.

Antifatigue medicine; also used against toothache, headache, and asthma.
    Hallucinogenic intoxication (uncertain)
	Chewing of the rootstalk.	The active principles are α-asarone and β-asarone.
		    In large doses, visual hallucinations and other effects similar to those of LSD may occur.

Syrian Rue has many uses in folk medicine, as well as being valued as an aphrodisiac. Often used as incense.	The dried seeds constitute the Indian drug Harmal.	The plant possesses undoubted hallucinogenic principles: β-carboline alkaloids—harmine, harmaline, tetrahydroharmine, and related bases known to occur in at least eight families of higher plants. These constituents are found in the seeds.
Known to be employed as a hallucinogen, it has been suggested that *Pernettya* has played a role in magico-religious ceremonies in South America—a still unproven claim.	Eating of the fruit.	The chemistry of the toxic fruits of both *P. furens* and *P. parvifolia*, which cause mental confusion and even insanity, is not yet elucidated.
Medicine men of the Kamsá tribe drink a tea from the leaves for the purpose of diagnosing disease or when they "want to dream."	Tea made from the leaves or fruit.	Nothing is as yet known of the chemistry of *D. spinosa*. Visions are experienced and some of the medicine men assert that they temporarily "go crazy" under its influence.

REF. NUMBER	COMMON NAME	TYPE OF PLANT	BOTANICAL NAME	USAGE: HISTORY AND ETHNOGRAPHY
38	Takini		*Helicostylis pedunculata* Benoist; *H. tomentosa* (P. et E.) Macbride	In the Guianas, Takini is a sacred tree.
22 64 76 78	Teonanácatl Tamu Hongo de San Isidro She-to To-shka (see also pages 156–163)		*Conocybe siligineoides* Heim; *Panaeolus sphinctrinus* (Fr.) Quélet; *Psilocybe acutissima* Heim; *P. aztecorum* Heim; *P. caerulescens* Murr.; *P. caerulescens* Murr. var. *albida* Heim; *P. caerulescens* Murr. var. *mazatecorum* Heim; *P. caerulescens* Murr. var. *nigripes* Heim; *P. caerulescens* Murr. var. *ombrophila* Heim; *P. mexicana* Heim; *P. mixaeensis* Heim; *P. semperviva* Heim et Cailleux; *P. wassonii* Heim; *P. yungensis* Singer; *P. zapotecorum* Heim; *Psilocybe cubensis* Earle	Mushroom worship seems to be rooted in centuries of native Indian tradition of Middle America. The Aztec Indians called the sacred mushrooms Teonanácatl; the Mazatec and Chinantec in northeastern Oaxaca, Mexico, refer to *Panaeolus sphinctrinus* as T-ha-na-sa, To-shka ("intoxicating mushroom"), and She-to ("pasture mushrooms"). While in Oaxaca *Psilocybe cubensis* is named Hongo de San Isidro, in the Mazatec language it is called Di-shi-tjo-le-rra-ja ("divine mushroom of manure").
29	Thorn Apple Jimsonweed (see also pages 106–111)		*Datura stramonium* L.	Reportedly employed by the Algonquin and others. Ingredient of the witches' brews of medieval Europe. Used in both the Old and New World, the geographic origin of Jimsonweed is uncertain.
27	Toloache Toloatzin (see also pages 106–111)		*Datura innoxia* Mill.; *D. discolor* Bernh. ex Tromms.; *D. kymatocarpa* A. S. Barclay; *D. pruinosa* Greenm.; *D. quercifolia* HBK; *D. reburra* A. S. Barclay; *D. stramonium* L.; *D. wrightii* Regel.	Known also as *D. meteloides*, *D. innoxia* is used in Mexico and the American Southwest.
50	Tupa Tabaco del Diablo		*Lobelia tupa* L.	Recognizing *L. tupa* as toxic, the Mapuche Indians of Chile value the leaves for their intoxicating properties. Other Andean Indians take it as an emetic and purgative.
46	Turkestan Mint		*Lagochilus inebrians* Bunge	The Tajik, Tatar, Turkoman, and Uzbek tribesman on the dry steppes of Turkestan have for centuries prepared a tea made from *L. inebrians*.
97	Voacanga		*Voacanga africana* Stapf; *V. bracteata* Stapf; *V. dregei* E. Mey. *V. grandiflora* (Miq.) Rolfe.	In Africa, a number of varieties of the genus *Voacanga* have been used as hallucinogens, aphrodisiacs, and medicines.
53	Wichuriki Hikuli Rosapara Hikuri Peyote de San Pedro Mammillaria		*Mammillaria craigii* Lindsay; *M. grahamii* Engelm.; *M. senilis* (Lodd.) Weber	The Tarahumara Indians of Mexico value several species of *Mammillaria* among the most important "false Peyotes."
6	Wood Rose Hawaiian Wood Rose		*Argyreia nervosa* (Burman f.) Bojer	The Wood Rose has been used since ancient times in Ayurvedic medicine. A traditional use as a hallucinogen has been discovered in Nepal.
91	Yauhtli		*Tagetes lucida* Cav.	*Tagetes* is used by the Huichol of Mexico and valued ceremonially for its hallucinatory effects.
15	Yün-Shih		*Caesalpinia sepiaria* Roxb. [= *C. decapetala* (Roth) Alston]	China; used medicinally in Tibet and Nepal.
16	Zacatechichi Thle-Pelakano Aztec Dream Grass		*Calea zacatechichi* Schlecht.	Seems to be used only by the Chontal Indians of Oaxaca, even though it ranges from Mexico to Costa Rica.

USAGE: CONTEXT AND PURPOSE	PREPARATION	CHEMICAL COMPONENTS AND EFFECTS
Little is known of the use.	A mildly poisonous intoxicant is prepared from the red "sap" of the bark.	No specific hallucinogenic constituents have been identified. Extracts from the inner bark of both species have pharmacologically been shown to elicit depressant effects similar to those produced by Marijuana.
Mythological and sacramental use. Employed today in divination and healing ceremonies. Contacts with Christianity or modern ideas do not seem to have influenced the deep spirit of reverence characteristic of the mushroom ritual. It has been suggested that *Psilocybe* species may be employed for hallucinogenic inebriation also by the Yurimagua Indians of Amazonian Peru.	Personal preference, purpose of use, and seasonal availability determine the kinds of mushrooms used by different shamans. *P. mexicana,* one of the most widely used, may perhaps be considered the most typical sacred mushroom. Anywhere from 2 to 30 mushrooms (depending on the type used) are eaten during a typical ceremony. They may be consumed either fresh or ground and made into an infusion.	The indolic alkaloids psilocybine and psilocine are the main hallucinogenic principles of the sacred mushrooms. The content varies from species to species between 0.2 and 0.6% of psilocybine and small amounts of psilocine in dried mushroom material. The mushrooms cause both visual and auditory hallucinations, with the dreamlike state becoming reality.
Initiation rites. Ingredient of the witches' brews.	The roots of the Thorn Apple may have been used in the hallucinogenic Algonquin drink *wysoccan.*	See Toloache.
D. innoxia was employed medicinally and as a sacred hallucinogen by the Aztec and other Indians. The Zuni Indians value the plant as an analgesic and as a poultice to cure wounds and bruises. Toloache is said to be the exclusive property of the rain priests. Valued in initiation rituals.	The Tarahumara add *D. innoxia* to their maize beer and use the roots, seeds, and leaves. The Zuni chew the roots and put powder prepared from them into the eyes. Among the Yokut Indians, the seeds are said to be taken only once during a man's lifetime.	All species of the genus *Datura* are chemically similar with the active principles tropane alkaloids, especially hyoscyamine and scopolamine, the latter being the main component.
Hallucinogenic intoxication; folk medicine.	Smoking of the leaves and taken internally.	Tupa leaves contain the piperidine alkaloid lobeline, a respiratory stimulant, as well as the diketo- and dihydroxy-derivatives lobelamidine and nor-lobelamidine, which are not known to be hallucinogenic.
Hallucinogenic intoxication.	The leaves are toasted to produce a tea. Drying and storage increases the aromatic fragrance. Stems, fruiting tops, and flowers may be added.	The presence of a crystalline compound called lagochiline—a diterpene of the grindelian type—is known. This compound is not known to be hallucinogenic.
The seeds of various *Voacanga* varieties are taken by African magic men to create visual hallucinations.	The seeds or the bark of various *Voacanga* varieties can be taken.	Many varieties of *Voacanga* contain psychoactive indole alkaloids, especially voacangine and voccamine, both of which are chemically related to ibogaine.
Used as a visual hallucinogen. *M. grahamii* is taken by shamans in special ceremonies.	*M. craigii* is split open, sometimes roasted, and the central tissue is used. The top of the plant, divested of its spines, is the most powerful part; the fruit and upper part of *M. grahamii* are said to have similar effects.	N-methyl-3, 4-di-methoxyphenylethylamine has been isolated from *M. heyderii,* a close relative to *M. craigii.* Deep sleep, during which a person is said to travel great distances, and brilliant colors characterize the intoxication.
In Ayurvedic medicine, Wood Rose is used as a tonic and as an aphrodisiac, and it is also used to increase intelligence and to slow down the aging process. Today, the seeds are of interest in Western society for their psychoactive properties.	The seeds are ground and mixed with water. Four to 8 seeds (approximately 2 g) are sufficient for a medium psychoactive dose.	The seeds contain 0.3% ergot alkaloids (especially chanoclavin-I, also ergine (LSA), ergonovine, and isolysergic acid amide).
Used to induce or enhance visions.	*T. lucida* is occasionally smoked alone but is sometimes mixed with tobacco (*Nicotiana rustica*).	No alkaloids have been isolated from *Tagetes,* but the genus is rich in essential oils and thiophene derivatives.
If consumed over a long period, the flowers are said to induce levitation and "communication with the spirits." Folk medicine.	Roots, flowers, and seeds.	An unknown alkaloid has been reported. The earliest Chinese herbal stated: the "flowers enable one to see spirits and cause one to stagger madly."
Used in folk medicine, especially as an apéritif, a febrifuge, and an astringent for treating diarrhea. The Chontal take Zacatechichi to clarify the senses.	Tea is made of the crushed dried leaves and used as a hallucinogen. After drinking Zacatechichi, the Indians recline quietly to smoke a cigarette of the dried leaves.	There is an as yet unidentified alkaloid. Also contains sesquiterpene-lactone. Restful and drowsy condition during which the Indians say that one's own heart and pulse can be felt.

TAB.III

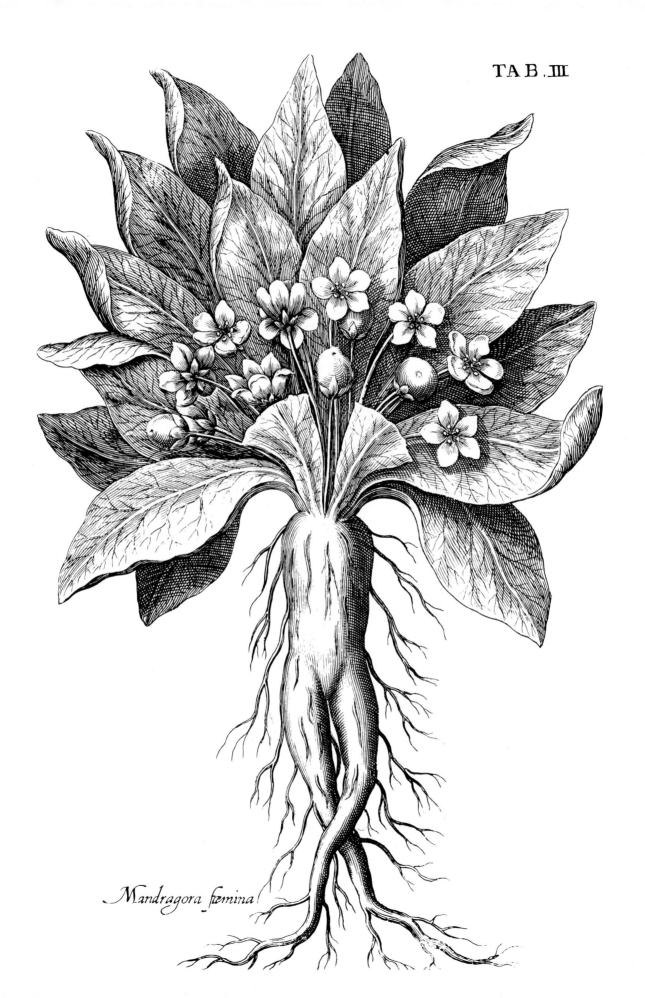

Mandragora fœmina

THE MOST IMPORTANT HALLUCINOGENIC PLANTS

Of the ninety-seven hallucinogens in the lexicon, the most important are discussed in detail in the ensuing chapters. Several reasons underlie our selection. Most of these plants are or have been so culturally and materially important in aboriginal societies that they cannot be overlooked. A few are of special botanical or chemical interest. Others are of great antiquity. Still others have recently been discovered or identified. And the use of one has spread throughout the modern world and is now of vital importance.

Amanita muscaria (Fly Agaric), one of the oldest hallucinogens, is employed in both hemispheres and is biochemically significant, since its active principle is atypically excreted unmetabolized.

The use of Peyote (*Lophophora williamsii*), of great antiquity, has now spread from its original Mexican homeland to Texas in the United States, where it is the basis of a new Indian religion. Its main psychoactive alkaloid, mescaline, is utilized in psychiatry.

The religious use of mushrooms—known as Teonanácatl—in Mexico and Guatemala is ancient and was firmly established among the Aztec Indians at the time of the Conquest. Their psychoactive constituents are novel structures not known in any other plants.

Of similar importance, and as ancient, are the seeds of several Morning Glories. Their use has persisted until the present in southern Mexico. Of great chemo-taxonomic interest, their psychoactive constituents are found only in an unrelated group of fungi, containing Ergot, which may have been hallucinogenically important in ancient Greece.

Deadly Nightshade, Henbane, and Mandrake were the main ingredients of the witches' brews of medieval Europe, where they long exerted a great cultural and historical influence.

In both hemispheres, *Datura* played highly significant roles in native cultures. The related *Brugmansia* is still employed as one of the principal hallucinogens in South America.

Archaeology indicates that the South American cactus *Trichocereus pachanoi* has a long history, although it has only recently been identified as a principal hallucinogen of the central Andes.

The most significant African hallucinogen is Iboga, employed in initiation rituals and to communicate with ancestors. Spreading today in Gabon and the Congo, it is a unifying culture trait deterring the intrusion of foreign customs from Western society.

The intoxicating drink prepared from *Banisteriopsis* holds a place of cultural primacy throughout the western Amazon. Known in Peru as Ayahuasca ("vine of the soul"), it allows the soul to leave the body and wander freely, communicating with the spirit world. Its psychoactive principles are β-carbolines and tryptamines.

Three snuffs are of importance in certain South American cultures. One, in the western Amazon, is prepared from a resin like liquid produced in the bark of several species of *Virola*. The others, made from the beans of a species of *Anadenanthera* and used in the Orinoco, adjacent Amazon, and Argentina, was formerly also valued in the West Indies. Both snuffs play significant roles in the life of many Indian groups and are of chemical interest, since their active principles are tryptamines.

Pituri is the most important psychoactive substance in Australia. *Cannabis,* an ancient Asiatic hallucinogen, is now used in nearly all parts of the world. An understanding of its roles in primitive societies may help elucidate its popularity in Western culture. Some of the fifty chemical structures found in *Cannabis* are medically promising.

A long chapter could well be written about any of the more than ninety species which have been enumerated in the plant lexicon. But in the interest of space, the following have been treated in greater detail for the reasons outlined.

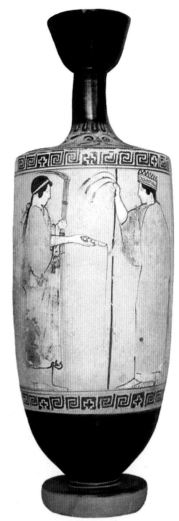

The Greek lecythus is a sacramental vessel filled with fragrant oils and placed next to a death bed or grave. On this lecythus (450–425 B.C.), a crowned Triptolemus holds the Eleusinian grain, a grass probably infected with Ergot; while Demeter or Persephone pours a sacred libation, prepared presumably from the infected grain. The two figures are separated by the staff of Triptolemus and united into one field by the grain and poured libation.

Page 80: Mandrake *(Mandragora officinarum),* "the man-like plant," has a complex history of usage. In Europe, it was employed as a stupefacient in addition to being one of the strongest ingredients added to the brews concocted by witches of the Middle Ages. The root of the Mandrake was likened to the form of a man or woman, and according to superstition, if the plant were pulled from the earth, its shrieks could drive the collectors mad. This image of *Mandragora* was engraved by the well-known artist Matthäus Merian in the early eighteenth century.

Page 83 top: Cliff drawing of a shaman in the Altai mountains of Asia.

Page 83 right: Fly Agaric (*Amanita muscaria)* is found around the world and is associated nearly everywhere with fairy worlds, alternative realities, and shamanic practices.

Soma, the god-narcotic of ancient India, attained an exalted place in magico-religious ceremonies of the Aryans, who 3,500 years ago swept down from the north into the Indus Valley, bringing with them the cult of Soma. These early invaders of India worshiped the holy inebriant and drank an extract of it in their most sacred rites. Whereas most hallucinogenic plants were considered merely as sacred mediators, Soma became a god in its own right. An ancient Indian tradition recorded in the Rig-Veda asserts that "Parjanya, the god of thunder, was the father of Soma" (Indra).

"Enter into the heart of Indra, receptacle

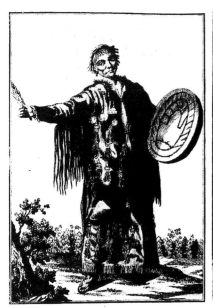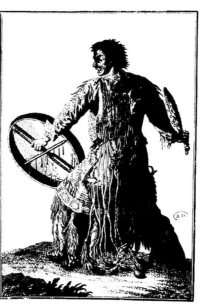

Siberian shamans use elaborate symbolic costumes and decorated drums in their ceremonies. The left figure is a shaman from Krasnojarsk District; at right, the Kamtchatka District.

of Soma, like rivers into the ocean, thou who pleasest Mitra, Varuna, Vaya, mainstay of heaven! ... Father of the gods, progenitor of the moving force, mainstay of the sky, foundation of the earth."

Of the more than 1,000 holy hymns in the Rig-Veda, 120 are devoted exclusively to Soma, and references to this vegetal sacrament run through many of the other hymns. The cult was suppressed, and the original holy plant was forgotten; other plant surrogates—with little

or no psychoactivity—were substituted. Yet the identity of Soma remained one of the enigmas of ethnobotany for two thousand years. Only in 1968 did the interdisciplinary research of Gordon Wasson provide persuasive evidence that the sacred narcotic was a mushroom, *Amanita muscaria,* the Fly Agaric. *Amanita muscaria* may be the oldest of the hallucinogens and perhaps was once the most widely used.

The curious hallucinogenic use of *Amanita muscaria* has been documented since 1730. It was then that a Swedish military officer, a prisoner of war in Siberia for twelve years, reported that primitive tribesmen there employed the Fly Agaric as a shamanistic inebriant. The custom persisted among scattered groups of Finno-Ugrian peoples of Siberia. Traditions suggest that other groups in this vast northern region also used the mushroom.

A Koryak legend tells us that the culture hero, Big Raven, caught a whale but was unable to put such a heavy animal back into the sea. The god Vahiyinin (Existence) told him to eat *wapaq* spirits to get the strength that he needed. Vahiyinin spat upon the earth, and little white plants—the *wapaq* spirits—appeared: they had red hats and Vahiyinin's spittle congealed as white flecks. When he had eaten *wapaq,* Big Raven became exceedingly strong, and he pleaded: "O *wapaq,* grow forever on earth." Whereupon he commanded his people to learn what *wapaq* could teach them. *Wapaq* is the Fly Agaric, a gift directly from Vahiyinin.

These Siberian mushroom users had no other intoxicants, until the Russians introduced alcohol. They dried the mushrooms in the sun and ingested them either alone or as an extract in water, reindeer milk, or the juice of several sweet plants. When the mushroom was swallowed as a solid, it was first moistened in the mouth, or a woman rolled it in her mouth into a moistened pellet for the men to swallow. The ceremonial use of the Fly Agaric developed a ritualistic practice of urine-drinking, since these tribesmen learned

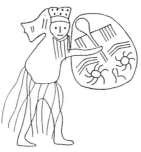

that the psychoactive principles of the mushroom pass through the body unmetabolized, or in the form of still active metabolites—most unusual for hallucinogenic compounds in plants. An early account, referring to the Koryak, reported that "they pour water on some of the mushrooms and boil them. They then drink the liquor, which intoxicates them; the poorer sort, who cannot afford to lay in a store of the mushrooms, post themselves on these occasions round the huts of the rich and watch the opportunity of the guests coming down to make water and then hold a wooden bowl to receive the urine, which they drink off greedily, as having still some virtue of the mushroom in it, and by this way, they also get drunk."

The Rig-Veda definitely refers to urine-drinking in the Soma ritual: "The swollen men piss the flowing Soma. The lords, with full bladders, piss Soma quick with movement." The priests impersonating Indra and Vayu, having drunk Soma in milk, urinate Soma. In the Vedic poems, urine is not offensive but is an ennobling metaphor to describe rain: the blessings of rain are likened to showers of urine, and the clouds fertilize the earth with their urine.

A traveler among the Koryak in the early twentieth century offered one of the few descriptions of intoxication in aboriginal use of the mushroom. He wrote that the "Fly Agaric produces intoxication, hallucinations, and delirium. Light forms of intoxication are accompanied by a certain degree of animation and some spontaneity of movements. Many shamans, previous to their séances, eat Fly Agaric to get into ecstatic states . . . Under strong intoxication, the senses become deranged, surrounding objects appear either very large or very small, hallucinations set in, spontaneous movements and convulsions. So far as I could observe, attacks of great animation alternate with moments of deep depression. The person intoxicated by Fly Agaric sits quietly rocking from side to side, even taking part in conversations with his family. Suddenly, his eyes dilate, he begins to gesticulate convulsively,

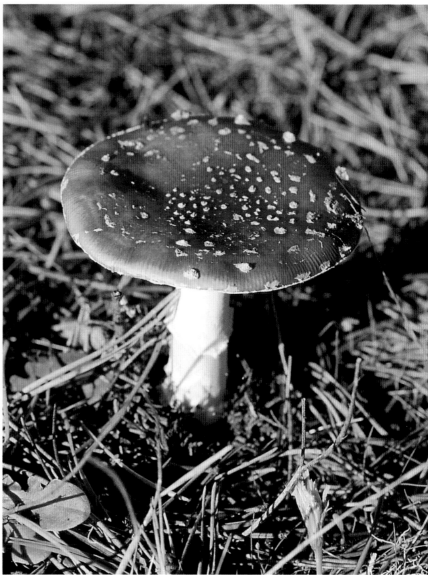

The Chemistry of Fly Agaric

The active principle of *Amanita muscaria* was thought once, a century ago, to have been muscarine when Schmiedeberg and Koppe isolated this substance. This belief has been proved erroneous. Recently Eugster in Switzerland and Takemoto in Japan isolated ibotenic acid and the alkaloid muscimole as being responsible for the Fly Agaric's psychotropic effects. The mushroom is taken usually dried. The drying process induces the chemical transformation of ibotenic acid to muscimole, the most active constituent.

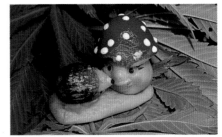

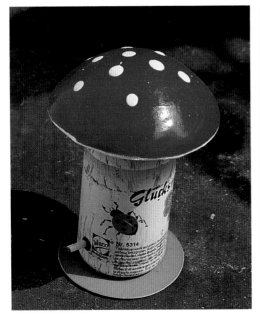

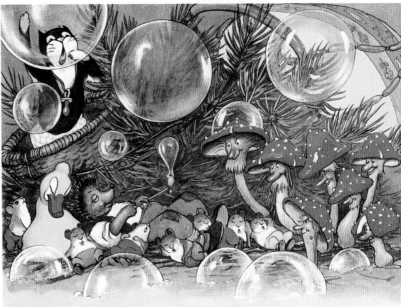

Above left: To bring good luck into the coming year, fireworks in the shape of Fly Agaric are set off on New Year's Eve.

Above right: The results of smoking Fly Agaric are depicted in the German children's book *Mecki and the Dwarves.*

Below right: It is possible that Fly Agaric is identical to the Vedic wonder-drug Soma. Today Ephedra *(Ephedra gerardiana)* is called *somalata,* "soma plant." In Nepal Ephedra is not hallucinogenic or psychedelic but is a very strong stimulant.

converses with persons whom he imagines he sees, sings and dances. Then an interval of rest sets in again."

The Fly Agaric was apparently employed hallucinogenically in Mesoamerica. It occurs naturally in highland areas in southern Mexico and Guatemala. The Maya of highland Guatemala, for example, recognize *Amanita muscaria* as having special properties, for they call it Kakuljá-ikox ("lightning mushroom"), relating it to one of the gods, Rajaw Kakuljá or Lord of Lightning. It is this god who directs the operating of *chacs,* dwarf rain-bringers now usually known by their Christian designation, *angelitos.* The Quiche name of the *Amanita muscaria,* Kaquljá, refers to its legendary origin, whereas the term *Itzelo-cox* refers to its sacred power as "evil or diabolical mushroom." Thunder and lightning have widely and anciently been associated with mushrooms, in both hemispheres, especially with *Amanita muscaria.* "In any event, the Quiche-Maya . . . are evidently well aware the *Amanita muscaria* is no ordinary mushroom but relates to the supernatural."

The first settlers of the Americas came from Asia, slowly crossing the region of the Bering Strait. Anthropologists have found many Asia-related or remnant culture traits that persist in the Americas. Recent discoveries have uncovered vestiges of the magico-religious importance of the Fly Agaric that have indeed survived in North American cultures. Indications of undoubted

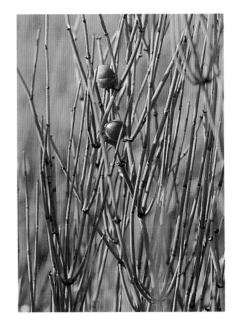

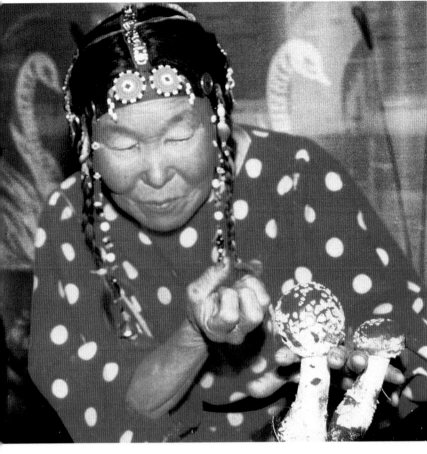

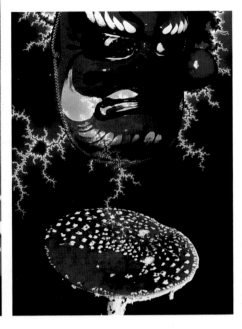

hallucinogenic use of the Fly Agaric have been discovered among the Dogrib Athabascan peoples, who live on the Mackenzie Mountain range in northwestern Canada. Here *Amanita muscaria* is employed as a sacrament in shamanism. A young neophyte reported that whatever the shaman had done to him, "he had snatched me. I had no volition, I had no power of my own. I didn't eat, didn't sleep, I didn't think—I wasn't in my body any longer." After a later séance, he wrote: "Cleansed and ripe for vision, I rise, a bursting ball of seeds in space . . . I have sung the note that shatters structure. And the note that shatters chaos, and been bloody . . . I have been with the dead and attempted the labyrinth." His first mushroom experience represented dismemberment; his second, meeting with the spirit.

More recently, the religious use of *Amanita muscaria* as a sacred hallucinogen has been discovered in an ancient annual ceremony practiced by the Ojibwa Indians or Ahnishinaubeg who live on Lake Superior in Michigan. The mushroom is known in the Ojibwa language as Oshtimisk Wajashkwedo ("Red-top mushroom").

THE HEXING HERBS

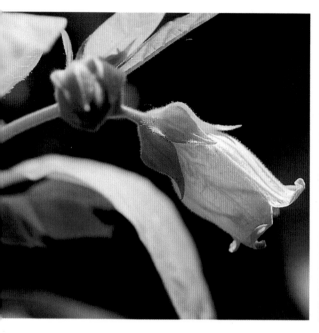

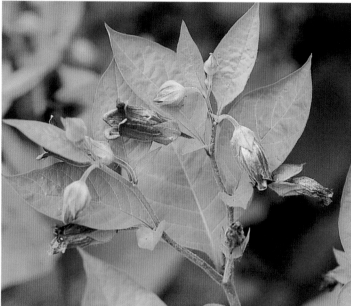

Above left: The yellow blossom of the rare variety of *Atropa belladonna* var. *lutea*. The yellow Deadly Nightshade is regarded as particularly potent for magic and witchcraft.

Above right: The bell-shaped flowers of the Deadly Nightshade clearly show its membership in the Nightshade family.

Page 87 above left: The flowers of the Mandrake *(Mandragora officinarum)* are rarely seen, as they bloom very briefly and then quickly vanish.

Page 87 above right: The flowers of the Black Henbane *(Hyoscyamus niger)* have a characteristic coloring and an unforgettable pattern on the petals. In earlier times, it was thought to be the eye of the devil.

Since antiquity several members of the Nightshade family have been associated with witchcraft in Europe. These plants enable witches to perform feats of occult wonder and prophecy, to hex through hallucinogenic communication with the supernatural and transport themselves to far-off places for the practice of their nefarious skills. These inebriating plants were mainly Henbane, *Hyoscyamus albus* and *H. niger;* Belladonna, *Atropa belladonna;* and Mandrake, *Mandragora officinarum.* All four species have long histories of use as hallucinogens and magic plants connected with sorcery, witchcraft, and superstition. The extraordinary reputation of these plants is due primarily to the bizarre psychoactivity that they possess. Their similarity in effects is the result of similarity in chemical constitution.

These four solanaceous plants contain relatively high concentrations of tropane alkaloids, primarily atropine, hyoscyamine, and scopolamine; other bases are found in trace amounts. It is apparently scopolamine, not atropine or hyoscyamine, that produces the hallucinogenic effects. It induces an intoxication fol-lowed by narcosis in which hallucinations occur during the transition state between consciousness and sleep.

Atropine has served chemists as a model for the synthesis of several hallucinogenic compounds. Their effects—and those of scopolamine—differ from those of the usual natural hallucinogens: they are extremely toxic; and the user remembers nothing experienced during the intoxication, losing all sense of reality and falling into a deep sleep like an alcoholic delirium.

Hyoscyamus has been known and feared from earliest classical periods, when it was recognized that there were several kinds and that the black variety was the most potent, capable of causing insanity. The ancient Egyptians recorded their knowledge of Henbane in the Ebers Papyrus, written in 1500 B.C. Homer described magic drinks with effects indicative of Henbane as a major ingredient. In ancient Greece it served as a poison, to mimic insanity, and to enable man to prophesy. It has been suggested that the priestesses at the Oracle of Delphi made their prophetic utterances while intoxicated with the smoke from Henbane seeds. In the

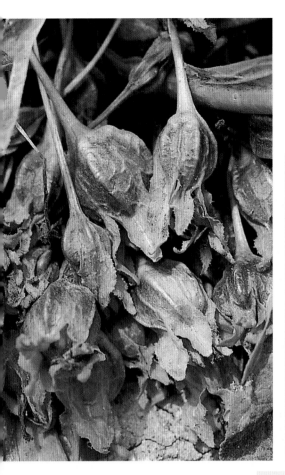

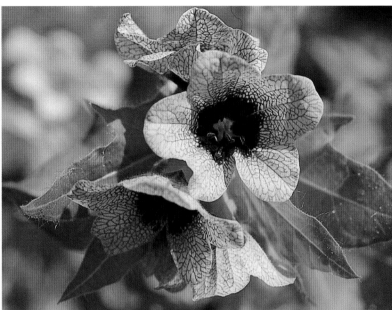

thirteenth century, Bishop Albertus the Great reported that Henbane was employed by necromancers to conjure up demons.

From earliest times, the painkilling properties of Henbane have been recognized, and it has been employed to relieve the suffering of those sentenced to torture and death. Its great advantage lies in its ability not only to allay pain but also to induce a state of complete oblivion.

Henbane is best known as an ingredient of the so-called "witch's salve."

When young people were to be inducted into membership in groups dedicated to witchcraft, for example, they were often given a drink of Henbane so that they could easily be persuaded to engage in the sabbat rituals preparatory to the acceptance officially of a place in witchcraft circles.

Those experiencing intoxication with Henbane feel a pressure in the head, a sensation as if someone were closing the eyelids by force; sight becomes unclear, objects are distorted in shape, and the most unusual visual hallucinations are induced. Gustatory and olfactory hallucinations frequently accompany the

The Chemistry of Deadly Nightshade, Henbane, and Mandrake

The three solanaceous plants *Atropa, Hyoscyamus,* and *Mandragora* contain the same active principles: primarily the alkaloids hyoscyamine, atropine, and scopolamine. The difference is only one of relative concentration. Belladonna contains little scopolamine, but this alkaloid is the main component of Mandrake and especially of Henbane.

The alkaloids are found in the entire plant, with the highest concentration in the seeds and roots. The hallucinogenic effects are due essentially to scopolamine. Atropine and hyosyamine are less active under these circumstances.

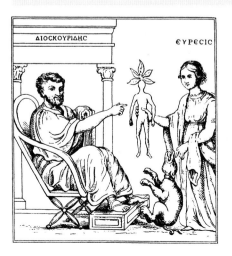

Left: According to this illustration from the *Juliana Codex,* the Greek herbalist Dioscorides received the Mandrake plant from Heuresis, goddess of discovery, illustrating the belief that this medicine was a plant of the gods.

87

"The Mandrake is the 'Tree of Knowledge'
and the burning love ignited by its pleasure
is the origin of the human race."
—Hugo Rahner
Greek Myths in Christian Meaning (1957)

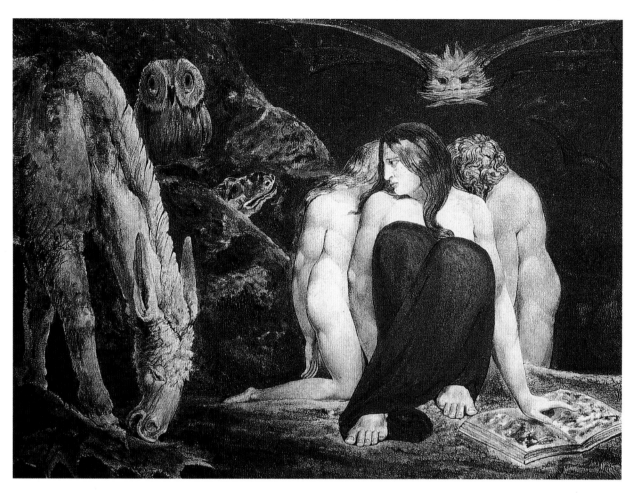

Above: The ancient goddess of witches, Hecate, lords over the psychoactive and magical herbs, particularly those in the Nightshade family. In this colored print by William Blake, she is depicted with her shamanic animals.

Page 89 below right: The design for the cover of a book about medicinal plants depicts the anthropomorphic Mandrake.

intoxication. Eventually sleep, disturbed by dreams and hallucinations, ends the inebriation.

Other species of *Hyoscyamus* have similar properties and are occasionally used in similar ways. Indian Henbane or Egyptian Henbane, or *H. muticus,* occurring from the deserts of Egypt east to Afghanistan and India, is employed in India as an intoxicant, the dried leaves being smoked. The Bedouins particularly employ this intoxicant to become drunk, and in some parts of Asia and Africa it is smoked with *Cannabis* as an inebriant.

Belladonna or Deadly Nightshade is native to Europe but is now spontaneous as an escape from cultivation in the United States and India. Its generic name, *Atropa,* comes from the Greek

Fate Atropos, the inflexible one who cuts the thread of life. The specific epithet, meaning "beautiful lady," recalls the use of sap of the plant to dilate the pupils of the eyes among the fine ladies of Italy who believed that the dreamy, intoxicated stare thus produced was the height of fetching beauty. Many vernacular names of the plant refer to its intoxicating properties: Sorcerer's Cherry, Witch's Berry, Devil's Herb, Murderer's Berry, Dwaleberry (*dwale* in English deriving from the Scandinavian root meaning "trance").

The maenads of the orgies of Dionysus in Greek mythology dilated their eyes and threw themselves into the arms of male worshipers of this god or, with "flaming eyes," they fell upon men to tear them apart and eat them. The wine

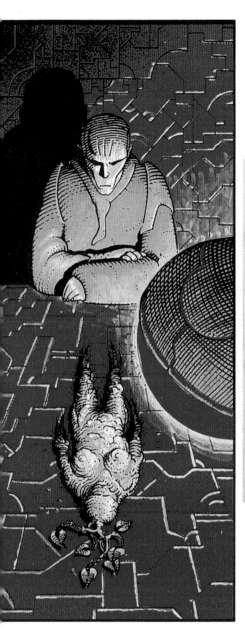

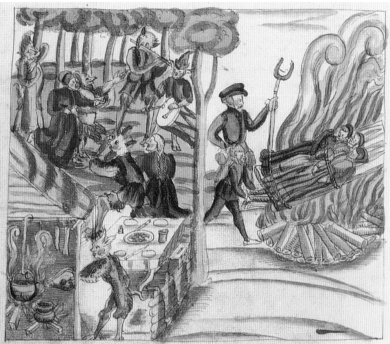

Left: The magical conjuration of the Mandrake is a durable theme in European literature and art history. Here is a scene from a modern comic, *Caza.*

Below right: "Witches" persecuted during the Inquisition were often accused of using hallucinogenic plants of the Nightshade family, in particular, Henbane and Mandrake. For this many were tortured, murdered, and burned.

of Bacchanals was possibly adulterated with juice of the Nightshade. Another belief from classical times maintained that Roman priests drank Belladonna before their supplications to the goddess of war for victory.

It was during the early Modern period, however, that Belladonna assumed its greatest importance in witchcraft and magic. It was one of the primary ingredients of the brews and ointments employed by witches and sorcerers. One such potent mixture, containing Belladonna, Henbane, Mandrake, and the fat of a stillborn child, was rubbed over the skin or inserted into the vagina for absorption. The familiar witch's broomstick goes far back in European magic beliefs. An investigation into witchcraft in 1324 reported that "in rifleing the

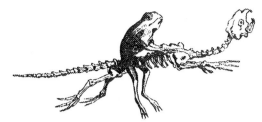

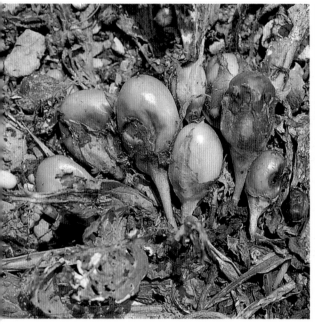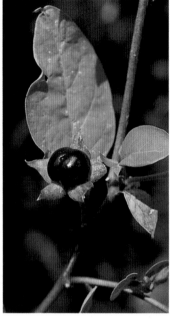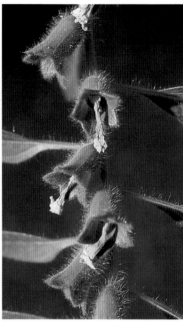

closet of the ladie, they found a Pipe of ointment, wherewith she greased a staffe, upon which she ambled and galloped through thick and thin, when and in what manner she listed." Later, in the fifteenth century, a similar account stated: "But the vulgar believe and the witches confess, that on certain days and nights they anoint a staff and ride on it to the appointed place or anoint themselves under the arms and in other hairy places and sometimes carry charms under the hair." Porta, a contemporary of Galileo, wrote in 1589 that under the effects of a potion of these solanaceous plants a "man would seem sometimes to be changed into a fish; and flinging out his arms, would swim on the ground; sometimes he would seem to skip up and then to dive down again. Another would believe himself turned into a goose and would eat grass, and beat the ground with his teeth like a goose; now and then sing and . . . clap his wings."

Mandrake became famous in magic and witchcraft because of its powerful narcotic effects and the bizarre form of its root. It would be difficult to find a better example of the application of the philosophy of the Doctrine of Signa-

tures. For the root of this herbaceous perennial, unassuming in its growth appearance, is so twisted and branched that it occasionally resembles the human body. This extraordinary resemblance led early to the belief that it exercised great supernatural powers over the human body and mind, even though actually its chemical composition gave it no greater psychoactivity than some other solanaceous species.

From earliest times, curious beliefs about the need to exercise great care in harvesting the root grew up. Theophrastus in the third century B.C. wrote that collectors of medicinal plants drew circles around Mandrake, and they cut off the top part of the root while facing west; the remainder of the root was gathered after the collectors had performed certain dances and recited special formulas. Two centuries earlier, the Greek Pythagoras had described Mandrake root as an anthropomorph, or tiny human being. In Roman times that magic began extensively to be associated with the psychoactive properties of the plant. In the first century A.D., Josephus Flavius wrote that there grew a plant in the Dead Sea area that glowed

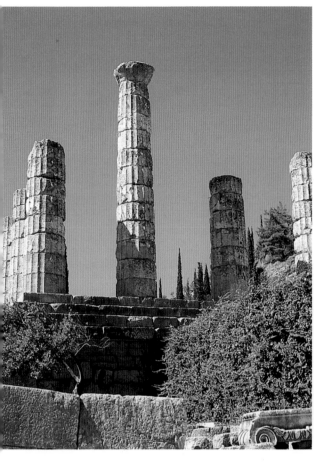

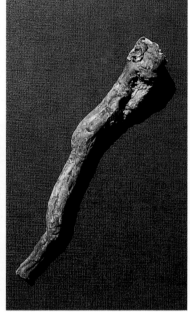

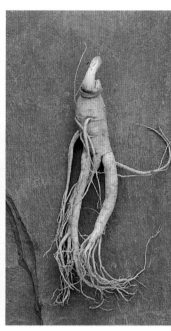

red at night and that it was difficult to approach the plant, which hid when a man drew near it; but it could be tamed if urine and menstrual blood were sprinkled on it. It was physically dangerous to pull the plant from the earth, but a dog, tied to the root, was employed to extract the root, after which, according to belief, the animal usually died. The myths surrounding Mandrake grew, until it was said that the plant hid by day but shone like a star at night, and that when being pulled from the ground the plant let out such unearthly shrieks that whoever heard the noise might die. Eventually, only black dogs—a color denoting evil and death—were employed. Early Christians believed that the Mandrake root was originally created by God as an experiment before he created man in the Garden of Eden.

When, later in the Dark Ages, Mandrake began to be cultivated in central Europe, it was thought that the plant would grow only under gallows where urine or semen from the condemned man fell—hence the common German names meaning "gallows man" and "dragon doll."

The apogee of Mandrake's fame seems to have occurred in the late sixteenth century. At this time, the herbalists began to doubt many of the tales associated with the plant. As early as 1526 the English herbalist Turner had denied that all Mandrake roots had a human form and protested against the beliefs connected with its anthropomorphism. Another English herbalist, Gerard, for example, wrote in 1597: "All which dreams and old wives tales you shall henceforth cast out of your books and memory; knowing this, that they are all and everie part of them false and most untrue. For I my selfe and my servants also have digged up, planted and replanted very many . . ." But many superstitions surrounding Mandrake persisted in European folklore even into the nineteenth century.

Above left: In the Temple of Apollo at Delphi, the "navel of the world," the Sibyl and prophetess informed the Pythia of her oracle after she had inhaled the smoke of Henbane.

Above middle: The root of the Mandrake *(Mandragora officinarum).*

Above right: The Ginseng's *(Panax ginseng)* root is not only similar to the Mandrake, but in Korea, Ginseng root is also attributed with secret and magical powers.

Below left: The sun and oracle god Apollo at a libation in front of a raven. (Discovered at Delphi).

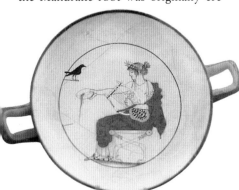

91

THE NECTAR OF DELIGHT

Tradition in India maintains that the gods sent man the Hemp plant so that he might attain delight and courage, and have heightened sexual desires. When nectar or Amrita dropped down from heaven, *Cannabis* sprouted from it. Another story tells how, when the gods, helped by demons, churned the milk ocean to obtain Amrita, one of the resulting nectars was *Cannabis*. It was consecrated to Shiva and was Indra's favorite drink. After the churning of the

"seeds," consumed by man for food; for its narcotic properties; and therapeutically to treat a wide spectrum of ills in folk medicine and in modern pharmacopoeias.

Mainly because of its various uses, *Cannabis* has been taken to many regions around the world. Unusual things happen to plants after long association with man and agriculture. They are grown in new and strange environments and often have opportunities to

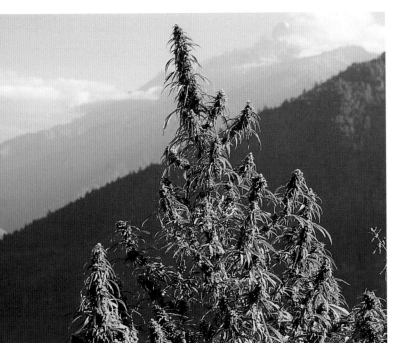

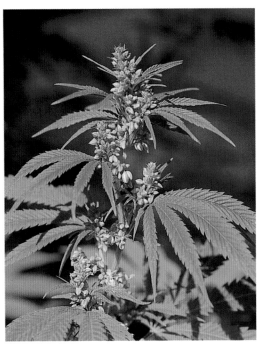

Above left: Wild Hemp plants *(Cannabis indica)* with splendid white flowers in the Langtang region of the Himalayas (Nepal).

Above right: Masculine plant of a Hemp cross-breed *(Cannabis indica x sativa).*

ocean, demons attempted to gain control of Amrita, but the gods were able to prevent this seizure, giving *Cannabis* the name Vijaya ("victory") to commemorate their success. Ever since, this plant of the gods has been held in India to bestow supernatural powers on its users.

The partnership of *Cannabis* and man has existed now probably for ten thousand years—since the discovery of agriculture in the Old World. One of our oldest cultivars, *Cannabis* has been a five-purpose plant: as a source of hempen fibers; for its oil; for its akenes or

hybridize that are not offered in their native habitats. They escape from cultivation and frequently become aggressive weeds. They may be changed through human selection for characteristics associated with a specific use. Many cultivated plants are so changed from their ancestral types that it is not possible to unravel their evolutionary history. Such is not the case, however, with *Cannabis*. Yet despite its long history as a major crop plant, *Cannabis* is still characterized more by what is not known about its biology than by what is known.

Below left: The blue-skinned Hindu god Shiva takes great pleasure in Hemp. Because of this, it is a sacred plant of the gods and is used for rituals and Tantric practices.

Right: The long-haired Sadhus or "holy men" of India devote their lives to the god Shiva. They have no property and practice yoga and meditation. In addition they often smoke a large amount of *charas* (handmade hash) and *ganja* (Marijuana) sometimes mixed with *Datura* leaves and other psychoac-tive plants (Sadhu at a Shiva temple, Pashupatinath, Kathmandu Valley, Nepal).

Bottom right: Cannabis is consumed in many countries, usually illegally. It is often smoked in hand-rolled cigarettes. There are countless products for the consumption of marijuana for everyone from beginners to the specialists—for instance, large-format rolling papers, preferably out of Hemp. Also shown here are a metal cigarette box and lighter.

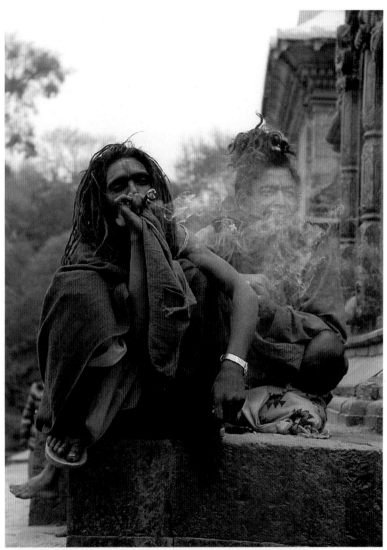

The botanical classification of *Cannabis* has long been uncertain. Botanists have not agreed on the family to which *Cannabis* belongs: early investigators put it in the Nettle family (Urticaceae); later it was accommodated in the Fig family (Moraceae); the general trend today is to assign it to a special family, Cannabaceae, in which only *Cannabis* and *Humulus,* the genus of Hops, are members. There has even been disagreement as to how many species of *Cannabis* exist:

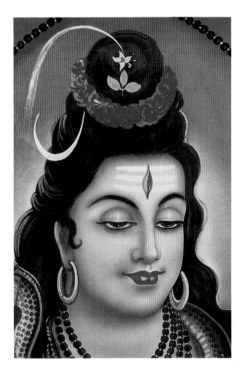

whether the genus comprises one highly variable species or several distinct species. Evidence now strongly indicates that three species can be recognized: *C. indica, C. ruderalis,* and *C. sativa.* These species are distinguished by different growth habits, characters of the akenes, and especially by major differences in structure of the wood. Although all species possess cannabinols, there may possibly be significant chemical differences, but the evidence is not yet available.

The Indian vedas sang of *Cannabis* as one of the divine nectars, able to give

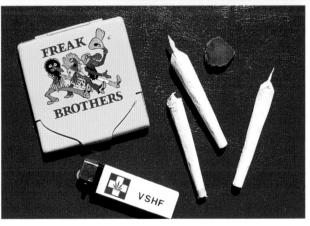

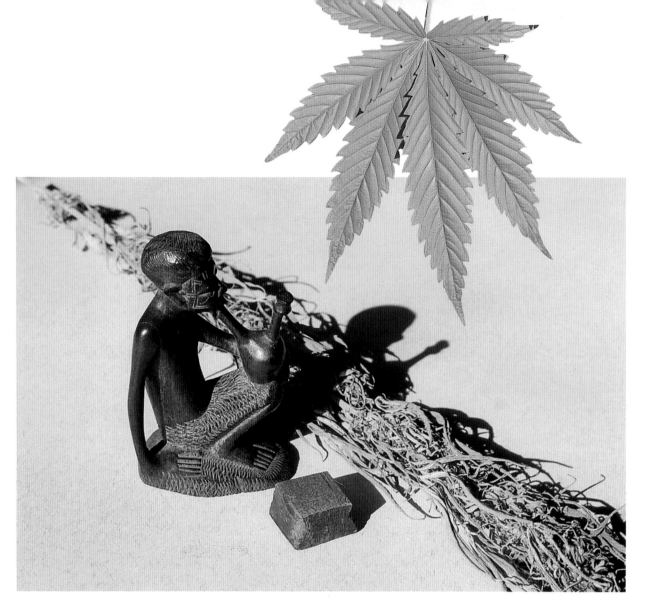

Above: In Africa Hemp is smoked for medicinal and pleasurable purposes, as this wood carving shows.

Top: The characteristic Hemp leaf *(Cannabis indica)* was formerly a symbol of the subculture and rebellion. Today, it has become a symbol of ecological awareness.

man anything from good health and long life to visions of the gods. The Zend-Avesta of 600 B.C. mentions an intoxicating resin, and the Assyrians used *Cannabis* as an incense as early as the ninth century B.C.

Inscriptions from the Chou dynasty in China, dated 700–500 B.C., have a "negative" connotation that accompanies the ancient character for *Cannabis, Ma,* implying its stupefying properties. Since this idea obviously predated writing, the Pen Tsao Ching, written in A.D. 100 but going back to a legendary emperor, Shen-Nung, 2000 B.C., maybe taken as evidence that the Chinese knew and probably used the psychoactive properties at very early dates. It was said that *Ma-fen* ("Hemp fruit") "if taken to excess, will produce hallucinations [literally, "seeing devils"]. If taken over a long term, it makes one communicate with spirits and lightens one's

body." A Taoist priest wrote in the fifth century B.C. that *Cannabis* was employed by "necromancers, in combination with Ginseng, to set forward time and reveal future events." In these early periods, use of *Cannabis* as a hallucinogen was undoubtedly associated with Chinese shamanism, but by the time of European contact 1,500 years later, shamanism had fallen into decline, and the use of the plant for inebriation seems to have ceased and been forgotten. Its value in China then was primarily as a fiber source. There was, however, a continuous record of Hemp cultivation in China from Neolithic times, and it has been suggested that *Cannabis* may have originated in China, not in central Asia.

About 500 B.C. the Greek writer Herodotus described a marvelous steam bath of the Scythians, aggressive horsemen who swept out of the Transcaucasus eastward and westward. He

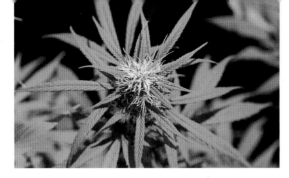

reported that "they make a booth by fixing in the ground three sticks inclined toward one another, and stretching around them woollen pelts which they arrange so as to fit as close as possible: inside the booth a dish is placed upon the ground into which they put a number of red hot stones and then add some Hemp seed ... immediately it smokes and gives out such a vapor as no Grecian vapor bath can exceed; the Scyths, delighted, shout for joy ..." Only recently, archaeologists have excavated frozen Scythian tombs in central Asia, dated between 500 and 300 B.C., and have found tripods and pelts, braziers, and charcoal with remains of *Cannabis* leaves and fruit. It has generally been accepted that *Cannabis* originated in central Asia and that it was the Scythians who spread the plant westward to Europe.

While the Greeks and Romans may not generally have taken *Cannabis* for inebriation, they were aware of the psychoactive effects of the drug. Democritus reported that it was occasionally drunk with wine and myrrh to produce visionary states, and Galen, about A.D. 200, wrote that it was sometimes customary to give Hemp to guests to promote hilarity and enjoyment.

Cannabis arrived in Europe from the north. The Roman writer Lucilius mentioned it in 120 B.C. Pliny the Elder outlined the preparation and grades of hempen fibers in the first century A.D., and hempen rope was found in a Roman site in England dated A.D. 140–180. Whether or not the Vikings used Hemp rope is not known, but palynological evidence indicates that Hemp cultivation had a tremendous increment in England from the early Anglo-Saxon period to late Saxon and Norman times—from 400 to 1100.

Henry VIII fostered the cultivation of Hemp in England. The maritime supremacy of England during Elizabethan times greatly increased the demand. Hemp cultivation began in the British colonies in the New World: first in Canada in 1606, then in Virginia in 1611; the Pilgrims took the crop to New Eng-

land in 1632. In pre-Revolutionary North America, Hemp was employed even for making work clothes.

Hemp was introduced quite independently into Spanish colonies in South America: Chile, 1545; Peru, 1554.

There is no doubt that hempen fiber production represents an early use of *Cannabis,* but perhaps consumption of its edible akenes as food predated the discovery of the useful fiber. These akenes are very nutritious, and it is difficult to imagine that early man, constantly searching for food, would have missed this opportunity. Archaeological finds of Hemp akenes in Germany, dated at 500 B.C., indicate the nutritional use of these plant products. From early times to the present, Hemp akenes have been used as food in eastern Europe, and in the United States as a major ingredient of bird food.

The folk-medicinal value of Hemp—frequently indistinguishable from its psychoactive properties—may even be its earliest role as an economic plant. The earliest record of the medicinal use of the plant is that of the Chinese emperor-herbalist Shen-Nung who, five thousand years ago, recommended *Cannabis* for malaria, beri-beri, constipation, rheumatic pains, absent-mindedness, and female disorders. Hoa-Glio, another ancient Chinese herbalist, recommended a mixture of Hemp resin and wine as an analgesic during surgery.

It was in ancient India that this "gift of the gods" found excessive use in folk medicine. It was believed to quicken the mind, prolong life, improve judgment, lower fevers, induce sleep, cure dysentery. Because of its psychoactive properties it was more highly valued than medicines with only physical activity. Several systems of Indian medicine esteemed *Cannabis.* The medical work *Sushrata* states that it cured leprosy. The *Bharaprakasha,* of about A.D. 1600, described it as antiphlegmatic, digestive, bile affecting, pungent, and astringent, prescribing it to stimulate the appetite, improve digestion, and better the voice. The spectrum of medicinal uses in India covered control of

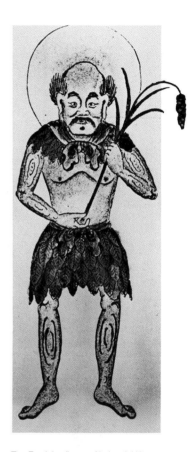

Top: Feminine flower of industrial Hemp *(Cannabis sativa).*

Above: The Chinese emperor Shen-Nung is said to have discovered the medicinal properties of many plants. His pharmacopoeia, believed to have been first compiled in 2737 B.C., notes that *Cannabis sativa* has both male and female plants.

95

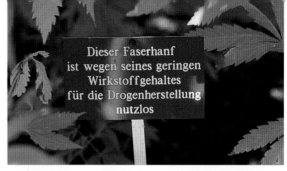

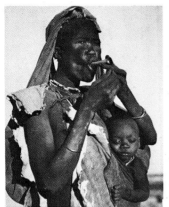
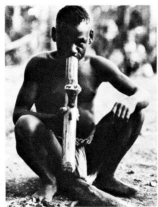
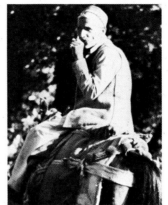
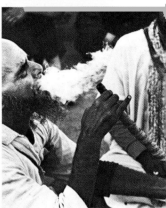

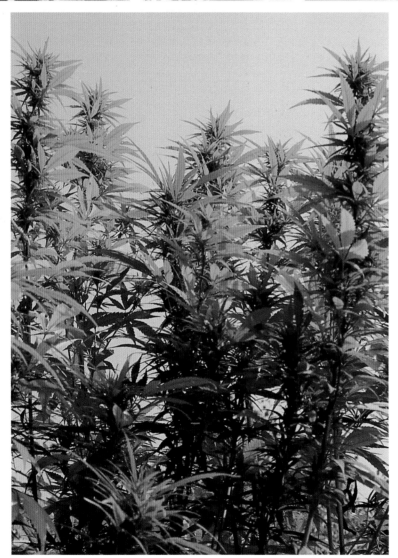

dandruff and relief of headache, mania, insomnia, venereal disease, whooping cough, earache, and tuberculosis!

The fame of *Cannabis* as a medicine spread with the plant. In parts of Africa, it was valued in treating dysentery, malaria, anthrax, and fevers. Even today the Hottentots and Mfengu claim its efficacy in treating snakebites, and Sotho women induce partial stupefaction by smoking Hemp before childbirth.

Cannabis was highly valued in medicine, and its therapeutic uses can be traced back to early classical physicians Dioscorides and Galen. Medieval herbalists distinguished "manured hempe" (cultivated) from "bastard hempe" (weedy), recommending the latter "against nodes and wennes and other hard tumors," the former for a host of uses from curing cough to jaundice. They cautioned, however, that in excess it might cause sterility, that "it drieth up . . . the seeds of generation" in men "and the milke of women's breasts." An interesting use in the sixteenth century—source of the name Angler's Weed in England—was locally important: "poured into the holes of earthwormes [it] will draw them forth and . . . fishermen and anglers have used this feate to baite their hooks."

The value of *Cannabis* in folk medicine has clearly been closely tied with its euphoric and psychoactive properties; knowledge of these effects may be as old as its use as a source of fiber. Primitive man, trying all sorts of plant

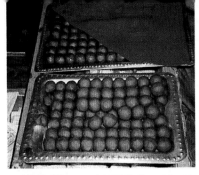
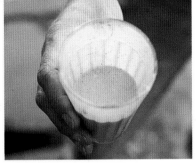

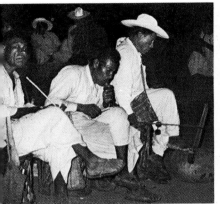
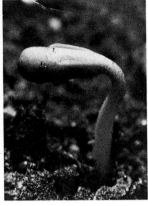
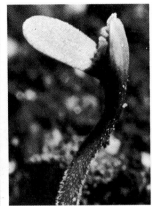
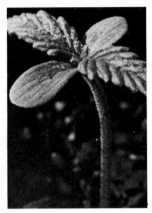

materials as food, must have known the ecstatic euphoria-inducing effects of Hemp, an intoxication introducing him to an otherworldly plane leading to religious beliefs. Thus the plant early was viewed as a special gift of the gods, a sacred medium for communion with the spirit world.

Although *Cannabis* today is the most widely employed psychoactive substance, its use purely as a narcotic, except in Asia, appears not to be ancient. In classical times its euphoric properties were, however, recognized. In Thebes, Hemp was made into a drink said to have opium-like properties. Galen reported that cakes with Hemp, if eaten to excess, were intoxicating. The use as an inebriant seems to have been spread east and west by barbarian hordes of central Asia, especially the Scythians, who had a profound cultural influence on early Greece and eastern Europe. And knowledge of the psychoactive effects of Hemp goes far back in Indian history, as indicated by the deep mythological and spiritual beliefs about the plant. One preparation, Bhang, was so sacred that it was thought to deter evil, bring luck, and cleanse man of sin. Those treading upon the leaves of this holy plant would suffer harm or disaster, and sacred oaths were sealed over Hemp. The favorite drink of Indra, god of the firmament, was made from *Cannabis,* and the Hindu god Shiva commanded that the word *Ghangi* be chanted repeatedly in hymns during

sowing, weeding, and harvesting of the holy plant. Knowledge and use of the intoxicating properties eventually spread to Asia Minor. Hemp was employed as an incense in Assyria in the first millennium B.C., suggesting its use as an inebriant. While there is no direct mention of Hemp in the Bible, several obscure passages may refer tangentially to the effects of *Cannabis* resin or Hashish.

It is perhaps in the Himalayas of India and the Tibetan plateau that *Cannabis* preparations assumed their greatest importance in religious contexts. Bhang is a mild preparation: dried leaves or flowering shoots are pounded with spices into a paste and consumed as candy—known as *maa-jun*—or in tea form. Ganja is made from the resin-rich dried pistillate flowering tops of cultivated plants that are pressed into a compacted mass and kept under pressure for several days to induce chemical changes; most Ganja is smoked, often with Tobacco or *Datura*. Charas consists of the resin itself, a brownish mass that is employed generally in smoking mixtures.

The Tibetans considered *Cannabis* sacred. A Mahayana Buddhist tradition maintains that during the six steps of asceticism leading to his enlightenment, Buddha lived on one Hemp seed a day. He is often depicted with "Soma leaves" in his begging bowl and the mysterious god-narcotic Soma has occasionally been identified with Hemp. In Tantric

The Chemistry of Marijuana

Whereas the psychoactive principles of most hallucinogenic plants are alkaloids, the active constituents of *Cannabis* are non-nitrogenous and occur in a resinous oil. The psychoactive properties are due to cannabinoids, of which the most effective is tetrahydrocannabinol, or THC—chemically: $(-)\Delta^1$-3,4-transtetrahydrocannabinol. The highest concentration is found in the resin of the unfertilized pistillate inflorescence. Even though less potent, the dried leaves are also employed for their psychoactive effects.

Following the elucidation of the chemical structure (see molecular model on page 184), it has recently been possible to synthesize THC.

Psychoactive Plants that are used as a Marijuana Substitute

Botanical Name	Common Name	Part of Plant Used
Alchornea floribunda	Niando	Roots
Argemone mexicana	Prickly Poppy	Leaves
Artemisia mexicana	Mexican Mugwort	Herbage
Calea zacatechichi	Dog Grass	Herbage
Canavalia maritima	Sea Bean	Leaves
Catharanthus roseus	Madagascar Periwinkle	Leaves
Cecropia mexicana	Chancarro	Leaves
Cestrum laevigatum	Lady of the Night	Leaves
Cestrum parqui	Palqui	Leaves
Cymbopogon densiflorus	Lemongrass	Flower extract
Helichrysum foetidum	Everlasting	Herbage
Helichrysum stenopterum	Everlasting	Herbage
Hieracium pilocella	Hawkweed	Herbage
Leonotis leonurus	Wild Dagga	Herbage
Leonurus sibiricus	Siberian Motherwort	Herbage
Nepeta cataria	Catnip	Herbage
Piper auritum	Root Beer Plant	Leaves
Sceletium tortuosum	Kougued	Herbage, Roots
Sida acuta	Common Wireweed	Herbage
Sida rhombifolia	Escobilla	Herbage
Turnera diffusa	Damiana	Herbage
Zornia diphylla	Maconha Brava	Leaves
Zornia latifolia	Maconha Brava	Dried leaves

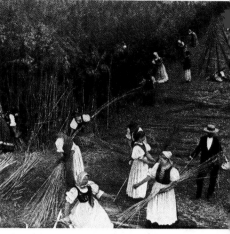

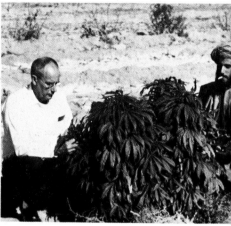

Buddhism of the Himalayas of Tibet, *Cannabis* plays a very significant role in the meditative ritual used to facilitate deep meditation and heighten awareness. Both medicinal and recreational secular use of Hemp is likewise so common now in this region that the plant is taken for granted as an everyday necessity.

Folklore maintains that the use of Hemp was introduced to Persia by an Indian pilgrim during the reign of Khursu (A. D. 531–579), but it is known that the Assyrians used Hemp as an incense during the first millennium B. C. Although at first prohibited among Islamic peoples, Hashish spread widely west throughout Asia Minor. In 1378, authorities tried to extirpate Hemp from Arabian territory by the imposition of harsh punishments.

Cannabis extended early and widely from Asia Minor into Africa, partly under the pressure of Islamic influence, but the use of Hemp transcends Islamic areas. It is widely believed that Hemp was introduced also with slaves from Malaya. Commonly known in Africa as Kif or Dagga, the plant has

> "Hemp is the 'giver of joy,' 'heaven's pilot,' 'the heavenly guide,'
> 'the heaven of the poor man,' 'the soother of sorrows.'
> No god, no man is as good as the religious hemp drinker."
> —Hemp Drug
> Commission Report (1884)

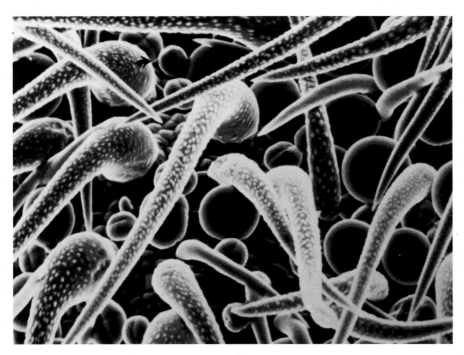

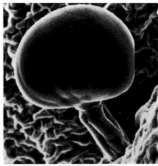

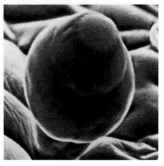

entered into archaic native cultures in social and religious contexts. The Hottentots, Bushmen, and Kaffirs used Hemp for centuries as a medicine and as an intoxicant. In an ancient tribal ceremony in the Zambesi Valley, participants inhaled vapors from a pile of smoldering Hemp; later, reed tubes and pipes were employed, and the plant material was burned on an altar. The Kasai tribes of the Congo have revived an old Riamba cult in which Hemp, replacing ancient fetishes and symbols, was elevated to a god—a protector against physical and spiritual harm. Treaties are sealed with puffs of smoke from calabash pipes. Hemp-smoking and Hashish-snuffing cults exist in many parts of east Africa, especially near Lake Victoria.

Hemp has spread to many areas of the New World, but with few exceptions the plant has not penetrated significantly into many Native American religious beliefs and ceremonies. There are, however, exceptions, such as its use under the name Rosa María, by the Tepecano Indians of northwest Mexico, who occasionally employ Hemp when Peyote is not available. It has recently been learned that Indians in the Mexican states of Veracruz, Hidalgo, and Puebla practice a communal curing ceremony with a plant called Santa Rosa, identified as *Cannabis sativa*, which is considered both a plant and a sacred intercessor with the Virgin. Although the ceremony is based mainly on Christian elements, the plant is worshiped as an Earth deity and is thought to be alive and to represent a part of the heart of God. The participants in this cult believe that the plant can be dangerous and that it can assume the form of a man's soul, make him ill, enrage him, and even cause death.

Sixty years ago, when Mexican laborers introduced the smoking of Marijuana to the United States, it spread across the South, and by the 1920s its use was established in New Orleans, confined primarily among the poor and minority groups. The continued spread of the custom in the United States and Europe has resulted in a still unresolved controversy.

Cannabis sativa was officially in the U.S. Pharmacopoeia until 1937, recom-

Scanning Electron Microscopy

Above left: In *C. sativa*, well-developed hairs of glandular and non-glandular kinds are shown in various stages of development.

Top right: Different types of glandular hairs of *Cannabis*. The capitate gland with a prominent pseudo-stalk on the surface of the anther wall that faces the center of the flower.

Bottom right: Bulbous gland from adaxial leaf surface. The stalk and head are made up of two cells each. The tip of the gland possesses a small, disk-shaped region below which resin accumulates in the extended membrane.

Page 98: Above, *Cannabis sativa* is being harvested for Hemp at the turn of the century. This species attains a height of 18 feet (6 m). Below, an extremely potent Hashish is produced from *Cannabis indica*, a low, pyramidal, densely branched species, as shown above growing wild near Kandahar, Afghanistan.

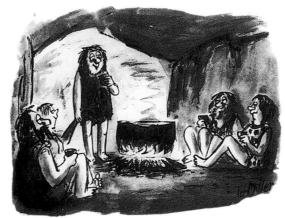

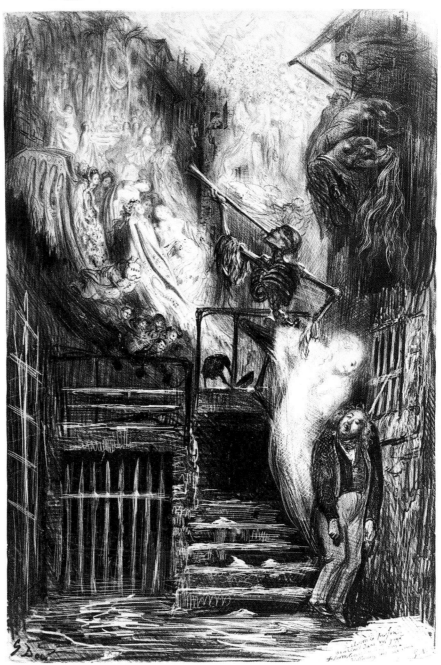

Top: Drawing by W. Miller. Copyright 1978 *The New Yorker* Magazine, Inc. "Hey, what is this stuff? It makes everything I think seem profound."

Below: Gustave Doré's painting "Composition of the Death of Gérard de Nerval," for which he may have used *Cannabis* and Opium for inspiration. The contemporary American cartoon shows in a humorous way the resurrection of this belief.

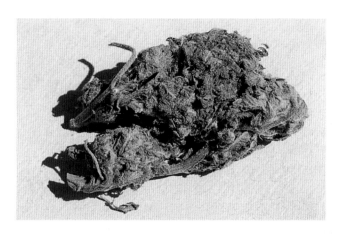

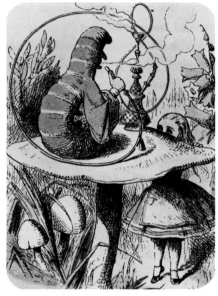

Above: Marijuana is made from the dried and slightly fermented blossoms of the feminine Hemp plant.

Left: In Lewis Carroll's *Alice in Wonderland,* the encounter between Alice and the languorous caterpillar is as follows: "She stretched herself up on tiptoe, and peeped over the edge of the mushroom, and her eyes immediately met those of a large blue caterpillar that was sitting on the top, with its arms folded, quietly smoking a long hookah, and taking not the slightest notice of her or anything else."

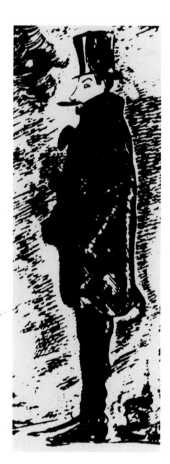

Above: In the nineteenth century, a select group of European artists and writers turned to psychoactive agents in an attempt to achieve what has come to be regarded as "mind-expansion" or "mind-alteration." Many people, such as the French poet Baudelaire (below), believed that creative ability could be greatly enhanced by the use of *Cannabis.* In fact, Baudelaire wrote vivid descriptions of his personal experiences under the influence of *Cannabis.*

mended for a wide variety of disorders, especially as a mild sedative. It is no longer an official drug, although research in the medical potential of some of the cannabinolic constituents or their semi-synthetic analogs is at present very active, particularly in relation to the side effects of cancer therapy.

The psychoactive effects of *Cannabis* preparations vary widely, depending on dosage, the preparation and the type of plant used, the method of administration, the personality of the user, and the social and cultural background. Perhaps the most frequent characteristic is a dreamy state. Long forgotten events are often recalled and thoughts occur in unrelated sequences. Perception of time, and occasionally of space, is altered. Visual and auditory hallucinations sometimes follow the use of large doses. Euphoria, excitement, inner happiness—often with hilarity and laughter—are typical. In some cases, a final mood of depression may be experienced.

"This marvelous experience often
occurs as if it were the effect of a
superior and invisible power acting
on the person from without . . .
This delightful and singular state . . .
gives no advance warning.
It is as unexpected as a ghost,
an intermittent haunting
from which we must draw,
if we are wise,
the certainly of a better existence.
This acuteness of thought,
this enthusiasm of the senses and
the spirit must have appeared to
man through the ages
as the first blessing."

—Charles Baudelaire
Les Paradis Artificiels

ST. ANTHONY'S FIRE

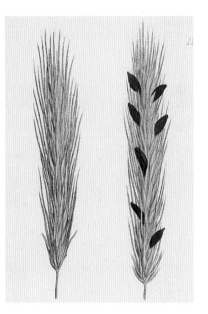

Above: While Ergot infects a number of different grasses, it is best known as a parasite on the inflorescence of rye.

Page 103 top: The Ergot of rye are considerably bigger than those of the Paspalum grass.

Page 103 left: Fruiting bodies of *Claviceps purpurea*. The specific name of this fungus means "purple," a color that in antiquity was linked with powers of the underworld.

Page 103 right: When grain is infected by Ergot, long black growths appear on the heads, called sclerotium.

"The ancient testimony about Eleusis is unanimous and unambiguous. Eleusis was the supreme experience in an initiate's life. It was both physical and mystical: trembling, vertigo, cold sweat, and then a sight that made all previous seeing seem like blindness, a sense of awe and wonder at a brilliance that caused a profound silence, since what had just been seen and felt could never be communicated; words were unequal to the task. These symptoms are unmistakably the experience induced by a hallucinogen. Greeks, and indeed some of the most famous and intelligent among them, could experience and enter fully into such irrationality . . .

"Eleusis was different from the convivial inebriation of friends . . . In their various ways, other Greek cults too enacted aspects of the ancient communion practiced between gods and men, between the living and the dead, but it was at Eleusis alone that the experience occurred with overwhelming finality . . .

"For close on to two thousand years, a few of the ancient Greeks passed each year through the portals of Eleusis. There they celebrated the divine gift to mankind of the cultivated grain, and they were also initiated into the awesome powers of the nether world through the purple dark of the grain's sibling . . ."

Thus in an interdisciplinary study based on three different approaches, ethnomycology, classical studies, and chemistry, the secret rites of ancient Greece, which have remained a puzzle for four thousand years, are associated with intoxication caused by the fungus *Claviceps,* which grows parasitically on certain cereals.

It is now believed that the intoxicant underlying the ecstasy experienced in the mysteries was induced by *Claviceps paspali,* and possibly other species, growing on various Loliums and other cereal grasses native to Greece. The biodynamic principles characteristic of the well-known Ergot, or *Claviceps purpurea,* have been isolated from some of the other species of this fungal parasite.

The reasons for considering the Eleusian mysteries to be associated with the use of *Claviceps* are long and complex, but the arguments are most convincing and apparently from several disciplines sound. Basically, it has now been shown that several species of *Claviceps* can infect a number of wild grasses in Greece.

By far the most important species of *Claviceps* is *C. purpurea,* the Ergot of rye *(Secale cereale).* This hard, brown or purplish black sclerotium of a fungus originating in the caryopsis of rye is exceedingly common in Europe. The native nomenclature of *Claviceps purpurea* is indeed complex. *Ergot,* the French word for "spur" of a cock, now generally employed in numerous languages, was first applied to the fungus in a region not far from Paris. There are, however, two dozen other words for the sclerotium in French; sixty-two vernacular names in German, *Mutterkorn* being the most commonly used. There are twenty-one in Dutch, fifteen in the Scandinavian languages, fourteen in Italian, and seven in English in addition to the borrowed word *Ergot.* This proliferation of vernacular terminology indicates the importance of the fungus in European countries.

Although its medicinal use was unknown in classical times, it was early recognized as a poison. As far back as 600 B.C., the Assyrians called the spurlike growth or Ergot a "noxious pustule in the ear of the grain." The sacred books of the Parsees (about 350 B.C.) reported: "Among the evil things created by Angro Maynes are noxious grasses that cause pregnant women to drop the womb and die in childbed." Although the ancient Greeks apparently employed the fungus in their religious rituals, they did not eat rye because of the "black malodorous produce of Thrace and Macedonia." Rye was not introduced into classical Europe until the beginning of the Christian era, so Ergot poisoning did not enter into Roman pharmaceutical literature.

The earliest undoubted reports of Ergot poisoning appeared during the Middle Ages, when bizarre epidemics broke

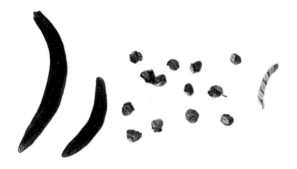

out in various parts of Europe, taking thousands of lives and causing untold agony and suffering. These epidemics manifested themselves in two forms: those with nervous convulsions and epileptic symptoms; those with gangrene, mummifications, atrophy, and occasional loss of extremities—noses, earlobes, fingers, toes, and feet. Delirium

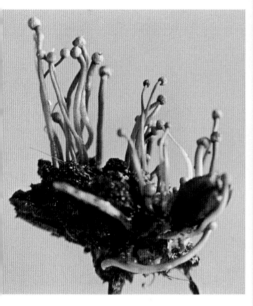

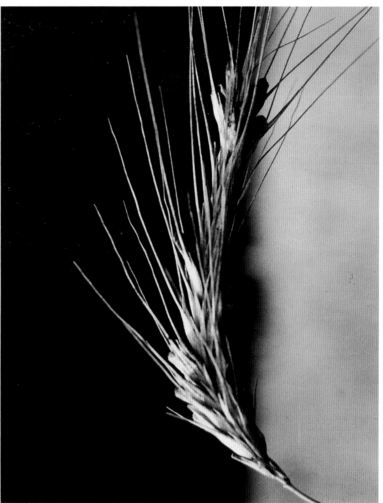

and hallucinations were common symptoms of the intoxication, which was frequently fatal. An early European visitation of ergotism described it as "a great plague of swollen blisters [that] consumed the people by a loathsome rot." Abortions of women were general during these attacks. The "Holy Fire" was always characterized by a feeling of burning in the feet and hands.

St. Anthony, after whom the "fire" was named, lived as a religious hermit in Egypt; he died at the age of 105 in A.D. 356. He is the protecting saint against fire, epilepsy, and infection. During the Crusades, the knights brought back his remains to Dauphiné, in France, for burial. It was here in Dauphiné that the earliest recognized plague of "Holy Fire" occurred in 1039. A wealthy citizen, Gaston, and his son were among the afflicted, and Gaston

The Chemistry of Ergot

The active ingredients in Ergot are indole alkaloids, all derived from the same basic compound, lysergic acid. The most important alkaloids in Ergot of rye are ergotamine and ergotoxine, in which lysergic acid is connected with a peptide radical consisting of three amino acids. These alkaloids and their derivatives have various medicinal uses.

In toxic doses they cause gangrene because of their vasoconstricting properties. Ergot from wild grasses, however, contains essentially simple lysergic acid amides, ergine, and lysergic acid-hydroxyethylamide (found only in traces in Ergot of rye). These psychotropic alkaloids may have played a role in the convulsive form of ergotism. They occur as the main active principles in the Mexican Morning Glory Ololiuqui *(Turbina corymbosa)* [see page 187 for the molecular model of the chemical structure] and other Bindweeds *(Ipomoea violacea, Argyreia nervosa)*.

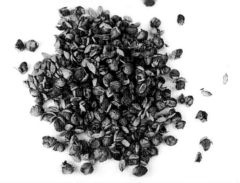

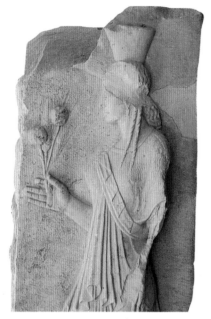

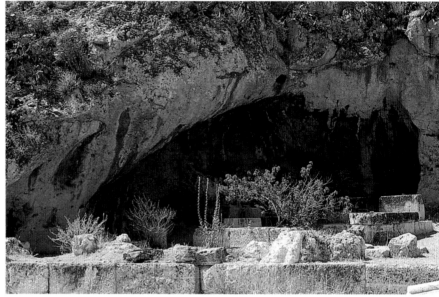

Above left: The goddess Demeter with sheaves of grain and opium pods in her hand.

Above right: The Plutoniuon of Eleusis.

Page 105 bottom: One of the rare outbreaks of ergotism in England attacked one family in Wattisham in 1762. So unusual was this plague that it has been memorialized with a plaque in the parish church.

promised to give all his wealth to aid other victims if St. Anthony would cure him and his son. Thus it was that in this French town a hospital to care for sufferers was founded and the Order of St. Anthony was also established.

A pilgrimage to shrines consecrated to St. Anthony was believed to cure the disease. But a change in diet—bread free of Ergot—may have had a beneficial effect. It was not until 1676—some five hundred years after the height of St. Anthony's fire—that the real cause of ergotism was discovered, whereupon measures of control were set up. Millers in the Middle Ages frequently kept clean rye flour for the affluent, selling flour made from "spurred rye"—that infected with Ergot—to poorer customers. Once the cause was known, vigilance in the mills quickly reduced the epidemics of St. Anthony's fire.

Even today, however, there are occasional outbreaks of epidemics in which whole villages are affected. The most notorious recent attacks have occurred in France and Belgium in 1953 and in the Ukraine and Ireland in 1929. There are suggestions that the alleged outbreaks of witchcraft in colonial New England, especially in Salem, Massachu-

setts, may have been due to Ergot poisoning.

European midwives had long known that Ergot could aid in cases of difficult childbirth and had used the fungus for that purpose. Chemicals isolated from Ergot are still official drugs to induce contraction of involuntary muscles in stubborn childbirth. The earliest medical report of the obstetric value of Ergot was published in 1582 by Lonicer of Frankfurt, who stated that Ergot-parasitized rye is of sovereign efficiency in pregnancy pains. Although widely employed by midwives, Ergot was first employed by a physician when Desgranges of Lyons experimented with it and published his observations in 1818. The Swiss botanist Bauhin described Ergot in 1595, and his son later produced the first illustration of Ergot in 1658. In 1676, the French physician-botanist Dodart added much scientific knowledge to the story of Ergot. He advised the French Academy that the only way to control plagues of ergotism was to sift the rye to extract the Ergot spores from it. But even as late as 1750, botanists still were uncertain how Ergot grew and why it was toxic. In 1711 and again in 1761, learned botanists accepted

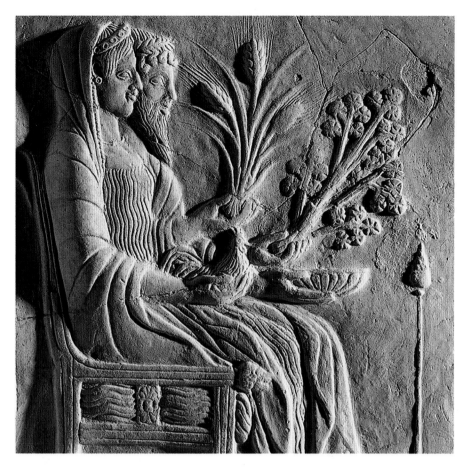

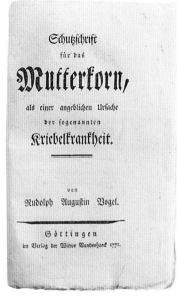

the view that the black spur was formed by the germinating embryo, which caused a hypertrophied growth in place of a normal caryopsis. Only in 1764 did the German botanist von Münchhausen declare that Ergot was a fungal infection, but his opinion was not accepted until the famous botanist A. P. de Candolle proved it in 1815. A widely acclaimed report of Ergot efficacy was published by Dr. John Stearns in 1808. A few years later, a Massachusetts doctor, Prescott, gave a dissertation on the "natural history and medicinal effects" of Ergot, which, when published in 1813, called the attention of medical science in the New World to the re-

markable properties of the fungus. From that time on, Ergot was increasingly employed in medicine, although it was not accepted in the Pharmacopoeia until 1836.

It was not, however, until the 1920s that the active principles of *Claviceps purpurea* were known: ergotamine in 1921; ergonovine in 1935. Subsequently, a number of other related alkaloids have been discovered in the plant. Even though this dangerous infection of rye never had a major magico-religious role in European culture, it did earn a special place as a plant having connections with spiritual forces—a kind of malevolent plant of the gods.

Above left: Persephone, the Queen of the Dead, making an offering of shafts of grain, is enthroned beside her husband, Hades, Lord of the Underworld. Originally a goddess associated with grain, she was abducted to the Underworld by Hades, and her return from the realm of the dead was connected with symbolic rebirth experiences in the Eleusinian mysteries, where the worshipers believed that the restoration of the goddess to the upper world ensured the faithful a resurrection. It is possible that these amazing events in Persephone's life might have been linked with intoxication from Ergot, since Greek sophistication in the chemical properties of plants was well developed.

Above right: The title page of a German book from 1771, *Ergot: An Alleged Cause of the So-called St. Anthony's Fire.*

This Inscription Serves to Authenticate the Truth of a Singular Calamity, Which Suddenly Happened to a poor Family in this Parish, Of which Six Persons lost their Feet by a Mortification not to be accounted for. A full Narrative of their Case is recorded In the Parish Register & Philos: Transactions for 1762.

HOLY FLOWER
OF THE NORTH STAR

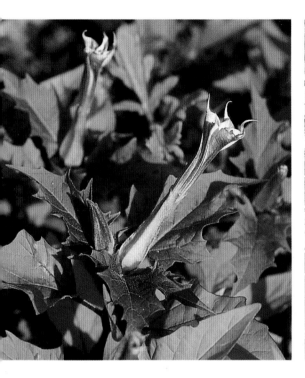

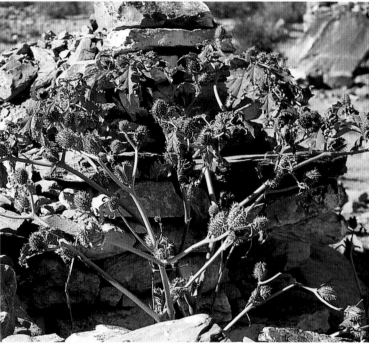

Above left: The *Datura stramonium* var. *tatula* is the most common in the Himalayas. It is easily recognized by the violet color of the flower.

Above right: The sacred Thorn Apple (*Datura metel*) is often found in the Himalayas on altars to the gods of the mountains (photo taken in Tukche, Nepal).

Below right: A yellow-flowered *Datura metel* in full bloom.

A beautiful Zuñi Indian legend tells of the divine origin of Aneglakya, *Datura innoxia*, their most sacred plant:

"In the olden time a boy and a girl, brother and sister (the boy's name was A'neglakya and the girl's name A'neglakyatsi'tsa), lived in the interior of the earth, but they often came to the outer world and walked about a great deal, observing closely everything they saw and heard and repeating all to their mother. This constant talking did not please the Divine Ones (twin sons of the Sun Father). On meeting the boy and the girl the Divine Ones asked, 'How are you?' and the brother and sister answered, 'We are happy.' (Sometimes A'neglakya and A'neglakyatsi'tsa appeared on Earth as old people.) They told the Divine Ones how they could make one sleep and see ghosts, and how they could make one walk about a little and see one who had committed theft. After this meeting the Divine Ones concluded that A'neglakya and A'neglakyatsi'tsa knew too much and that they should be banished for all time from this world; so the Divine Ones caused the brother and sister to disappear into the earth forever. Flowers sprang up at the spot where the two descended—flowers exactly like those that they wore on each side of their heads when visiting the earth. The Divine Ones called the plant 'a'neglakya' after the boy's name. The original plant has many children scattered over the earth; some of the blossoms are tinged with yellow, some with blue, some with red, some are all white—the colors belonging to the four cardinal points."

This and related species of *Datura*

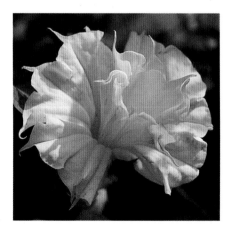

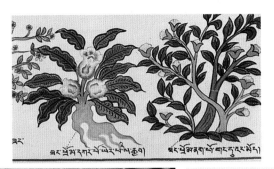

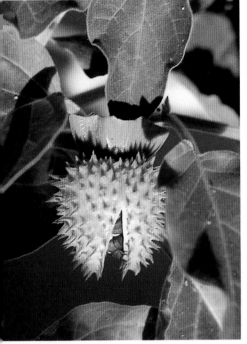

The Chemistry of *Datura*

The various species of *Datura* contain the same major alkaloids as related solanaceous plants (Angel's Trumpet, Belladonna, Henbane, and Mandrake) hyoscyamine and, in greatest concentration, scopolamine. Meteloidine is a characteristic secondary alkaloid of *D. metel*.

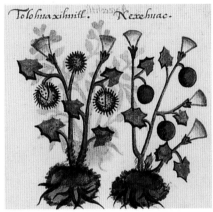

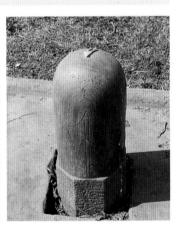

have long been employed as sacred hallucinogens, especially in Mexico and the American Southwest, and have played major roles in native medicine and magico-religious rites. Their undoubted danger as potent narcotics, however, has never been challenged, even from earliest times.

In the Old World, *Datura* has had a long history as a medicine and sacred hallucinogen, although the genus has apparently never enjoyed the ceremonial role that it has had in the New World. Early Sanskrit and Chinese writings mention *Datura metel*. It was undoubtedly this species that the Arabian doctor Avicenna reported in the eleventh century under the name *Jouzmathal* ("metel nut"); this report was repeated in Dioscorides' writings. The name *metel* is taken from this Arabic term, while the generic epithet *Datura* was adapted to Latin by Linnaeus from the Sanskrit *Dhatura*. In China, the plant was considered sacred: when Buddha was preaching, heaven sprinkled the plant with dew or raindrops. A Taoist legend maintains that *Datura metel* is

one of the circumpolar stars and that envoys to earth from this star carry a flower of the plant in their hand. Several species of *Datura* were introduced into China from India between the Sung and Ming dynasties—that is, between A. D. 960 and 1644—so they were not recorded in earlier herbals. The herbalist Li Shih-chen reported the medicinal uses of one of the species known as Man-t'o-lo in 1596: the flowers and seeds were employed to treat eruptions on the face, and the plant was prescribed internally for colds, nervous disorders, and other problems. It was taken together with *Cannabis* in wine as an anesthesia for minor surgical operations. Its narcotic properties were known to the Chinese, for Li Shih-chen personally experimented on himself and wrote: "According to traditions, it is alleged that when the flowers are picked for use with wine while one is laughing, the wine will cause one to produce laughing movements; and when the flowers are picked while one is dancing, the wine will cause one to produce dancing movements. [I have found out] that

Top: Traditional depiction of the Thorn Apple on a Tibetan medicinal painting.

Above left: The hanging fruit of *Datura innoxia*. The seeds that are chewed by shamans to induce a clairvoyant trance are clearly visible.

Above middle: Many species of *Datura* have played a vital medicinal and inebriant role in Mexico since early times. This page from the "Badianus Manuscript" (*Codex Berberini Latina* 241, Folio 29) depicts two species of *Datura* and describes their therapeutic uses. This document of 1542 is the first herbal to be written in the New World.

Above right: A *Datura* flower is left as an offering on a Shiva Lingam at Pashupatinath (Nepal).

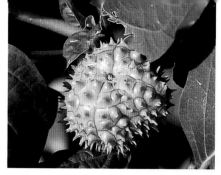

Right: The typical fruit of the *Datura metel*. In India it is given to the god Shiva as an offering.

Below: It was believed that when Buddha preached, dew or raindrops fell from heaven on *Datura*. This bronze shrine from the Sui period of China depicts Amitabha Buddha seated under the jeweled trees of Paradise.

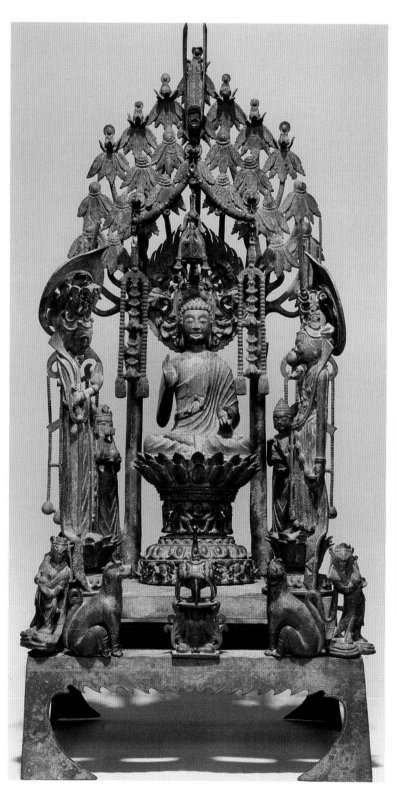

such movements will be produced when one becomes half-drunk with the wine and someone else laughs or dances to induce these actions."

In India, it was called tuft of Shiva, the god of destruction. Dancing girls sometimes drugged wine with its seeds, and whoever drank of the potion, appearing in possession of his senses, gave answers to questions, although he had no control of his will, was ignorant of whom he was addressing, and lost all memory of what he did when the intoxication wore off. For this reason, many Indians called the plant "drunkard," "madman," "deceiver," and "foolmaker." The British traveler Hardwicke found this plant common in mountain villages in India in 1796 and reported that an infusion of the seeds was used to increase the intoxication from alcoholic drinks. During the Sanskritic period, Indian medicine

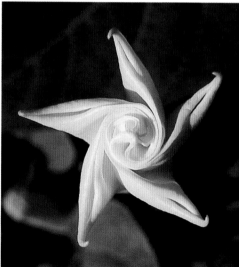

valued *Datura metel* for treating mental disorders, various fevers, tumors, breast inflammations, skin diseases, and diarrhea.

In other parts of Asia, *D. metel* was valued and similarly employed in native medicine and as an intoxicant. Even today, seeds or powdered leaves of this plant are often mixed with *Cannabis* or Tobacco and smoked in Indochina. In

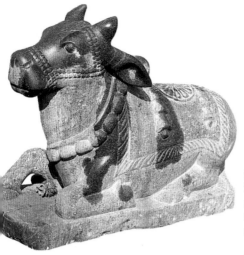

1578, its use as an aphrodisiac in the East Indies was reported. From earliest classical times, the dangers of *Datura* were recognized. The English herbalist Gerard believed that *Datura* was the *Hippomanes* that the Greek writer Theocritus mentioned as driving horses mad.

Datura stramonium var. *ferox,* a species now widely distributed in the warmer parts of both hemispheres, has uses almost identical with those of *D. metel.* It is employed especially in parts of Africa. In Tanzania, it is added to Pombe, a kind of beer, for its inebriating

to induce visual hallucinations but also for a great variety of medicinal uses, especially when applied to the body to relieve rheumatic pains and to reduce swellings.

Writing shortly after the conquest of Mexico, Hernández mentioned its medicinal value but warned that excessive use would drive patients to madness with "various and vain imaginations." Neither its magico-religious nor its therapeutic use has diminished in Mexico. Among the Yaqui, for example, it is taken by women to lessen the pain of childbirth. It is considered so powerful that it can be handled only by "someone of authority." One ethnobotanist wrote: "My collecting these plants was often accompanied with warnings that I would go crazy and die because I was mistreating them. Some Indians refused to talk to me for several days afterward."

Page 108 bottom right: The opening blossom of a *Datura innoxia.* The Mayans call it *xtohk'uh,* "toward the gods," and still use it for shamanic purposes such as divination and medicinal healing.

Above left: A *Datura* fruit has been left as an offering at the image of Nandi, Shiva's sacred steer.

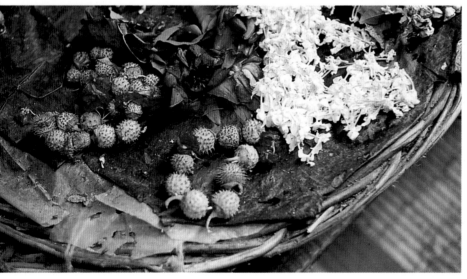

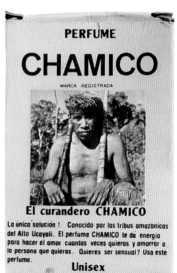

effects. A common medical use in Africa is smoking the leaves to relieve asthma and pulmonary problems.

In the New World, the Mexicans call *Datura* Toloache, a modern version of the ancient Aztec Toloatzin (that is, "inclined head," in reference to its nodding fruit). It was also known in the Nahuatl language as Tolohuaxihuitl and Tlapatl. It was employed not only

Toloache is rather widely added to mescal, a distilled liquor from *Agave,* or to Tesguino, a fermented maize drink, as an added intoxicant—"as a catalyst and to induce a good feeling and visions." Some Mexicans prepare a fatty ointment containing seeds and leaves of Toloache, which is rubbed over the abdomen to induce visual hallucinations.

Among the Indians of the Southwest,

Bottom left: In northern India *Datura* fruit is threaded into garlands and offered to the Hindu god Shiva.

Bottom right: The *Curanderos* (local healers) of northern Peru enjoy using a perfume that is named *Chamico* (Thorn Apple).

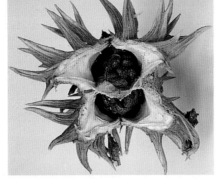

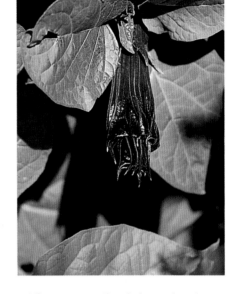

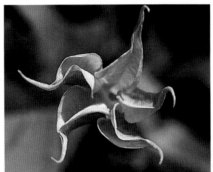

"I ate the thorn apple leaves
And the leaves made me
dizzy.

I ate the thorn apple leaves
And the leaves made me
dizzy.

I ate the thorn apple flowers
And the drink made me
stagger.

The hunter's bow remaining
He overtook and killed me.

Cut and threw my horns
away,
The hunter, reed remaining.

He overtook and killed me
Cut and threw my feet away.

Now the flies become crazy
And drop with flapping
wings.

No drunken butterflies sit
With opening and shutting
wings."

—F. Russel
Pima hunting song

D. innoxia has assumed extraordinary importance as a sacred element and is the most widely used plant to induce hallucinations. The Zuñis believe that the plant belongs to the Rain Priest Fraternity and rain priests alone may collect its roots. These priests put the powdered root into their eyes to commune with the Feathered Kingdom at night, and they chew the roots to ask the dead to intercede with the spirits for rain. These priests further use *D. innoxia* for its analgesic effects, to deaden pain during simple operations, bone-setting, and cleaning ulcerated wounds. The Yokut, who call the plant Tanayin, take the drug only during the spring, since it is considered to be poisonous in the summer; it is given to adolescent boys and girls only once in a lifetime to ensure a good and a long life.

Boys and girls of the Tubatulobal tribe drink *Datura* after puberty to "obtain life," and adults use it to obtain visions. The roots are macerated and soaked in water for ten hours; after drinking large amounts of this liquor, the youths fall into a stupor accompanied by hallucinations that may last up to twenty-four hours. If an animal—an eagle, a hawk, for example—is seen during the visions, it becomes the child's "pet" or spiritual mascot for life: if "life" is seen, the child acquires a ghost. The ghost is the ideal object to appear, since it cannot die. Children never may kill the animal "pet" that they see in their *Datura* vision, for these "pets" may visit during serious illness and effect a cure.

The Yuman tribes believe that the reaction of braves under the influence of Toloache may foretell their future. These people use the plant to gain occult power. If birds sing to a man in a *Datura* trance, he acquires the power to cure.

The Navajo take *Datura* for its visionary properties, valuing it for diagnosis, healing, and purely intoxicating use. Navajo use is magic-oriented. Visions induced by this drug are especially valued, since they reveal certain animals possessing special significance. Upon learning from these visions the cause of a disease, a chant may be prescribed. If a man be repulsed in love by a girl, he seeks revenge by putting her saliva or dust from her moccasins on a *Datura,* then the singing of a chant will immediately drive the girl mad.

Datura stramonium is now believed to be native to eastern America, where the Algonquins and other tribes may have employed it as a ceremonial hallucinogen. Indians of Virginia used a toxic medicine called *wysoccan* in initiatory rites: the Huskanawing ceremony. The active ingredient was probably *Datura stramonium.* Youths were confined for long periods, given "no other substance but the infusion or decoction of some poisonous, intoxicating roots" and "they became stark, staring mad, in which raving condition they were kept eighteen or twenty days." During the ordeal, they "unlive their former lives" and begin manhood by losing all memory of ever having been boys.

There is in Mexico a curious species

Right: A magician of Kuma in northeast Africa leads entranced women in a ritual dance. The substance that they ingest consists of a secret mixture of many different plants, most of which are unknown. Evidence suggests that *Datura* is among them. The women are possessed by the spirits who use them as their medium.

Left: The illustration from the early writings of Sahagun, the Spanish friar who wrote shortly after the conquest of Mexico, pictures the utilization of an infusion of *Datura* to relieve rheumatism. This use is still found recommended in modern pharmacopoeias.

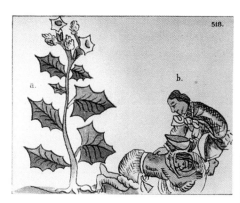

of *Datura,* so distinct that a separate section of the genus has been set up for its classification. It is *D. ceratocaula,* a fleshy plant with thick, forking stems of bogs, or growing in water. Known as Torna Loco ("maddening plant"), it is powerfully narcotic. In ancient Mexico, it was considered "sister of Ololiuqui" and was held in great veneration. Little is known concerning its use today for hallucinogenic purposes.

The effects of all species are similar, since their constituents are so much alike. Physiological activity begins with a feeling of lassitude and progresses into a period of hallucinations followed by deep sleep and loss of consciousness. In excessive doses, death or permanent insanity may occur. So potent is the psychoactivity of all species of *Datura* that it is patently clear why peoples in indigenous cultures around the world have classed them as plants of the gods.

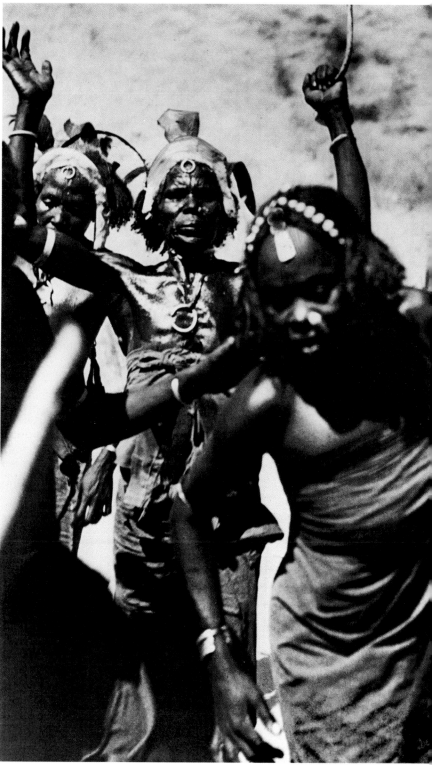

GUIDE TO THE ANCESTORS

"Zame ye Mebege [the last of the creator gods] gave us Eboka. One day . . . he saw . . . the Pygmy Bitamu, high in an Atanga tree, gathering its fruit. He made him fall. He died, and Zame brought his spirit to him. Zame cut off the little fingers and the little toes of the cadaver of the Pygmy and planted them in various parts of the forest. They grew into the Eboka bush."

open the head," thus inducing a contact with the ancestors through collapse and hallucinations."

The drug has far-reaching social influence. According to the natives, the initiate cannot enter the cult until he has seen Bwiti, and the only way to see Bwiti is to eat Iboga. The complex ceremonies and tribal dances associated with consumption of Iboga vary greatly

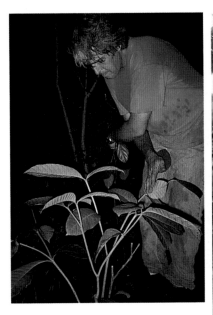

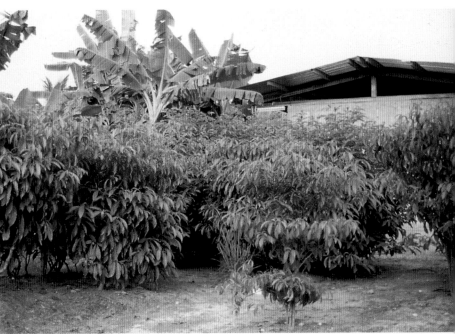

Left: The roots of the Iboga bush are ritually eaten by the Bwiti cult in order to call forth the ancestors.

Right: Iboga, necessary for rituals, is grown at the temple of the Bwiti cult.

One of the few members of the Apocynaceae utilized as a hallucinogen, this shrub attains a height of 4 to 6 feet (1.5–2 m). Its yellowish root is the active part of the plant, containing the psychoactive alkaloids. The root bark is rasped and eaten directly as raspings or as a powder or is drunk as an infusion.

Iboga is basic to the Bwiti cult and other secret societies in Gabon and Zaire. The drug is taken in two ways: regularly in limited doses before and in the early part of the ceremonies, followed after midnight by a smaller dose; and once or twice during the initiation to the cult in excessive doses of one to three basketfuls over an eight- to twenty-four-hour period, to "break

from locality to locality. Iboga enters also other aspects of Bwiti's control of events. Sorcerers take the drug to seek information from the spirit world, and leaders of the cult may consume Iboga for a full day before asking advice from ancestors.

Iboga is intimately associated with death: the plant is frequently anthropomorphized as a supernatural being, a "generic ancestor," which can so highly value or despise an individual that it can carry him away to the realm of the dead. There are sometimes deaths from the excessive doses taken during initiations, but the intoxication usually so interferes with motor activity that the initiates must sit gazing intently into space,

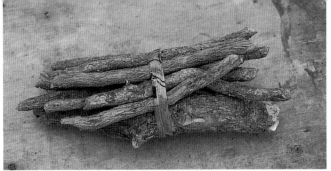

eventually collapsing and having to be carried to a special house or forest hideout. During this almost comatose period, the "shadow" (soul) leaves the body to wander with the ancestors in the land of the dead. The *banzie* (angels)—the initiates—relate their visions as follows: "A dead relative came to me in my sleep and told me to eat it"; "I was sick and was counseled to eat Iboga to cure

The Chemistry of Iboga

As with other hallucinogens, especially Teonanácatl (*Psilocybe* spp.) and Ololiuqui, the active principles of *Tabernanthe iboga* belong to the large class of indole alkaloids. Ibogaine, which can be produced synthetically, is the main alkaloid of *T. iboga*. Its hallucinogenic effects are accompanied by strong stimulation of the central nervous system.

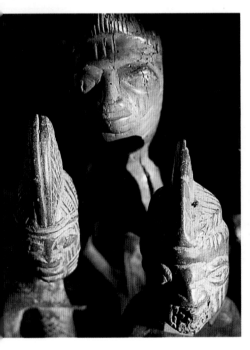

myself"; "I wanted to know God—to know things of the dead and the land beyond"; "I walked or flew over a long, multicolored road or over many rivers which led me to my ancestors, who then took me to the great gods."

Iboga may act as a powerful stimulant, enabling the partaker to maintain extraordinary physical exertion without fatigue over a long period. The body may feel lighter, and levitation—a feeling of floating—is often experienced. Spectrums or rainbowlike effects are seen in surrounding objects, indications to the *banzie* that the initiate is approaching the realms of the ancestors and of the gods. Time perception is altered; time is lengthened, and initiates

Addiction Therapy with Ibogaine

Iboga roots contain an alkaloid known as ibogaine. This substance was first introduced in the 1960s by the Chilean psychiatrist Claudio Naranjo as a "fantasy-enhancing drug" for psychotherapy. Today, ibogaine is in the spotlight of neuropsychological research, which has shown that the alkaloid can ease drug addiction (to such drugs as heroin and cocaine) and make way for a cure. Ibogaine calms the motor activity that is present when under the influence of an opiate. The chiropractor Karl Naeher says that "Ibogaine, when taken in one high dose by an opiate addict, drastically reduces withdrawal symptoms and, at the same time, causes a 'trip' that reveals such deep insights into the personal causes of the addiction that the majority of those who undergo this type of therapy can go for months without a relapse. But several additional sessions are required before a lasting stabilization is evident."

Research into the potential use of ibogaine as a treatment for substance abuse is being carried out by Deborah Mash and her team in Miami.

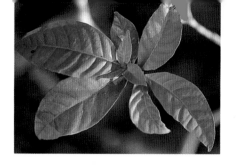

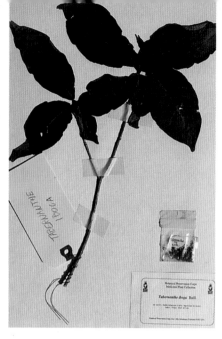

Page 115 top: The seeds of the Iboga bush can germinate only under particular conditions. They themselves contain no active compounds.

Page 115 right: Music plays a central role in the Bwiti cult. The harp player not only allows the strings to resonate, but also sings liturgies in which the cosmology and worldview of the tribe are expressed.

Top left: The typical leaves of the Iboga bush.

Top right: A herbarium specimen of *Tabernanthe iboga* in a comparative botanical collection.

feel that their spiritual trip has taken many hours or even days. The body is seen as detached: one user reported, "Here I am, and there is my body going through its action." Large doses induce auditory, olfactory, and gustatory synesthesia. Mood may vary greatly from fear to euphoria.

An Englishman writing on Gabon mentioned *"Eroga"* under "fetish plants" as early as 1819. Describing it as a "favorite but violent medicine," he undoubtedly saw it powdered and assumed that it represented a charred fungus. French and Belgian explorers encountered this remarkable drug and the cults using it a little over a century ago. They stated that the drug greatly increased muscular strength and endurance and that it had aphrodisiac properties. An early report, in 1864, insisted that Iboga is not toxic except in high doses, that "warriors and hunters use it constantly to keep themselves awake

description of the experiences of an initiate under high dosage of the drug: "Soon all his sinews stretch out in an extraordinary fashion. An epileptic madness seizes him, during which, unconscious, he mouths words which, when heard by the initiated ones, have a prophetic meaning and prove that the fetish has entered him."

Other plants of reputed narcotic properties are involved in the Iboga

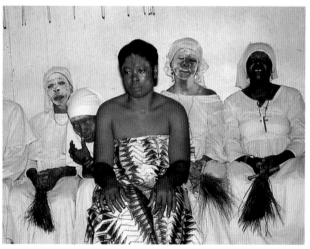

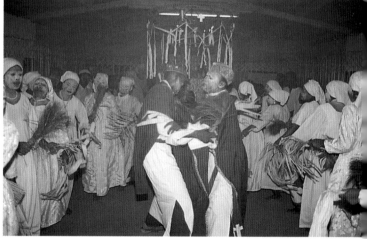

Above left and right: During the initiation rites of the Bwiti cult, the novices ingest extremely high doses of the Iboga root in order to attain contact with the ancestors during the powerful ritual.

during night watches . . ." In the 1880s, the Germans met it in Cameroon (northern Gabon), and in 1898 it was reported that the root had an "exciting effect on the nervous system so that its use is highly valued on long, tiring marches, on lengthy canoe voyages, and on difficult night watches."

The earliest report of its hallucinogenic effects dates from 1903, with the

cults, sometimes used alone, sometimes as admixtures with *Tabernanthe iboga* itself. *Cannabis sativa*—known as Yama or Beyama—may often be smoked following ingestion of small doses of Iboga. In Gabon, *Cannabis* resin may on occasion be eaten with Iboga. Alan, the euphorbiaceous *Alchornea floribunda*, is often consumed in large amounts to help produce the collapse experienced

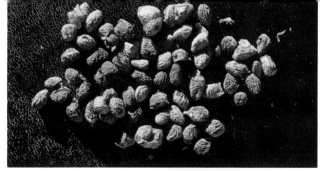

in Bwiti initiations; in southern Gabon, it is mixed with Iboga. Another euphorbiaceous plant—Ayan-beyem or *Elaeophorbia drupifera*—may be taken during Bwiti initiations, when Alan is slow to take effect; the latex is applied directly to the eyes with a parrot feather, affecting the optical nerve and inducing visions.

The Bwiti cult has been growing in number of converts and in social strength, not waning, in recent decades. It represents a strong native element in a changing society being rapidly engulfed in foreign cultural influences. They consider that the drug and its associated cults enable them more easily to resist the vertiginous transition from the individualism of traditional tribal life to the collectivism and loss of identity in the encroaching Western civilization. It may well offer the strongest single force against the missionary spread of Christianity and Islam, since it unifies many of the once hostile, warring tribes in resistance to European innovations. As one initiate stated: "Catholicism and Protestantism is not our religion. I am not happy in the mission churches."

The cultural importance of the drug is everywhere seen. The name *Iboga* is used for the whole Bwiti cult; *ndzieboka* ("eater of Iboga") means a member of the cult; *nyiba-eboka* signifies the religion surrounding the narcotic plant.

Iboga in every sense of the term is indeed a plant of the gods. It appears to be here to stay in the native cultures of west-central Africa.

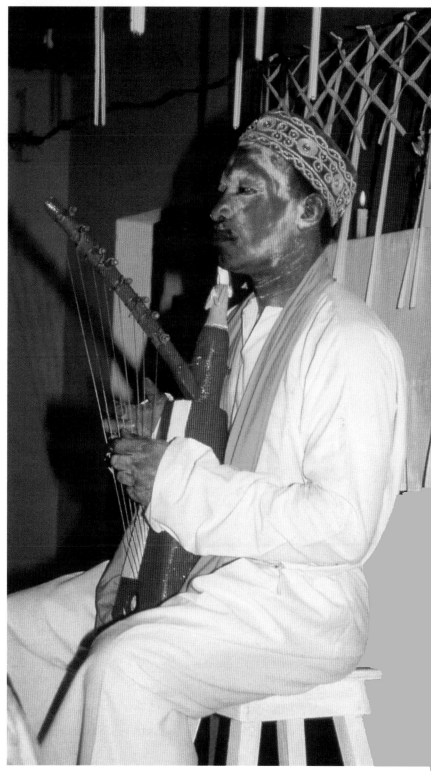

BEANS OF THE HEKULA SPIRIT

In the beginning, the Sun created various beings to serve as intermediaries between Him and Earth. He created hallucinogenic snuff powder so that man could contact supernatural beings. The Sun had kept this powder in His navel, but the Daughter of the Sun found it. Thus it became available to man—a vegetal product acquired directly from the gods.

center of use of this snuff is and probably always has been the Orinoco. The West Indian tribes are thought to have been, in the main, invaders from northern South America. It is very probable that the custom of snuffing the drug, as well as the tree itself, was introduced by invaders from the Orinoco area.

It is now suspected that Yopo was

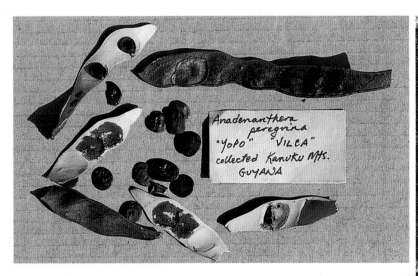

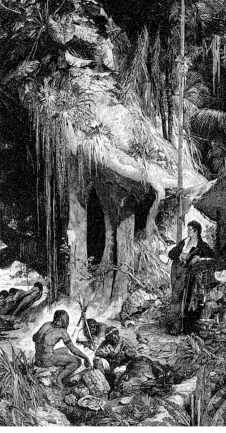

Left: The beans of the Yopo Tree *(Anadenanthera peregrina)* are used by many Indians as a shamanic snuff (specimen collected in Guyana).

Right: Baron Alexander von Humboldt and his co-collector Aimé Bonpland carefully explored the flora of the Orinoco River, the frontier between Colombia and Venezuela, and while there they encountered the preparation and use of Yopo snuff in 1801.

As far back as 1496, an early Spanish report mentioned that the Taino of Hispaniola inhaled a powder called Cohoba to communicate with the spirit world. It was so strong that those who took it lost consciousness; when the stupefying action began to wane, the arms and legs became loose and the head nodded, and almost immediately they believed that they saw the room turn upside-down so that men were walking with their heads downward. Mainly because of the disappearance of aboriginal peoples in the West Indies, this snuff is no longer employed anywhere in the Antilles.

In 1916, ethnobotanical research established the identity of this Cohoba—quite generally until then thought to have been a very potent kind of Tobacco snuff—with the hallucinogenic snuff of the Orinoco called Yopo and derived from the beans of *Anadenanthera peregrina,* better known in the literature as *Piptadenia peregrina.* The

used much more widely in earlier periods. There is evidence that in pre-Hispanic times, this snuff was used by Chibchan tribes from the Colombian Andes east across the *llanos,* or plains, to the upper Orinoco.

In 1560 a missionary in the Colombian *llanos* wrote that the Indians along the Rio Guaviare "are accustomed to take Yopa and Tobacco, and the former is a seed or pip of a tree . . . they become drowsy while the devil, in their dreams, shows them all the vanities and corruptions he wishes them to see and which they take to be true revelations in which they believe, even if told they will die. This habit of taking Yopa and Tobacco is general in the New Kingdom." Another chronicler wrote in 1599: "They chew Hayo or Coca and Jopa and

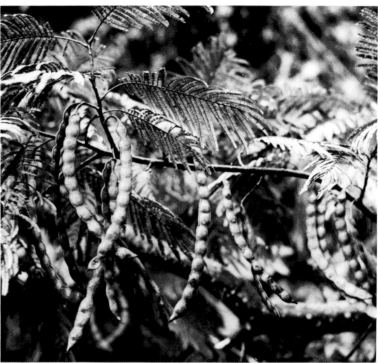

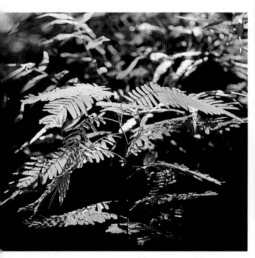

Tobacco ... going out of their minds, and then the devil speaks to them ... Jopa is a tree with small pods like those of vetches, and the seeds inside are similar but smaller." Yopo was so important in pre-Conquest Colombia that Indians of the highlands, where the tree will not grow, traded the drug up from the tropical lowlands: the Muisca of the Colombian Andes, according to an early Spanish historian, used the snuff: "Jop: herb of divination, used by the *mojas* or sun-priests in Tunja and Bogotá." The Muisca "will not travel nor wage war nor do any other thing of importance without learning beforehand what will be the outcome, or this they try to ascertain with two herbs which they consume, called Yop and Osca ..."

Yopo snuff may sometimes, as among the Guahibo, be taken daily as a stimulant. But it is more commonly employed by *payés* (shamans) to induce trances and visions and communicate with the

The Chemistry of Yopo

The active principles of *Anadenanthera peregrina* belong to both open-chained and ringed tryptamine derivatives and, therefore, to the important class of indole alkaloids. Tryptamine is also the basic compound of the amino acid tryptophane, widely distributed in the Animal Kingdom. Dimethyltryptamine (DMT) and 5-hydroxydimethyltryptamine (bufotenine) are representatives of the open-chained *Anadenanthera* tryptamines. Bufotenine has also been found in the skin secretion of a toad (*Bufo* sp.)—hence its name. Ringed tryptamine derivatives found in *Anadenanthera* are 2-methyl- and 1,2-dimethyl-6-methoxytetrahydro-β-carboline.

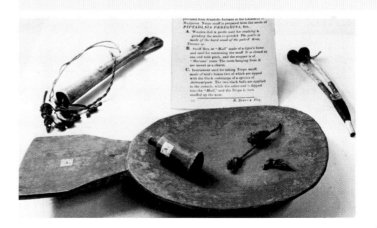

Drawings right (pages 118–19):
Countless artifacts related to the ritual
use of snuff have been discovered in
archaeological digs in the Caribbean
and in South America (for example,
Haiti, Costa Rica, Colombia, and
Brazil).

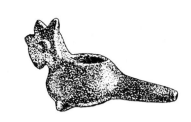

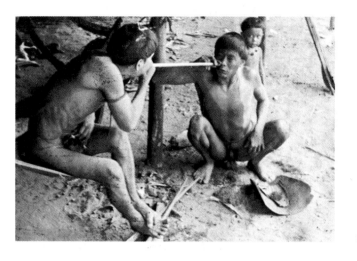

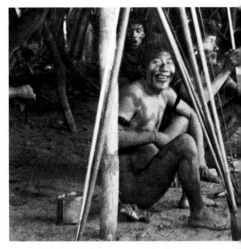

Photo sequence pages 118–19:
Undoubtedly the most intense use of
Yopo snuff prepared from *Anadenanthera peregrina* is found among the
various groups of Waiká living in
southernmost Venezuela and adjacent
parts of northernmost Brazil. These
peoples consume enormous amounts
of the hallucinogenic powder, blowing it
forcefully into the nostrils through long
tubes made from the stems of
maranthaceous plants.

Before snuffing Yopo, the Waiká shamans gather and chant, invoking the
Hekula spirits with whom they will be
communicating during the ensuing
intoxication.

The snuff acts rapidly, causing first a
profuse flow of mucus from the nasal
passages and occasionally a notable
quivering of the muscles, especially in
the arms, and a contorted expression
on the face.

This period quickly gives way to one
in which the shamans begin to prance,
gesticulating and shrieking violently,
calling on the Hekula.

The expenditure of energy lasts from
half an hour to an hour; eventually, fully
spent, they fall into a trancelike stupor,
during which visions are experienced.

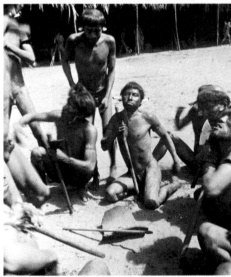

Hekula spirits; to prophesy or divine; to
protect the tribe against epidemics of
sickness; to make hunters and even their
dogs more alert. There has been a long
and complicated confusion between the
hallucinogenic snuff prepared from
Anadenanthera and that from *Virola*
and other plants. Consequently, the numerous distribution maps in anthropo-
logical literature showing immense
areas of South American using *Anadenanthera*-derived snuff must be used
with due caution.

In 1741, the Jesuit missionary Gumil-
la, who wrote extensively on the geography of the Orinoco, described the
use of Yopo by the Otomac: "They have
another abominable habit of intoxicating themselves through the nostrils with
certain malignant powders which they
call Yupa which quite takes away their
reason, and they will furiously take up
arms . . ." Following a description of the
preparation of the snuff and a custom of
adding lime from snail shells, he reported that "before a battle, they would
throw themselves into a frenzy with
Yupa, wound themselves and, full of
blood and rage, go forth to battle like
rabid jaguars."

The first scientific report of Yopo was
made by the explorer Baron von Humboldt, who botanically identified the
source and reported that the Maypure
Indians of the Orinoco, where he witnessed the preparation of the drug in

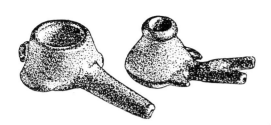

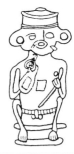

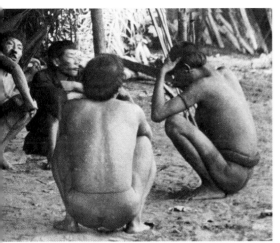

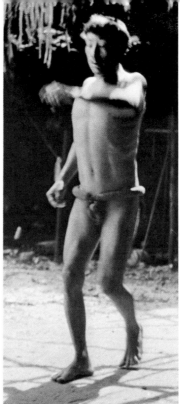

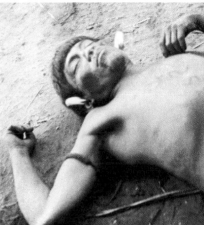

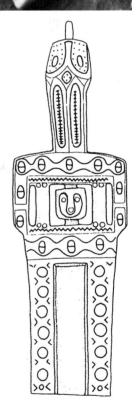

1801, broke the long pods, moistened them, and allowed them to ferment; when they turned black, the softened beans were kneaded into cakes with cassava flour and lime from snails. These cakes were crushed to make snuff. Humboldt, quite erroneously, believed that "it is not to be believed that the . . . pods are the chief cause of the . . . effects of the snuff . . . These effects are due to the freshly calcined lime."

Later, Spruce offered an extremely detailed report on the preparation and use of Yopo among the Guahibo of the Orinoco. He collected a complete set of ethnographic material connected with the substance, and seeds that he collected for chemical study in 1851 were chemically analyzed only in 1977.

"A wandering horde of Guahibo Indians . . . was encamped on the savannas of Maypures, and on a visit to their camp I saw an old man grinding Niopo seeds, and purchased of him his apparatus for making and taking the snuff . . . The seeds, being first roasted, are powdered on a wooden platter . . . It is held on the knees by a broad thin handle, which is grasped in the left hand, while the fingers of the right hold a small spatula or pestle . . . with which the seeds are crushed . . . The snuff is kept in a mull made of a bit of the leg-bone of the jaguar . . . For taking the snuff, they use an apparatus made of the leg bones

of herons or other long-shanked birds put together in the shape of the letter Y . . ."

A contemporary observer described the effects of Yopo snuffing as follows: "His eyes started from his head, his mouth contracted, his limbs trembled. It was fearful to see him. He was obliged to sit down or he would have fallen. He was drunk but only for about five minutes; he was then gayer."

There is appreciable variation from tribe to tribe and from one area to another in the preparation of Yopo. The seeds are usually toasted and pulverized. Lime from snails or the ashes of certain plants are normally added, but some Indians use the snuff without this alkaline admixture. It appears that other plant admixtures are never employed with *Anadenanthera* snuff.

Anadenanthera peregrina occurs naturally and sometimes apparently cultivated in the plains or grassland areas of the Orinoco basin of Colombia and Venezuela, in light forests in southern British Guyana, and in the Rio Branco area of the northern Amazonia of Brazil. It may occur also in isolated savanna areas in the Rio Medeira region. When it is found elsewhere, it may probably have been introduced by Indians. There is evidence that, a century ago, it was cultivated in more localities outside of its natural range than at present.

SEEDS OF CIVILIZATION

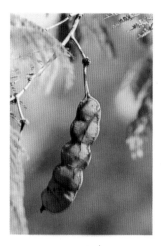 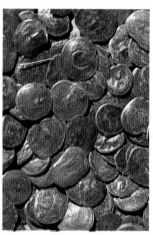 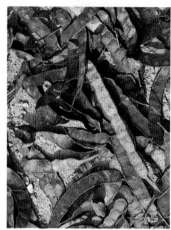 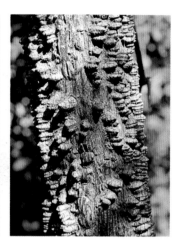

Above from left to right: The Mataco use a decoction of fresh (still green) Cebíl pods as a head wash for headaches.

Cebíl, the "Seeds of Civilization" (seeds of the *Anadenanthera colubrina*). Bufotenine is the main active constituent.

The ripe seed pods of the Cebíl tree (*Anadenanthera colubrina* var. *cebil*) collect underneath the leaf canopy. The knotty bark of the Argentinian Cebíl tree (*Anadenanthera colubrina* bvar. *cebil*).

Page 121: The Cebíl tree (*Anadenanthera colubrina* var. *cebil*) with ripe seed pods.

In the Atacama Desert of northern Chile there is an oasis called San Pedro de Atacama. The art historian and archaeologist C. Manuel Torres excavated and studied over six hundred prehistoric graves there. The results were astonishing. Nearly every interred person was accompanied for the last journey by numerous tools dedicated to the ritual sniffing of Cebíl.

The name Cebíl designates a tree (*Anadenanthera colubrina*) as well as its seeds, which can induce a strong psychoactive effect.

In the Puna region of northwest Argentina is the oldest archaeological proof of the ritual or shamanic use of Cebíl. They have been smoked there for over 4,500 years. Numerous ceramic pipes have been discovered in certain caves of this region. Occasionally the bowls of the pipe still contain Cebíl seeds. The psychoactive use seems in particular to have influenced the culture of Tiahuanaco (literally, "City of the Gods"). The Tiahuanaco culture is the "mother" of Andean civilizations. All subsequent high cultures of the region have been influenced by it.

Many examples of pre-Columbian snuff paraphernalia (snuff tablets, snuff pipes) displaying the iconography of the Tiahuanaco culture have been found in Puna and the Atacama Desert. They appear to be significantly inspired by the visions of the Cebíl seeds.

The use of Cebíl as a snuff powder in the southern Andean region is first mentioned in 1580 by the Spanish chronicler Cristobal de Albornoz in his work *Relacion*. A psychoactive substance cited in sources from colonial times called *Villca* is possibly identical to Cebíl.

The shamans of the Wichi (Mataco Indians) of northwest Argentina still use a snuff made of Cebíl today. The shamans of the Mataco smoke the dried or roasted seeds, preferably in a pipe or rolled in a cigarette. The Cebíl seeds are for them a means to enter and influence another reality. Cebíl is, in a manner of speaking, a gateway to a visionary world; this is how the shaman Fortunato Ruíz expresses it. He smokes the seeds with tobacco and Aromo—just as his ancestors did five thousand years ago. This makes the

The Chemistry of *Anadenanthera colubrina*

Some varieties of Cebíl seed contain exclusively bufotenin ($C_{12}H_{16}ON_2$) as the psychoactive ingredient. In tests of other seeds, 5-MeO-MMT, DMT, DMT-*N*-oxide, bufotenin, and 5-OH-DMT-*N*-oxide were found. Old tests of the seeds contained 15 mg/g of bufotenin.

In the dried seeds from the trees of northeast Argentina (Salta), there has been found mostly bufotenin (more than 4%), and a related substance (perhaps serotonin), but otherwise no other tryptamines or alkaloids. In tests of other seeds taken from the garden of a Mataco shaman, 12% bufotenin content was found. The ripe pods of the fruit also contain some bufotenin.

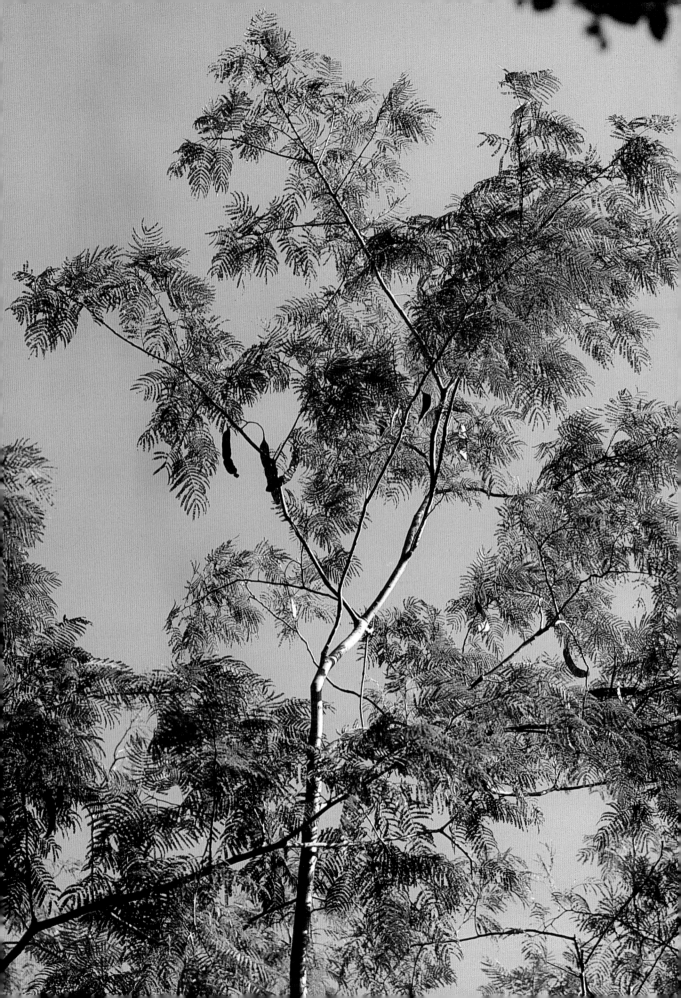

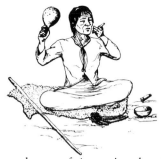

Below: The German artist Nana Nauwald depicted her experience with Cebíl seeds in a painting in 1996. The picture bears the title "Nothing is separate from me" and shows the typical "worm-like" visions.

Right: Recently it was reported that the Mataco in northern Argentina smoke and sniff *Anadenanthera colubrina.* With this, the Spaniards' assumption, that the snuffs Cebíl and Villca are made from this plant, is confirmed.

What Was Villca?

In the colonial literature of New Spain, there are numerous references to the psychoactive use of certain seeds or fruits that were known variously as Huilca, Huillca, Vilca, Vilcas, Villca, Wil'ka, Willca, or Willka. The ethnohistorically documented *villca* (fruit) is today known as the seed of *Anadenanthera colubrina.* Villca was of great ritual and religious significance in Peru in the time before the arrival of the Spaniards, and was known to the Incan high priests and soothsayers *(umu)* as *Villca* or *Villca camayo.* A holy Indian relic *(huaca)* was known as *Villca* or *Vilcacona* and an especially holy mountain is known as Villca Coto. On the peak of Villca Coto, it is said that a couple of humans saved themselves during the primeval deluge.

Villca seeds had a ceremonial significance for the Incas as a psychoactive subsitute for beer. The "juice" of Villca was added to a fermented corn beverage and taken by the soothsayer, who would then be able to look into the future.

Villca was also the name for enemas, which were used for medicinal or shamanic purposes.

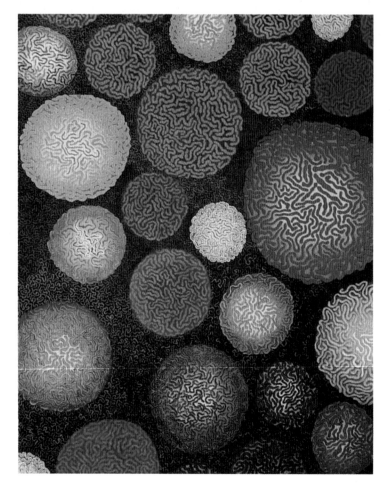

northwest of Argentina the place with the longest uninterrupted ritualistic or shamanic use of psychoactive substances in the world.

As some Matacos have converted to Christianity in recent years, they have come to identify Cebíl with the biblical Tree of Knowledge. But they do not see Cebíl as a "forbidden fruit"; rather, they see it as the fruit of a holy tree, which is used by shamans for healing.

The hallucinations triggered by Cebíl seem to have been very influential in the iconography of the so-called Tiahuanaco Style. The iconography of artist Chavín de Huantar is full of similar motifs: intertwined snakes coming out of the head of the oracle god are clearly Cebíl hallucinations.

The vision-inducing effects of Cebíl snuff last for roughly twenty minutes and include strong hallucinations, which are often only black and white, and seldom in color. They are not (or are only very rarely) geometric in nature, but are strongly flowing and "decentralized." They are very reminiscent of the images produced by the pre-Columbian Tiahuanaco culture.

Cebíl seeds also have psychoactive effects if they are smoked. The effects are very strong for about thirty minutes and then fade away. The effects begin with a feeling of heaviness in the body. After five to ten minutes, visual hallucinations begin with the eyes closed, often featuring worm- and snakelike images flowing into one another. Sometimes geometric, symmetrical, or crystallographic hallucinations can occur, but very seldom are there any strong visions of a realistic nature (such as the experience of flying, traveling in another world, transforming into an animal, contact with helping spirits, and so on).

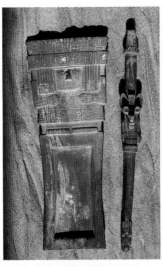

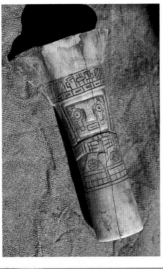

Far left: Pre-Columbian snuff tools from a grave at San Pedro de Atacama.

Left: Pre-Columbian snuff vessel made from a carved bone (San Pedro de Atacama, Chile).

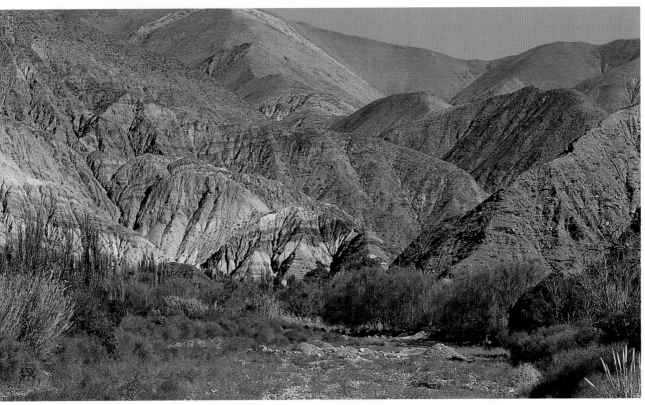

Above: The northwest Argentinian region of Puna is the area in which the longest continued use of visionary and shamanic plants can be proved. In this region the Cebíl seeds have been smoked or sniffed for 4,500 years for healing ceremonies.

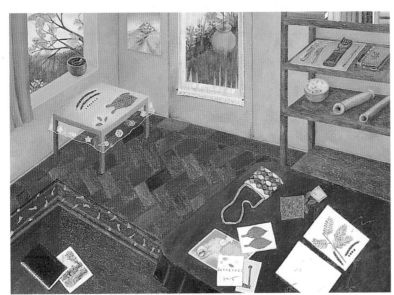

Left: The painting (oil on canvas, 1996) by the Columbian-American artist Donna Torres shows the study of an ethnobotanist who is researching *Anadenanthera colubrina*.

123

THE MAGIC DRINK
OF THE AMAZON

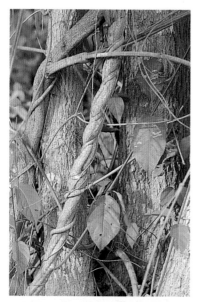

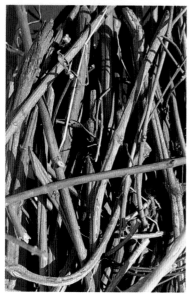

There is a magic intoxicant in northwesternmost South America that the Indians believe can free the soul from corporeal confinement, allowing it to wander free and return to the body at will. The soul, thus untrammeled, liberates its owner from the realities of everyday life and introduces him to wondrous realms of what he considers reality and permits him to communicate with his ancestors. The Quechua term for this inebriating drink—Ayahuasca ("vine of the soul")—refers to this freeing of the spirit. The plants involved are truly plants of the gods, for their power is laid to supernatural forces residing in their tissues, and they were divine gifts to the earliest Indians on earth.

Ayahuasca has many native names: Caapi, Dápa, Mihi, Kahí, Natema, Pindé, Yajé. The drink, employed for prophecy, divination, sorcery, and medical purposes, is so deeply rooted in native mythology and philosophy that there can be no doubt of its great age as a part of aboriginal life.

Two closely related species of the malpighiaceous genus *Banisteriopsis*— *B. caapi* and *B. inebrians*—are the most important plants used in preparing Ayahuasca. But other species are apparently used locally on occasion: *B. quitensis; Mascagnia glandulifera, M. psilophylla* var. *antifebrilis; Tetrapteris methystica* and *T. mucronata*. All of these plants are large forest lianas of the same family. *Banisteriopsis caapi* and *B. inebrians* are frequently cultivated in order to have a supply close at hand for use.

Many plants of diverse families are often added to the basic drink to alter the intoxicating effects. The most commonly used admixtures are leaves of *Diplopterys cabrerana* and of the rubiaceous *Psychotria carthaginensis* or *P. viridis*. Other known psychoactive plants, such as *Brugmansia suaveolens, Brunfelsia chiricaspi*, and *B. grandiflora*, may also be added. Among the many plants employed are Tobacco; *Malouetia tamaquarina* and a species of *Tabernaemontana* of the Apocynaceae; the acanthaceous *Teliostachya lanceolata* var. *crispa* or Toé negra; *Calathea veitchiana*

of the Maranthaceae; the amaranthaceous *Alternanthera lehmannii* and a species of *Iresine;* several ferns including *Lygodium venustum* and *Lomariopsis japurensis; Phrygylanthus eugenioides* of the Misteltoe family; the American Basil *Ocimum micranthum;* a species of the sedge genus *Cyperus;* several cacti including species of *Opuntia* and *Epiphyllum;* and members of the families Clusiaceae and Guttiferae.

The natives often have special names for diverse "kinds" of Ayahuasca, although the botanist frequently finds them all representative of the same species. It is usually difficult to understand the aboriginal method of classification; some may be age forms; others may come from different parts of the liana; still others may be ecological forms growing under varying conditions of soil, shade, moisture, and so on. The natives assert that these "kinds" have a variety of effects, and it is conceivable that they may actually have different chemical compositions. This possibility is one of the least investigated yet most significant aspects in the study of Ayahuasca.

Among the Tukano of the Colombia Vaupés, for example, six "kinds" of Ayahuasca or Kahi are recognized. Botanical identification has not yet been possible in all cases, but the "kinds" have definite native names. Kahi-riáma, the strongest, produces auditory hallucinations and announces future events. It is said to cause death if improperly employed. The second strongest, Méné-kahí-má, reputedly causes visions of green snakes. The bark is used, and it is also said to cause death, unless cautiously taken. These two "kinds" may not belong to *Banisteriopsis* or even to the family Malpighiaceae.

The third in strength is called Suána-Kahí-má ("Kahí of the red jaguar"), producing visions in red. Kahí-vaí Bucura-rijomá ("Kahí of the monkey head") causes monkeys to hallucinate and howl. The weakest of the hallucinogenic "kinds" of Kahí or Ajúwri-kahí-má has little effect but is used in the drink to help the Méné-Kahí-má. All of these "kinds" are referable probably to *Banis-*

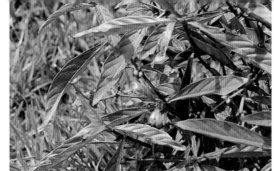

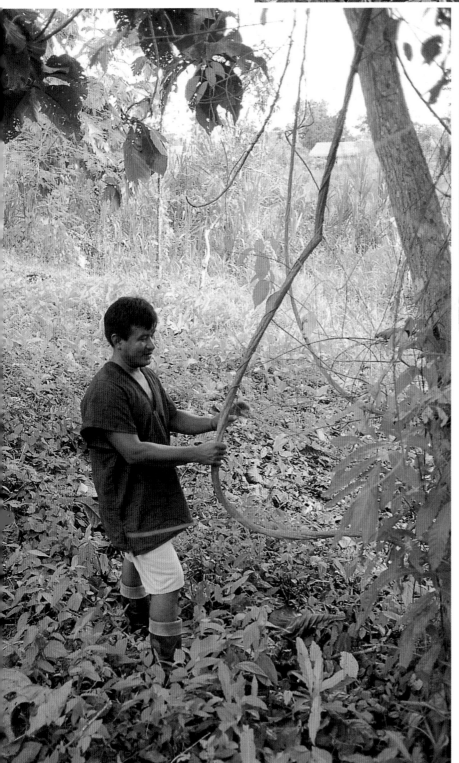

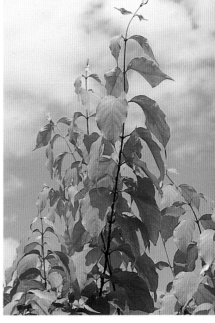

Top: The Chacruna shrub *(Psychotria viridis)* is the second most important ingredient in the Ayahuasca drink.

Above right: The shoots of the Ayahuasca liana.

Left: A Shipibo Indian with an Ayahuasca liana that he has cultivated in his garden.

Page 124 above: The Ayahuasca liana *(Banisteriopsis caapi)* is a powerful and vigorously growing tropical vine.

Page 124 below: The pieces of branch are the base of the Ayahuasca preparation.

"Ayahuasca, medicine, enrapture me fully!
Help me by opening your beautiful world to me!
You also are created by the god who created man!
Reveal to me completely your medicine worlds. I shall heal the sick bodies:
These sick children and this sick woman shall I heal by making everything good!"

—Ayahuasca Song of the Shipibo

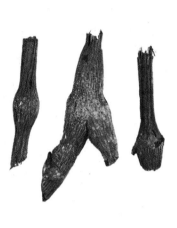

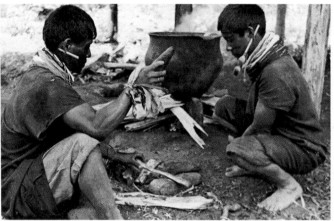

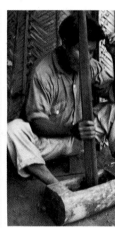

Above left: The British plant explorer Spruce collected the first botanical specimens of *Banisteriopsis caapi* in 1851. He sent material from the same plant for chemical analysis. The material was located in the Museum at the Royal Botanic Gardens at Kew in 1969.

Above right: Among the Kofán of Colombia and Ecuador, special medicine men prepare Curare and Yajé. There is an association between these two plant products, and Yajé is taken before hunting in the belief that the visions will reveal the hiding places of the animals to be sought.

Far right: To make Ayahuasca or Caapi, the freshly stripped bark must be vigorously pounded before being boiled in water or kneaded thoroughly in cold water.

Page 127 left: The numerous Tukanoan tribes of the Vaupés River basin in Colombia and Brazil practice a male-oriented ancestor ceremony. The Yuruparí dance, in which Caapi is a major element, enables the participants to communicate with spirits of the dead.

Page 127 right: Line dancing with intricate steps and gourd rattles accompanying chants is typical of Barasana ceremonies in which Caapi is taken, Piraparaná River.

teriopsis caapi. Kahí-somomá or Kahí-uco ("Kahí that makes you vomit"), a shrub, the leaves of which are added to the drink, an emetic agent, is undoubtedly *Diplopterys cabrerana,* the same plant known among the western Tukanoan Siona of the Colombian Putumayo as Oco-yajé.

Although not so famous as Peyote or the sacred Mexican mushrooms, Ayahuasca has received popular attention because of news articles extolling the so-called telepathic powers of the drink. In fact, in the chemical investigation of *Banisteriopsis,* the first alkaloid isolated was named *telepathine.*

The hallucinogen may be prepared in diverse ways. Usually, bark is scraped from freshly harvested pieces of the stem. In the western areas, the bark is boiled for several hours, and the bitter, thick liquid is taken in small doses. In other localities, the bark is pulverized and then kneaded in cold water; much larger doses must be taken, since it is less concentrated.

The effects of the drink vary according to the method of preparation, the setting in which it is taken, the amount ingested, the number and kinds of admixtures, and the purposes for which it is used, as well as the ceremonial control exercised by the shaman.

Ingestion of Ayahuasca usually induces nausea, dizziness, vomiting, and leads to either a euphoric or an aggressive state. Frequently the Indian sees overpowering attacks of huge snakes or jaguars. These animals often humiliate him because he is a mere man. The repetitiveness with which snakes and jaguars occur in Ayahuasca visions has intrigued psychologists. It is understandable that these animals play such a role, since they are the only beings respected and feared by the Indians of the tropical forest; because of their power and stealth, they have assumed a place of primacy in aboriginal religious beliefs. In many tribes, the shaman becomes a feline during the intoxication, exercising his powers as a wild cat. Yekwana medicine men mimic the roars of jaguars. Tukano Ayahuasca-takers may experience nightmares of jaguar jaws swallowing them or huge snakes approaching and coiling about their bodies. Snakes in bright colors climb up and down the house posts. Shamans of the Conibo-Shipibo tribe acquire great snakes as personal possessions to defend themselves in supernatural battles against other powerful shamans.

The drug may be the shaman's tool to diagnose illness or to ward off impending disaster, to guess the wiles of an enemy, to prophesy the future. But it is more than the shaman's tool. It enters into almost all aspects of the life of the people who use it, to an extent equaled by hardly any other hallucinogen. Partakers, shamans or not, see all the gods, the first human beings, and animals, and

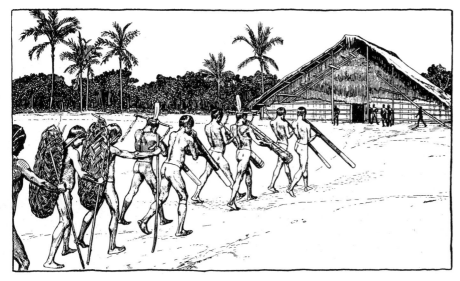

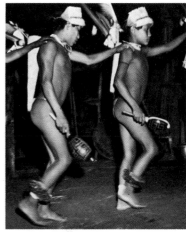

come to understand the establishment of their social order.

Ayahuasca is, above all, a medicine—the great medicine. The Ayahuasca leader among the Campa of Peru is a religious practitioner who, following a strict apprenticeship, maintains and increases his shamanistic power through the use of Tobacco and Ayahuasca. The Campa shaman under Ayahuasca acquires an eerie, distant voice and a quivering jaw that indicates the arrival of good spirits who, splendidly clad, sing and dance before him; the shaman's singing is merely his own voice echoing their song. During the singing, his soul may travel far and wide—a phenomenon not interfering with performance of the ceremony nor with the shaman's ability to communicate the wishes of the spirits to participants.

Among the Tukano, the partaker of the drug feels himself pulled along by powerful winds that the leading shaman explains as a trip to the Milky Way, the first stop on the way to heaven. Similarly, the Ecuadorean Zaparo experience a sensation of being lifted into the air. The souls of Peruvian Conibo-Shipibo shamans fly about in the form of a bird; or shamans may travel in a supernatural canoe manned by demons to reconquer lost or stolen souls.

The effects of the drink are greatly altered when leaves of *Diploterys cabrerana* or of *Psychotria* are added. The

The Chemistry of Ayahuasca

In the belief that they were new discoveries, the first alkaloids isolated from *Banisteriopsis* were called telepathine and banisterine. Further chemical investigations revealed that these preparations were identical with the alkaloid harmine, previously isolated from Syrian Rue, *Peganum harmala*. Furthermore, the secondary alkaloids of *Paganum,* harmaline and tetrahydroharmine, also occur in *Banisteriopsis*. The active principles are indole alkaloids found in several other hallucinogenic plants.

The drink made from Ayahuasca is a unique pharmacological combination of *Banisteriopsis caapi*, a liana that contains harmaline, and Chacruna *(Psychotria viridia)* leaves, which contain DMT. Harmaline is an MAO inhibitor; it reduces the body's production and distribution of monoamine oxidase (MAO). MAO normally breaks down the vision-inducing ingredient DMT before it can cross the blood-brain barrier into the central nervous system. Only with this combination of ingredients can the drink have its consciousness-expanding effects and trigger visions.

Plants Containing the MAO-Inhibiting β-Carboline Alkaloids:

Banisteriopsis spp.	Harmine
Kochia scoparia (L.) SCHRAD.	Harmine, Harmane
Passiflora involucrata	β-Carboline
Passiflora spp.	Harmine, Harmane, etc.
Peganum harmala L.	Harmine, Tetrahydroharmine, Dihydroharmaline, Harmane, Isoharmine, Tetrahydroharmol, Harmalol, Harmol, Norharmine, Harmaline
Strychnos usambarensis GILG	Harmane
Tribulus terrestris L.	Harmine, among others

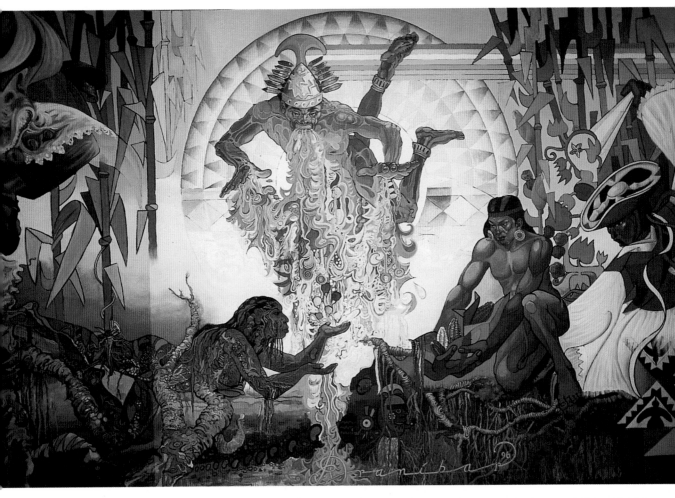

"Practically all decorative elements . . . are said . . . to be derived from hallucinatory imagery . . . The most outstanding examples are the paintings executed on the front walls of the malocas . . . sometimes . . . representing the Lord of Game Animals . . . When asked about these paintings, the Indians simply reply: 'This is what we see when we drink Yajé . . .'"

—G. Reichel-Dolmatoff

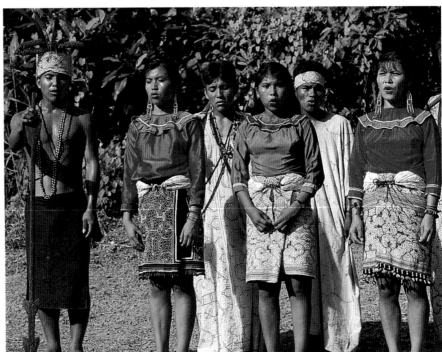

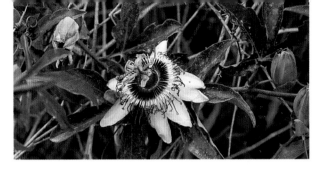

tryptamines in these additives are believed to be inactive when taken orally, unless monoamine oxidase inhibitors are present. The harmine and its derivatives in *B. caapi* and *B. inebrians* are inhibitors of this kind, potentiating the tryptamines. Both types of alkaloids, however, are hallucinogenic.

Length and vividness of the visual hallucinations are notably enhanced when these additives are present. Whereas visions with the basic drink are seen usually in blue, purple, or gray, those induced when the tryptaminic additives are used may be brightly colored in reds and yellows.

The Ayahuasca intoxication may be a very intense experience with visions of light setting in with the eyes closed after a period of giddiness, nervousness, profuse sweating, and sometimes nausea. A period of lassitude initiates the play of colors—at first white, then mainly a hazy, smoky blue that later increases in intensity; eventually sleep, interrupted by dreams and occasional feverishness, takes over. Serious diarrhea, which continues after the intoxication, is the uncomfortable effect most frequently experienced. With the tryptaminic additives, many of these effects are intensified, but trembling and convulsive shaking, mydriasis, and increase of pulse rate are also noted. Frequently, a show of recklessness, sometimes even aggressiveness, marks advanced states of the inebriation.

The famous Yuruparí ceremony of the Tukanoans is an ancestor-communication ritual, the basis of a man's tribal society and an adolescent male initiation rite. Its sacred bark trumpet, which calls the Yuruparí spirit, is taboo to the sight of women; it symbolizes the forces to whom the ceremony is holy, favorably influencing fertility spirits, effecting cures of prevalent illnesses, and improving the male prestige and power over women. The Yuruparí ceremony is now little practiced. One of the most detailed reports of a recent dance describes it as follows:

"A deep booming of drums from within the maloca heralded the appearance of the mystic Yuruparí horns. With only very slight urging from one of the older men, all females from babes in arms to withered, toothless hags betook themselves to the fringing forest, to hear only from afar the deep, mysterious notes of the trumpets, sight of which is believed to spell certain death for any woman . . . Payés shamans and older men are not above aiding the workings of the mystery by the judicious administration of poison to any overcurious female.

"Four pairs of horns had been taken from places of concealment, and the players now ranged themselves in a rough semi-circle, producing the first deep, lugubrious notes . . .

"Many of the older men had meanwhile opened their tangatara boxes of ceremonial feathers and were selecting with great care brilliant feather ruffs, which were bound to the mid-section of the longer horns . . .

"Four oldsters, with perfect rhythm and dramatic timing, paraded through the maloca, blowing the newly decorated horns, advancing and retreating with short dancing steps. At intervals, a couple danced out of the door, their horns raised high, and returned after a brief turn, the expanding and contracting feather ruffs producing a beautiful burst of translucent color against the stronger light. Younger men were beginning the first of the savage whippings, and the master of ceremonies appeared with the red, curiously shaped clay jar containing the powerful narcotic drink called Caapi. The thick, brown, bitter liquid was served in pairs of tiny round gourds; many drinkers promptly vomited . . .

"Whipping proceeded by pairs. The first lashes were applied to the legs and ankles, the whip flung far back in a deliberately calculated dramatic gesture; the blows resounded like pistol shots. Places were immediately exchanged. Soon the whips were being freely applied, and all the younger men were laced with bloody welts on all parts of the body. Tiny lads not more than six or seven years old would catch up the abandoned whips, merrily imitating their elders. Gradually the volume of sound diminished, until only two lone performers remained, enchanted with

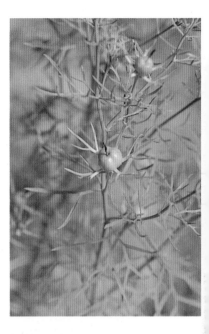

Top: Many species of Passion flower (*Passiflora* spp.) contain the active substances harmine and harmaline.

Above right: Syrian Rue (*Peganum harmala)* with fruit capsules.

Page 128 above: The mural in the Cuzco Airport (Peru) reveals the visionary world of Ayahuasca.

Page 128 below: Shipibo Indians in traditional costumes decorated with Ayahuasca patterns (Yarinacocha, Peru).

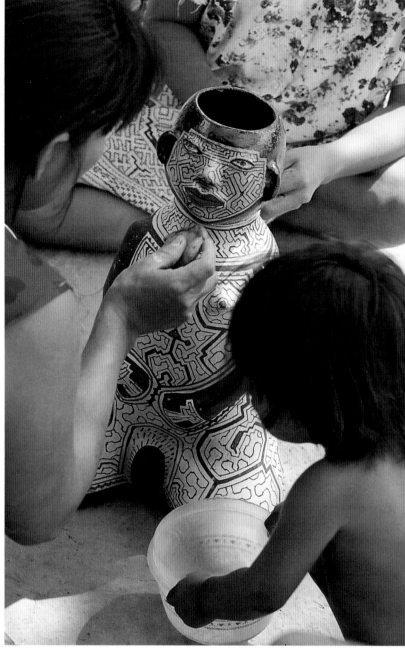

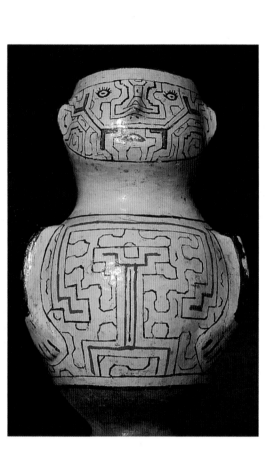

Left: A beer mug of the Conibo-Shipibo Indians that has been completely painted with the Ayahuasca pattern.

Right: Shipibo women communally paint a ceramic with Ayahuasca patterns.

their art, bowing, advancing, and retreating, with great delicacy and grace in the center of the maloca. About a dozen of the older men were outfitting themselves with their finest diadems of resplendent guacamayo feathers, tall, feathery egret plumes, oval pieces of the russet skin of the howler monkey, armadillo-hide disks, prized loops of monkey-hair cord, precious quartzite cylinders, and jaguar-tooth belts. Bedecked with these triumphs of savage art, the men formed a swaying, dancing semi-circle, each with his right hand resting on his neighbor's shoulder, all shifting and stamping in slow unison.

Leading the group was the ancient payé, blowing Tobacco smoke in benediction on his companions from the huge cigar in its engraved ceremonial fork, while his long, polished rattle-lance vibrated constantly. The familiar, dignified Cachirí ceremonial chant was intoned by the group; their deep voices rose and fell, mingling with the mysterious booming tones of the Yuruparí horns."

The Tukano believe that when, at the time of creation, humans arrived to populate the Vaupés region, many extraordinary happenings took place. People had to endure hardship before settling the new regions. Hideous snakes and

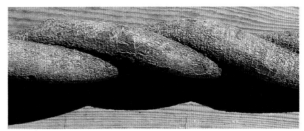

dangerous fish lived in the rivers; there were spirits with cannibalistic proclivities; and the Tukano received in trepidation the basic elements of their culture.

There lived among these early Tukano a woman—the first woman of creation—who "drowned" men in visions. Tukanoans believe that during coitus, a man "drowns"—the equivalent of seeing visions. The first woman found

the sensual, to a mystical union with the mythic era, the intrauterine stage, is the ultimate goal, attained by a mere handful but coveted by all."

All or much of Indian art, it has been proposed, is based on visionary experience. Colors, similarly, are symbolically significant: yellow or off-white has a seminal concept, indicating solar fertilization; red—color of the uterus, fire,

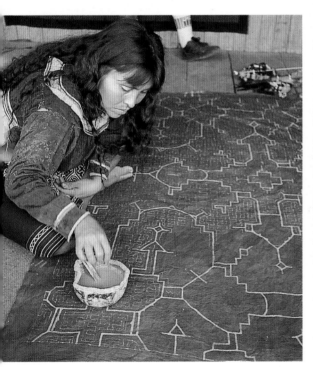

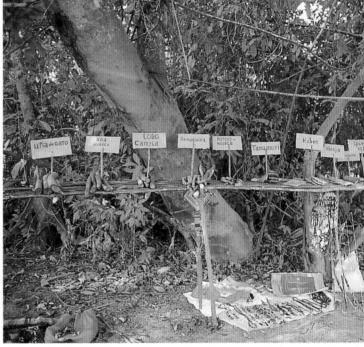

herself with child. The Sun-father had impregnated her through the eye. She gave birth to a child who became Caapi, the narcotic plant. The child was born during a brilliant flash of light. The woman—Yajé—cut the umbilical cord and, rubbing the child with magical plants, shaped its body. The Caapi-child lived to be an old man zealously guarding his hallucinogenic powers. From this aged child, owner of Caapi or the sexual act, the Tukanoan men received semen. For the Indians, wrote Gerardo Reichel-Dolmatoff, "the hallucinatory experience is essentially a sexual one ... to make it sublime, to pass from the erotic,

heat—symbolizes female fecundity; blue represents thought through Tobacco smoke. These colors accompany Ayahuasca intoxications and have precise interpretations. Many of the complicated rock engravings in the river valleys of the Vaupés region are undoubtedly based upon drug experiences. Likewise, the stereotyped paintings on the bark wall of Tukanoan communal houses represent themes from Ayahuasca hallucinations.

Pictures and decorations on pots, houses, basketry, and other household objects fall into two categories: abstract design and figurative motifs.

Above left: A Shipibo woman paints a piece of fabric with her traditional Ayahuasca pattern.

Above right: The jungle pharmacy of the Shipibo Indians. Countless medicinal plants are taken with Ayahuasca, which strengthen the effects.

The Indians know the difference between the two and say that it is due to Caapi intoxication. "Someone watching a man at work or finding a drawing would say: 'This is what one sees after three cups of Yajé,' occasionally specifying the kind of plant that had been used and thus giving an indication of the nature of the narcotic effects they attributed to different concoctions," speculated G. Reichel-Dolmatoff.

It would seem that such an important drug would have attracted the attention of Europeans at a very early date. Such was not the case. In 1851, however, the English botanist Spruce, who was collecting among Tukanoan tribes in the

Orinoco. Later, he encountered Ayahuasca among the Zaparo of Ecuador and identified it as the same hallucinogen as Caapi.

"In the course of the night," Spruce wrote of Caapi, "the young men partook of Caapi five or six times, in the intervals between the dances; but only a few of them at a time, and a very few drank of it twice. The cup-bearer—who must be a man, for no woman can touch or taste Caapi—starts at a short run from the opposite end of the house, with a small calabash containing about a teacupful of Caapi in each hand, muttering 'Mo-mo-mo-mo-mo' as he runs, and gradually sinking down until at last his chin nearly touches his knees, when he reaches out one of his cups to the man who stands ready to receive it . . . In two minutes or less after drinking it, the effects begin to be apparent. The Indian turns deadly pale, trembles in every limb, and horror is in his aspect. Suddenly contrary symptoms succeed; he bursts into perspiration and seems possessed with reckless fury, seizes whatever arms are at hand . . . and rushes to the door, while he inflicts violent blows on the ground and doorposts, calling out all the while: 'Thus would I do to mine enemy [naming him by name] were this he!' In about ten minutes, the excitement has passed off, and the Indian grows calm but appears exhausted."

Since Spruce's time, this drug has been mentioned often by many travelers and explorers, but little has been accomplished until recently. In fact, it was not until 1969 that chemical analysis of Spruce's material, collected for such examination in 1851, was carried out.

Much remains to be learned about Ayahuasca, Caapi, Yajé. There is little time before increasing acculturation and even extinction of whole tribes will make it forever impossible to learn about these age-old beliefs and uses.

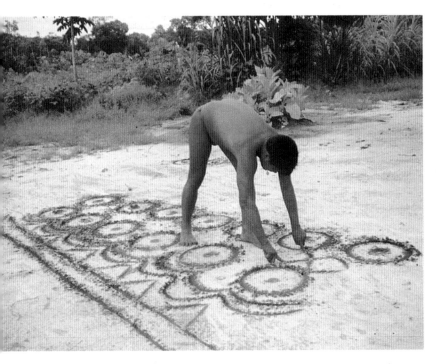

Above: A Barasana Indian traces in sand near his maloca patterns seen during the course of Caapi intoxication. It has been suggested that many of the design motifs induced by Caapi are, on the one hand, culture-bound and, on the other hand, controlled by specific biochemical effects of the active principles n the plant.

Rio Vaupés region of Brazil, met with Caapi and sent material for chemical study to England. Three years later, he observed Caapi use again among the Guahibo Indians along the upper

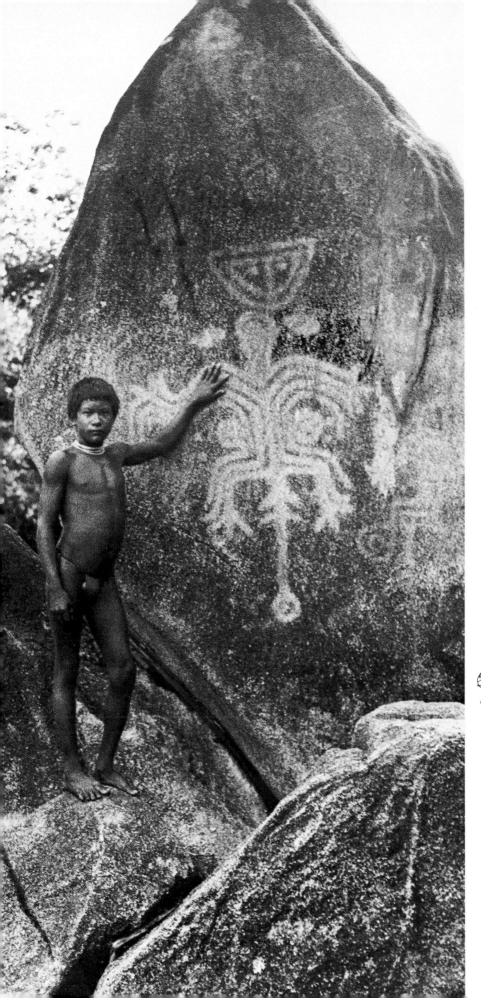

Left: This beautiful engraving on a granite rock at Nyí on the lower Piraparaná River in Colombia is obviously ancient. The rapids at this point on the river are at the earth's equator, a zone vertically related to the rising and setting constellations. It has been suggested that this turbulent area of the river was the place where the Sun Father married Earth Mother to create the first Tukanoans. The Indians interpret the triangular face as a vagina and the stylized human figure as a winged phallus.

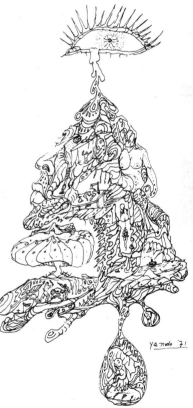

Above: The talented Peruvian artist Yando, the son of an Ayahuasquero from Pucallpa, drew this Ayahuasca vision. Notice that the complexities of the hallucinations are treated in an imagery in which microscopic and macroscopic dimensions are skillfully blended.

133

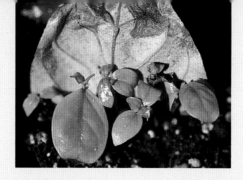

Right: Young cultivated Chacruna
(Psychotria viridis).

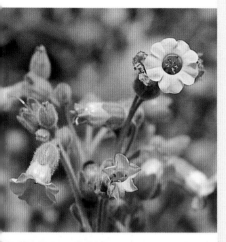

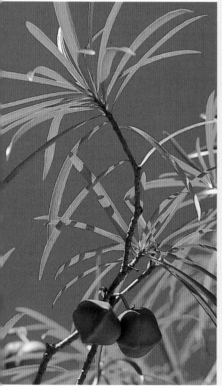

Above: Farmer's tobacco *(Nicotiana rustica)* is one of the most important shaman plants in South America.

Bottom: The fruit of a species of *Thevetia* called *Cabalonga blanca* is added to Ayahuasca to protect the drinker from malicious spirits.

Ayahuasca Ingredients

A selection of plants used in the preparation of the Ayahuasca drink to give it its desired healing powers or specific qualities:

Ai curo	*Euphorbia* sp.	for better singing
Ají	*Capsicum frutescens*	tonic
Amacisa	*Erythrina* spp.	purgative
Angel's Trumpet	*Brugmansia* spp.	to treat delusions, illnesses caused by magic arrows *(chonteado)*, and enchantment
Ayahuma	*Couroupita guianensis*	strengthens the body
Batsikawa	*Psychotria* sp.	for cooling and reduction of visions
Cabalonga	*Thevetia* sp.	protects against spirits
Catahua	*Hura crepitans*	purgative
Cat's claw	*Uncaria tomentosa*	strengthens; used to treat allergies, kidney problems, stomach ulcer, venereal disease
Chiricaspi	*Brunfelsia* spp.	for fever, rheumatism, and arthritis
Cuchura-caspi	*Malouetia tamaquarina*	to enable a better diagnosis
Cumala	*Virola* spp.	strengthens the vision
Guatillo	*Iochroma fuchsioides*	strengthens the vision
Guayusa	*Ilex guayusa*	for purification and treatment of vomiting
Hiporuru	*Alchornea castanaefolia*	to treat diarrhea
Kana	*Sabicea amazonensis*	"sweetens" the Ayahuasca drink
Kapok tree	*Ceiba pentandra*	diarrhea, intestinal problems
Lupuna	*Chorisia insignis*	to treat intestinal problems
Pfaffia	*Pfaffia iresinoides*	sexual weakness
Pichana	*Ocimum micranthum*	fever
Piri piri	*Cyperus* sp.	fright; promotes spiritual development; for abortions
Pulma	*Calathea veitchiana*	to stimulate visions
Rami	*Lygodium venustum*	to strengthen the Ayahuasca drink
Remo caspi	*Pithecellobium laetum*	strengthens the Ayahuasca drink
Sanango	*Tabernaemontana sananho*	poor memory; for spiritual development; arthritis, rheumatism
Sucuba	*Himatanthus sucuuba*	to extract magic arrows
Tobacco	*Nicotiana rustica*	for poisoning
Toé	*Ipomoea carnea*	strengthens the vision

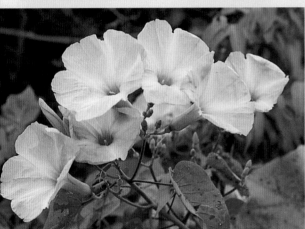

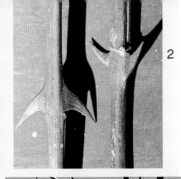

1: The Chiricaspi bush *(Brunfelsia grandiflora* spp. *schultesii)* is an important shaman plant in the northern regions of South America.

2: Cat's Claw *(Uncaria tomentosa)* is one of the important medicinal plants for treating chronic illnesses among the Peruvian Indians.

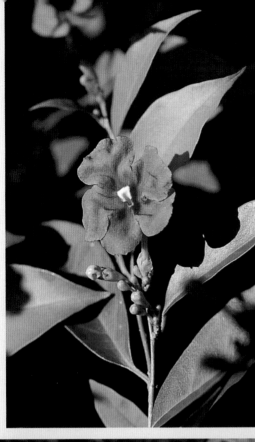

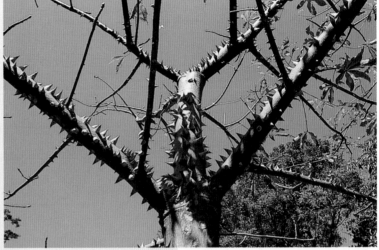

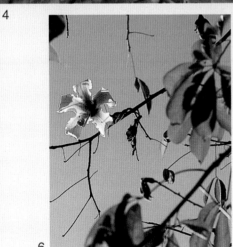

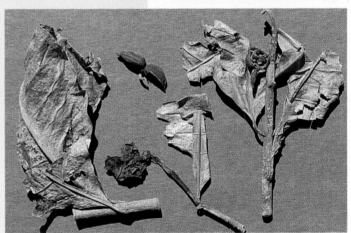

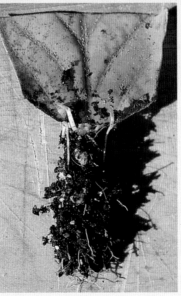

3: For many Indians, the Kapok tree *(Ceiba pentandra)* is the world tree.

4: The bindweed *Ipomea carnea* contains potent psychoactive alkaloids and is used in the Peruvian Amazon basin as an ingredient in Ayahuasca.

5: The Sanango leaves *(Tabernaemontana sananho)* strengthen the memory.

6: The Palo de Borracho "tree of drunkenness" *(Chorisia insignis)* is a world tree in the cosmology of the shaman. Its astringent bark is added to Ayahuasca.

7: A leaf cutting from *Psychotria viridis* (grown in California).

135

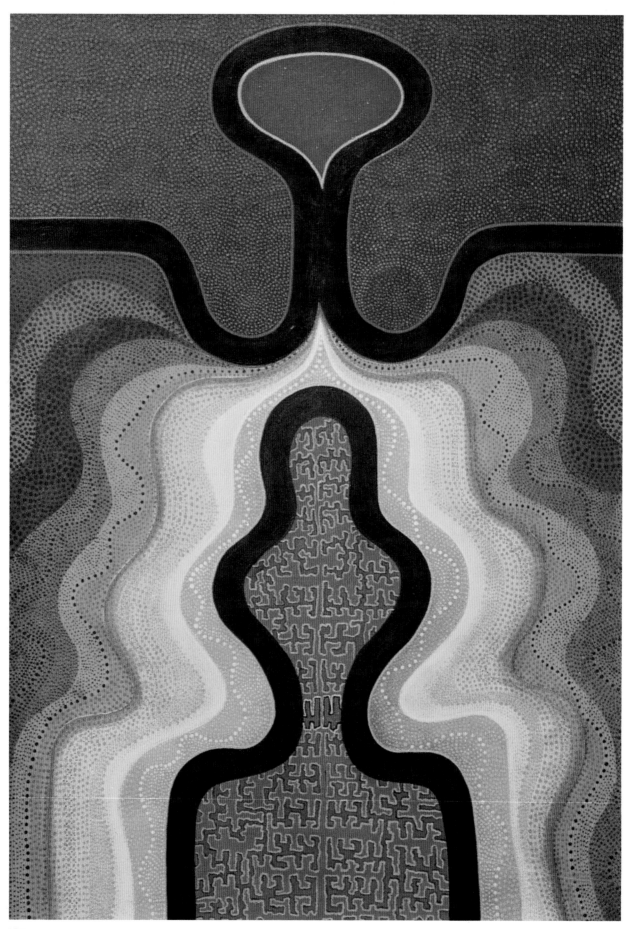

AYAHUASCA ANALOGS

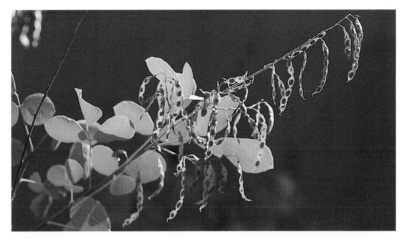

The pharmacological agent that has been identified in Ayahuasca can be imitated in plants with similar active ingredients (harmaline/harmine, DMT/5-MeO-DMT). Nontraditional combinations of plants with these ingredients are today known as "Ayahuasca analogs" or Anahuasca. Combinations made of the isolated of synthesized ingredients are called "pharmahuasca."

Jonathan Ott, a chemist specializing in natural substances, writes: "Psychonautic pharmahuasca research is so distant from the scientific mainstream that it took nearly three decades of no one supporting, or independent scientists doing 'underground' research before the enzyme inhibitor theory of Ayahuasca pharmacology was put to the test. Paradoxically, this research can rightfully claim that is stands exactly in the center of the research on the biochemistry of consciousness and the genetics of pathological brain functions! ... Ayahuasca research is not just on the vertex of neuro-scientific research, but it is possible that the reversible MAO-inhibiting effects of Ayahuasca could present a practical, less toxic alternative to the harmful substances that are finding medical uses!"

The value of these Ayahuasca analogs lies in the entheogenic effects that lead to a deeper spiritual ecology and an all-encompassing mystical insight. Ayahuasca and its analogs bring about—but only with the right dosage—a shamanic ecstasy:

"Shamanic ecstasy is the *true* ancient religion, of which modern churches are merely pale imitations. Our ancestors discovered in many places, and at many times, that suffering humanity could find in ecstatic entheogenic experiences the reconciliation between the cultivated intelligence that separates each human being from other creatures and even from other humans, and the wild, untamed, magnificent animal physical-

ity that we all possess ... It is not necessary to have faith because the ecstatic experience in and of itself *gives* one the belief in the true unity and integrity of the universe, and in ourselves as an integral part of the whole. Ecstatic experience is what reveals to us the sublime grandeur of our universe and the fluctuating, shimmering alchemical wonder that constitutes our everyday consciousness. Entheogens such as Ayahuasca could be the appropriate medicine for hypermaterialistic humanity on the threshold of the new millennium, where it will be decided if our way will be continuing to grow and progress or if we will be destroyed in a massive biological holocaust unparalleled by anything that has happened in our realm in the last 65 million years ... The entheogenic reformation is our greatest hope for healing our dear Mother Gaia, because it is bringing about a true religious revival that will help to bring in the new millennium."

All formulas for Ayahuasca analogs must contain an MAO inhibitor and a DMT supplier.

Until now, most experiments have been with *Banusteriopsis caapi, Banisteriopsis* spp., and *Peganum harmala*. But there are other MAO inhibitors in nature, such as caltrop *(Tribulus terrestris)*. Preferred DMT suppliers include *Psychotria viridis* and *Mimosa tenuiflora*, although there are numerous other possibilities (see tables).

Page 136: The German artist Nana Nauwald renders her Ayahuasca visions in this painting, allowing the viewer a glimpse into the "alternate reality."

Above: Many species of the North American plant genus *Desmodium* contain the potent substance DMT in their root bark, making them suited in the preparation of drinks similar to Ayahuasca.

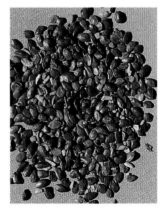

Above: The seeds of the *Mimosa scabrella* contain DMT and are usable in the preparation of Ayahuasca analogs.

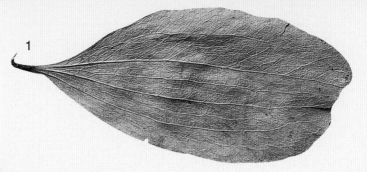

1: The leaf of the extremely rare *Acacia phlebophylla* is rich with DMT. It grows only on one mountain in Australia.

2: *The* Australian native *Acacia maidenii* contains a high concentration of DMT in its bark.

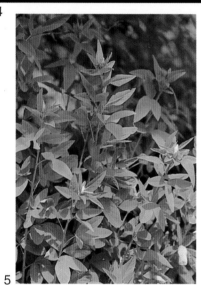

4

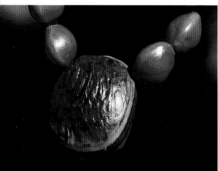

5

3: The seeds of the South American tree *Dictyloma incanescens*. This tree contains ample amounts of 5-MeO-DMT.

4: The seeds of the tropical *Mucuna pruriens* are preferred by the traditional people to make jewelry. In addition they contain high concentrations of DMT and 5-MeO-DMT.

5: A species of the DMT-containing genus *Desmodium*.

6: The Turkey Red variety of the grass *Phalaris arundinacea* contains liberal amounts of DMT.

7: The root bark of the Mexican *Mimosa tenuiflora (Mimosa hostillis)* is full of psychoactive alkaloids. The dried root bark contains about 1% DMT. It is well suited for the production of an Ayahuasca analog.

Ayahuasca Analogs: Plants that contain DMT

Plant Family	Drug	Tryptamine
Gramineae (Poaceae)		
Arundo donax L.	Rhizome	DMT
Phalaris arundinacea L.	Grass, root	DMT
Phalaris tuberosa L. (Italian strain)	Leaves	DMT
Phragmites australis (Cav.) TR. et ST.	Rhizome	DMT, 5-MeO-DMT
Leguminosae (Fabaceae)		
Acacia maidenii F.v. Muell.	Bark	0.36% DMT
Acacia phlebophylla F.v. Muell.	Leaves	0.3% DMT
Acacia simplicifolia Druce	Leaves, bark	0.81% DMT
Anadenanthera peregrina (L.) Spag.	Bark	DMT, 5-MeO-DMT
Desmanthus illinoensis (Michx.) Macm.	Root-bark	up to 0.34% DMT
Desmodium pulchellum Benth. ex. Bak.	Root bark	DMT
Desmodium spp.		DMT
Lespedeza capitata Michx.		DMT
Mimosa scabrella Benth.	Bark	DMT
Mimosa tenuiflora (Willd.) Poir.	Root bark	0.57–1% DMT
Mucuna pruriens DC.	Seeds	DMT, 5-MeO-DMT
Malpighiaceae		
Diplopterys cabrerana (Cuatr.) Gates	Leaves	DMT, 5-MeO-DMT
Myristicaceae		
Virola sebifera Aub.	Bark	DMT
Virola theiodora (Spruce ex Benth.) Warb.	Flowers	0.44% DMT
Virola spp.	Bark, resin	DMT, 5-MeO-DMT
Rubiaceae		
Psychotria poeppigiana MUELL. -ARG.	Leaves	DMT
Psychotria viridis R. et P.	Leaves	DMT
Rutaceae		
Dictyoloma incanescens DC	Bark	0.04% 5-MeO-DMT

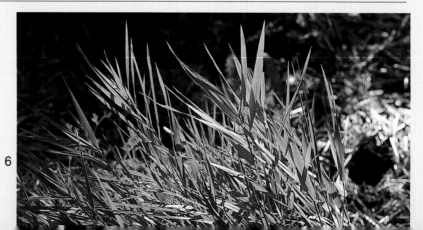

6

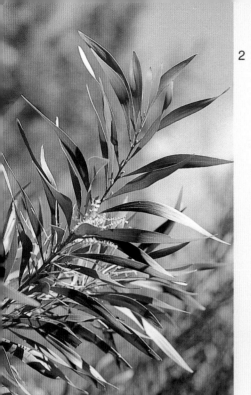

2

3

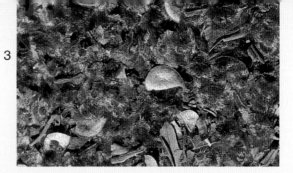

Juremahuasca or Mimohuasca

This Ayahuasca analog is known among people knowledgeable in the field as a preparation that is the most psychoactive and easiest to tolerate. Per person, prepare:

 3 g *Peganum harmala,* finely ground
 9 g root husk of *Mimosa tenuiflora*
 Lemon or lime juice

The ground seeds of Syrian Rue *(Peganum harmala)* are soaked in water and swallowed or taken in a gelatin capsule. Fifteen minutes later, drink the boiled mixture of lemon or lime juice and Mimosa husk.

 After 45 to 60 minutes—often after brief nausea or vomiting—the visions begin. They often take the form of fireworks or kaleidoscope-like designs, flashing colors, fantastic mandalas, or travels to another world. The effects are equal to the effects of the Ayahuasca preparations from the Amazon.

Ayahuasca Churches

In addition to the true shamanic use of Ayahuasca, recently various syncretic churches have been established that also use Ayahuasca as part of their religious rituals. The Santo Daime cult as well as the Ayahuasca church, *União do Vegetal,* hold regular meetings in which the members—the great majority of whom are mestizos from the lower classes—drink Ayahuasca together and sing pious songs. Led by a priest, the group travels to the spirits of the trees as well as to the Christian holy spirits. Many cult members discover a new meaning to life and find healing for the soul. For the members of these Brazilian churches, which have also made headway in Europe, the use of this magic potion is just as legal as it is for the shamans of the jungle.

 Santo Daime, the ritual drink of a cult, and *hoasca,* the sacrament of another church, are both made according to an original Indian recipe in which the *Banisteriopsis caapi* vine and the leaves of the charcruna shrub *(Psychotria viridis)* are boiled to make an extremely psychedelic mixture.

 The Santo Daime cult also has missionaries active in Europe, and this Brazilian group has been especially successful in Germany and the Netherlands. In Amsterdam, they have their own church. Also in the Netherlands, the potential use of Ayahuasca to treat addictions is being tested.

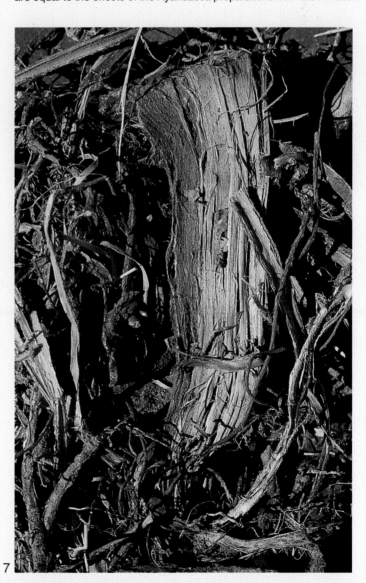

7

TRUMPETS OF THE ANGELS

1: The shamanic use of the gold-yellow flowering *Brugmansia* occurs primarily in Colombia and northern Peru.

2: The flowers and leaves are used by many Indian shamans for medicinal purposes.

3: The ripe fruit of the *Brugmansia sanguinea*. This Angel's Trumpet puts out far more fruit than does any other species.

4: The flower of *Brugmansia sanguinea*.

The Guambiano of southern Colombia say of *Brugmansia vulcanicola:* "How pleasant is the perfume of the long, bell-like flowers of the Yas, as one inhales it in the afternoon ... But the tree has a spirit in the form of an eagle which has been seen to come flying through the air and then to disappear ... The spirit is so evil that if a weak person stations himself at the foot of the tree, he will forget everything, ... feeling up in the air as if on wings of the spirit of the Yas ... If a girl ... sits resting in the tree's shade, she will dream about men of the Paez tribe, and later a figure will be left in her womb which will be borne six months later in the form of pips or seeds of the tree."

The species of *Brugmansia* are native to South America. *Brugmansia* in the past has usually been considered to represent a section of the genus *Datura.* Thorough studies of the biology of these plants have shown that they deserve to be classified in a distinct genus. The behavior of the species—as well as their location—indicates long association with man.

The hallucinogenic use of *Brugmansia* may have come from knowledge of the closely related *Datura,* knowledge that proto-Indian Mongoloids brought to the New World in late Paleolithic and Mesolithic times. As they migrated southward, they encountered other species of *Datura,* especially in Mexico, and bent them to shamanic use. Upon arriving in the Andes of South America, they recognized the resemblance of the Brugmansias to *Datura* and found their psychoactive properties very similar. At any rate, everything about the use of *Brugmansia* bespeaks great antiquity.

Little is known, however, of pre-Conquest use of *Brugmansia.* There are, nevertheless, scattered references to these hallucinogens. The French scientist de la Condamine mentioned its use among the Omagua of the Rio Marañón. The explorers von Humboldt and Bonpland remarked on Tonga, the red-flowered *B. sanguinea,* as a sacred plant of the priests in the Temple of the Sun at Sogamoza in Colombia.

Brugmansia arborea, B. aurea, and *B. sanguinea* usually occur above an altitude of six thousand feet. The seeds are widely employed as an additive to chicha. The crushed leaves and flowers are prepared in hot or cold water to be taken as a tea. Leaves can be mixed with an infusion of Tobacco. Some Indians may scrape off the soft green bark of the stems and soak it in water for use.

The *Brugmansia* intoxication varies but is always characterized by a violent phase. There is probably no more succinct description than that of Johann J. Tschudi in 1846, who saw the effects in

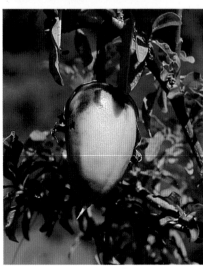

1

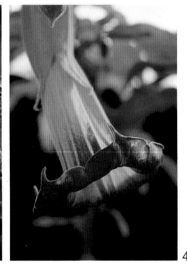

2

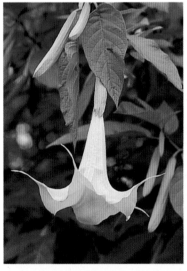

3

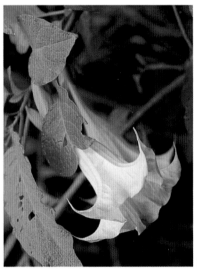

4

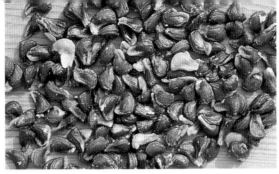

Peru. The native "fell into a heavy stupor, his eyes vacantly fixed on the ground, his mouth convulsively closed, and his nostrils dilated. In the course of a quarter of an hour, his eyes began to roll, foam issued from his mouth, and his whole body was agitated by frightful convulsions. After these violent symptoms had passed, a profound sleep of several hours' duration followed, and when the subject had recovered, he related the particulars of his visit with his forefathers."

At Tunja, among the Muisca, according to a report in 1589, a "dead chief was accompanied to the tomb by his women and slaves, who were buried in different layers of earth ... of which none was without gold. And so that the women and poor slaves should not fear their death before they saw the awful tomb, the nobles gave them things to drink of inebriating Tobacco and other leaves of the tree we call Borrachero, all mixed in their usual drink, so that of their senses none is left to foresee the harm soon to befall them." The species employed were undoubtedly *Brugmansia aurea* and *B. sanguinea*.

Among the Jívaro, recalcitrant children are given a drink of *B. sanguinea* with parched maize; when intoxicated, the children are lectured so that the spirits of the ancestors may admonish them. In the Chocó, *Brugmansia* seeds put into magic chicha beer were thought to produce in children an excitement during which they could discover gold.

Indians in Peru still call *Brugmansia sanguinea* by the name Huaca or Huacachaca ("plant of the tomb") from the belief that it reveals treasures anciently buried in graves.

In the warmer parts of the western Amazon, *Brugmansia suaveolens, B. versicolor,* and *B.* x *insignis* are employed as hallucinogens or as an admixture with Ayahuasca.

Perhaps no locality can equal the Valley of Sibundoy in the Andes of Colombia for *Brugmansia* use. The Kamsá and Ingano Indians use several species and a number of local cultivars as hallucinogens. The Indians of this region, espe-

cially shamans, have a developed knowledge of the effects of these plants and grow them as private possessions.

Usually the property of specific shamans, these cultivars have native names. The leaves of Buyés *(B. aurea)* are employed mainly to relieve rheumatism, an effective medicine with its high concentration of tropane alkaloids. Biangan was employed formerly by hunters: the leaves and flowers were mixed with dogs' food to enable them to find more game. The tongue-shaped leaf of Amarón is valued as a suppurant and in treating rheumatism. The rarest

Above: The seeds of *Brugmansia suaveolens* are used in Peru as an intoxicating additive to corn beer. They are taken by the shamans in higher doses and often produce a delirium that can last for days with the most powerful of hallucinations.

Below: The Blood-Red Angel's Trumpet is often planted in sacred places and cemeteries. Here is a large plant growing with an image of the Madonna in southern Chile.

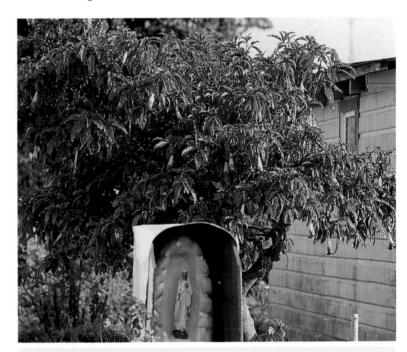

The Chemistry of *Brugmansia*

The solanaceous *Brugmansia arborea, B. aurea, B. sanguinea, B. suaveolens,* and *B. versicolor* contain the same tropane alkaloids as the Daturas: scopolamine, hyoscyamine, atropine, and the various secondary alkaloids of the tropane group, such as norscopolamine, aposcopolamine, meteloidine, etc. Scopolamine, responsible for the hallucinogenic effects, is always found in the largest quantity. The leaves and stems of *B. aurea,* for example, with a total alkaloid of 0.3 percent, contain 80 percent scopolamine, which is also the main alkaloid in the roots of *Brugmansia.*

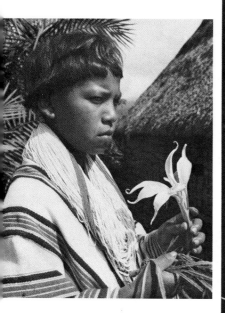

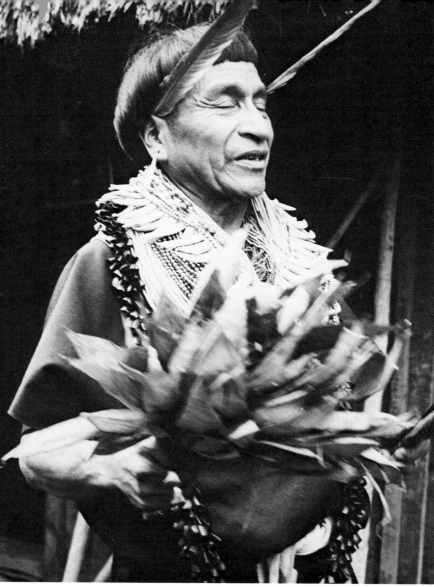

Right: The Valley of Sibundoy in southern Colombia is a location of intensive use of *Brugmansia.* One of the most renowned medicine men of the Kamsá tribe is Salvador Chindoy. Here he is pictured in his ceremonial garb at the beginning of a *Brugmansia*-induced intoxication for purposes of divination.

Left: A young Kamsá Indian boy of Sibundoy, Colombia, holds a flower and leaves of *Culebra Borrachera* prior to brewing a tea for the purpose of intoxication in preparation for learning the secrets of use of hallucinogens in magic and medicine.

cultivar is Salamán, with bizarrely atrophied leaves; it is employed both in treating rheumatism and as a hallucinogen. The extreme in aberration is found in Quinde and Munchira: these two are used as hallucinogens but also in the treatment of rheumatism and as emetics, carminatives, vermifuges, and suppurants; Munchira likewise is employed to treat erysipelas. Quinde is the most widely employed cultivar in Sibundoy; Munchira the most toxic. The rare Dientes and Ochre find their most important use in the treatment of rheumatic pains.

"A spirit so evil, our grandparents tell us, was in these trees with flowers like long bells, which give off their sweet perfume in the afternoon, that they were the food of those Indians at whose name people trembled: fierce Pijaos."

Culebra borrachero is thought by some botanists to be one of those monstrous cultivars. More potent than any

of the cultivars of *Brugmansia,* it is used hallucinogenically for the most difficult cases of divination and as an effective medicine for rheumatic or arthritic pains.

The cultivars Quinde and Munchira are most frequently used for their psychoactive effects. The juice of the crushed leaves or flowers is drunk either alone in a cold-water preparation or with aguardiente (an alcoholic distillate of sugar). In Sibundoy only shamans usually take *Brugmansia.* Most shamans "see" fearful visions of jaguars and poisonous snakes. Symptoms and unpleasant aftereffects probably have contributed to the limitation of *Brugmansia* as a hallucinogen.

The Jívaro believe that normal life is an illusion, that the true powers behind daily life are supernatural. The shaman, with his potent hallucinogenic plants, can cross over into the world of ethereal wonder and deal with the forces of

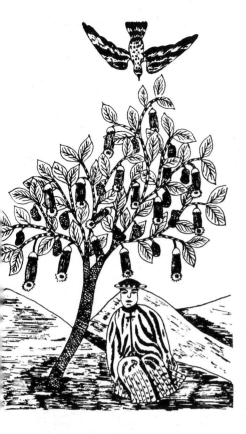

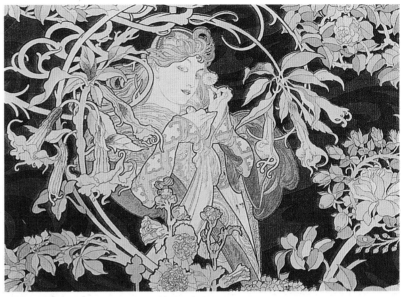

evil. A Jívaro boy at the age of six must acquire an external soul, an *arutam wakani,* the vision-producing soul that can allow him to communicate with ancestors. To get his *arutam* the boy and his father make a pilgrimage to a sacred waterfall, bathing, fasting, and drinking Tobacco water. Maikoa or *Brugmansia* juice may also be taken to effect contact with the supernatural during which the boy's *arutam* appears as jaguars and anacondas and enters his body.

The Jívaro frequently take Natema (Ayahuasca) or *Banisteriopsis* to acquire the *arutam,* since it is a strong intoxicant, but *Brugmansia* must be used if Natema is not successful. Maikoa intoxication, the Jívaro assert, may cause insanity.

From all viewpoints, species of *Brugmansia* have had a difficult time of it in spite of their great beauty. They are plants of the gods, but not the agreeable gifts of the gods, like Peyote, the mushrooms, Ayahuasca. Their powerful and wholly unpleasant effects, leading to periods of violence and even temporary insanity, together with their sickening aftereffects, have conspired to put them in a place of second category. They are plants of the gods, true, but the gods do not always strive to make life easy for man—so they gave man the Brugmansias, to which he must on occasion repair. The evil eagle hovers over man, and his Borrachero is an ever-present reminder that it is not always easy to attain an audience with the gods.

Right: The beautiful flowers of the Angel's Trumpet inspired the Symbolists (fabric printed after a design by Alphonse Mucha, Paris 1896; original is in the Württemburg State Museum, Stuttgart, Germany).

Left: This drawing by a Guambiano Indian of the southern Andes of Colombia depicts a native woman under a Borrachero tree, *Brugmansia vulcanicola.* The portrayal of an eagle associated with an evil spirit indicates the dangerous toxicity of this tree, which causes a person tarrying under it to become forgetful and to feel as if he were flying.

THE TRACKS OF THE LITTLE DEER

Page 145 top: The Peyote crowns take on many different forms, depending on age and growing conditions.

Page 145 below: A group of large Peyote cacti in their native habitat of southern Texas.

Ever since the arrival of the first Europeans in the New World, Peyote has provoked controversy, suppression, and persecution. Condemned by the Spanish conquerors for its "satanic trickery," and attacked again and again by local governments and religious groups, the plant has nevertheless continued to play a major sacramental role among the Indians of Mexico, while its use has spread to the northern tribes in the United States in the last hundred years. The persistence and growth of the Peyote cult constitute a fascinating chapter in the history of the New World—and a challenge to the anthropologists and psychologists, botanists and pharmacologists who continue to study the plant

lished in native religions, and their efforts to stamp out this practice drove it into hiding in the hills, where its sacramental use has persisted to the present time.

How old is the Peyote cult? An early Spanish chronicler, Fray Bernardino de Sahagún, estimated on the basis of several historical events recorded in Indian chronology that Peyote was known to the Chichimeca and Toltec at least 1,890 years before the arrival of the Europeans. This calculation would give the "divine plant" of Mexico an economic history extending over a period of some two millennia. Then Carl Lumholtz, the Danish ethnologist who did pioneer work among the Indians of Chihuahua,

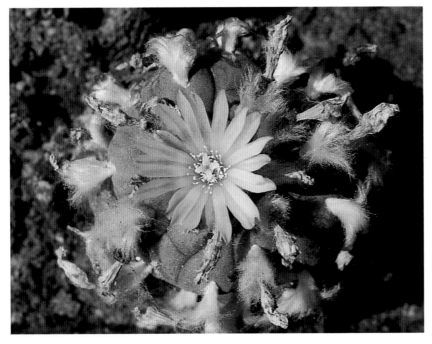

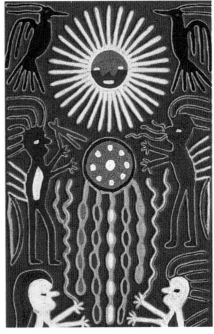

Left: The flowering Peyote cactus (*Lophophora williamsii*).

Right: A Huichol yarn painting shows the nurturing and fertile gifts of the Peyote cactus.

and its constituents in connection with human affairs.

We might logically call this needleless Mexican cactus the prototype of the New World hallucinogens. It was one of the first to be discovered by Europeans and was unquestionably the most spectacular vision-inducing plant encountered by the Spanish conquerors. They found Peyote firmly estab-

suggested that the Peyote cult is far older. He showed that a symbol employed in the Tarahumara Indian Peyote ceremony appeared in ancient ritualistic carvings preserved in Mesoamerican lava rocks. More recently, archaeological discoveries in dry caves and rock shelters in Texas have yielded specimens of Peyote. These specimens, found in a context suggesting ceremonial use, indi-

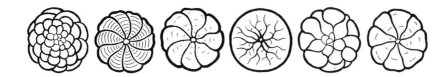

cate that its use is more than seven thousand years old.

The earliest European records concerning this sacred cactus are those of Sahagún, who lived from 1499 to 1590 and who dedicated most of his adult life to the Indians of Mexico. His precise, firsthand observations were not published until the nineteenth century. Consequently, credit for the earliest published account must go to Juan Cardenas, whose observations on the marvelous secrets of the Indies were published as early as 1591.

Sahagún's writings are among the most important of all the early chroniclers. He described Peyote use among the Chichimeca, of the primitive desert plateau of the north, recording for posterity: "There is another herb like tunas [*Opuntia* spp.] of the earth. It is called peiotl. It is white. It is found in the north country. Those who eat or drink it see visions either frightful or laughable. This intoxication lasts two or three days and then ceases. It is a common food of the Chichimeca, for it sustains them and gives them courage to fight and not feel fear nor hunger nor thirst. And they say that it protects them from all danger."

It is not known whether or not the Chichimeca were the first Indians to discover the psychoactive properties of Peyote. Some students believe that the Tarahumara Indians, living where Peyote grew, were the first to discover its use and that it spread from them to the Cora, the Huichol, and other tribes. Since the plant grows in many scattered localities in Mexico, it seems probable that its intoxicating properties were independently discovered by a number of tribes.

Several seventeenth-century Spanish Jesuits testified that the Mexican Indians used Peyote medicinally and ceremonially for many ills and that when intoxicated with the cactus they saw "horrible visions." Padre Andréa Pérez de Ribas, a seventeenth-century Jesuit who spent sixteen years in Sinaloa, reported that Peyote was usually drunk but that its use, even medicinally, was

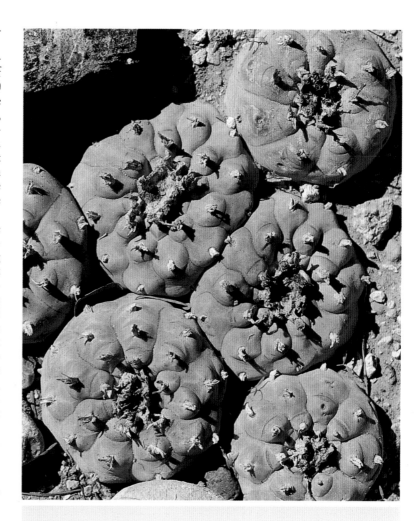

The Chemistry of Peyote

The active principle of *Lophophora williamsii,* the first hallucinogenic plant to be chemically analyzed, was already identified at the end of the nineteenth century as a crystallized alkaloid (see page 23). Because the dried cacti from which the alkaloid was extracted are called mescal buttons, it was named mescaline. In addition to mescaline, responsible for the visual hallucinogenic effects, several related alkaloids have been isolated from Peyote and related cacti.

When the chemical structure of mescaline was determined, it could be produced synthetically. The chemistry is relatively simple: 3,4,5,-trimethoxy-phenylethylamine. The model of this structure is shown on page 186.

Mescaline is chemically related to the neurotransmitter noradrenaline (norepinephrine), a brain hormone, also shown here. The active dose of mescaline is 0.5–0.8 gram when applied orally.

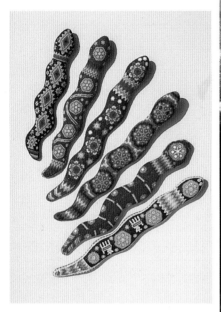

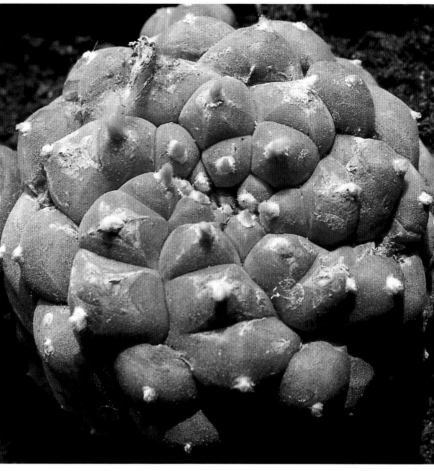

Left: Following visions received during the Peyote ritual, the Huichol bring beaded "Peyote snakes" decorated with designs of the Peyote to remote mountain shrines of Earth Mother as an offering of gratitude.

Right: An old and very large Peyote cactus that is addressed as "Grandfather" by the Indians. Notice the young crowns.

forbidden and punished, since it was connected with "heathen rituals and superstitions" to contact evil spirits through "diabolic fantasies."

The first full description of the living cactus was offered by Dr. Francisco Hernández, who as personal physician of King Philip II of Spain was sent to study Aztec medicine. In his ethnobotanical study of New Spain, Dr. Hernández described *peyotl,* as the plant was called in the Nahuatl language of the Aztecs: "The root is of nearly medium size, sending forth no branches or leaves above the ground, but with a certain woolliness adhering to it on account of which it could not aptly be figured by me. Both men and women are said to be harmed by it. It appears to be of a sweetish taste and moderately hot. Ground up and applied to painful joints, it is said to give relief. Wonderful properties are attributed to this root, if any faith can be given to what is commonly said among them on this point. It causes those devouring it to be able to foresee and to predict things . . ."

In the latter part of the seventeenth century, a Spanish missionary in Nayarit recorded the earliest account of a Peyote ritual. Of the Cora tribe, he reported: "Close to the musician was seated the leader of the singing, whose business it was to mark time. Each had his assistants to take his place when he should become fatigued. Nearby was placed a tray filled with Peyote, which is a diabolical root that is ground up and drunk by them so that they may not become weakened by the exhausting effects of so long a function, which they begin by forming as large a circle of men and women as could occupy the space that had been swept off for this purpose. One after the other, they went dancing in a ring or marking time with their feet, keeping in the middle the musician and choir-master whom they invited, and singing in the same unmusical tune that he set them. They would dance all night, from five o'clock in the evening to seven o'clock in the morning, without stopping nor leaving the circle. When the dance was ended, all stood who could hold themselves on their feet; for the majority, from the Peyote and wine which they

> "In consciousness dwells the wondrous,
> with it man attains the realm beyond the material,
> and the Peyote tells us,
> where to find it."
>
> —Antonin Artaud, *The Tarahumars* (1947)

drank, were unable to utilize their legs."

The ceremony among the Cora, Huichol, and Tarahumara Indians has probably changed little in content over the centuries: it still consists, in great part, of dancing.

The modern Huichol Peyote ritual is the closest to the pre-Columbian Mexican ceremonies. Sahagún's description of the Teochichimeca ritual could very well be a description of the contemporary Huichol ceremony, for these Indians still assemble together in the desert three hundred miles northeast of their homeland in the Sierra Madres of western Mexico, still sing all night, all day, still weep exceedingly, and still so esteem Peyote above any other psychotropic plant that the sacred mushrooms, Morning Glories, *Datura,* and other indigenous hallucinogens are consigned to the realm of sorcerers.

Most of the early records in Mexico were left by missionaries who opposed the use of Peyote in religious practice. To them Peyote had no place in Christianity because of its pagan associations. Since the Spanish ecclesiastics were intolerant of any cult but their own, fierce persecution resulted. But the Indians were reluctant to give up their Peyote cults established on centuries of tradition.

The suppression of Peyote, however, went to great lengths. For example, a

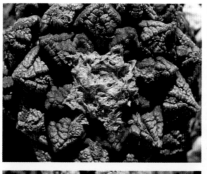
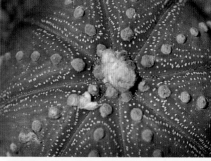
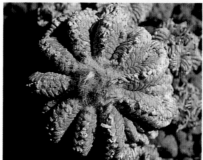
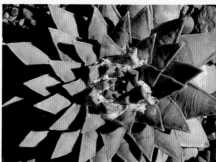

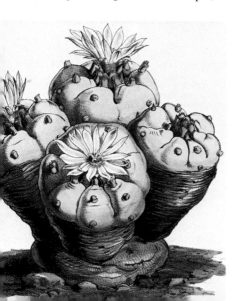

priest near San Antonio, Texas, published a manual in 1760 containing questions to be asked of converts. Included were the following: "Have you eaten the flesh of man? Have you eaten Peyote?" Another priest, Padre Nicolas de Leon, similarly examined potential converts: "Art thou a soothsayer? Dost thou foretell events by reading omens, interpreting dreams or by tracing circles and figures on water? Dost thou garnish with flower garlands the places where idols are kept? Dost thou suck the blood of others? Dost thou wander about at night, calling upon demons to help thee? Hast thou drunk Peyote or given it to others to drink, in order to discover secrets or to discover where stolen or lost articles were?"

During the last decade of the nineteenth century, the explorer Carl Lumholtz observed the use of Peyote among the Indians of the Sierra Madre Occidental of Mexico, primarily the Huichol and Tarahumara, and he reported on the Peyote ceremony and on various kinds of cacti employed with *Lophophora williamsii* or in its stead.

Above: Different cacti that are known in Mexico as Peyote, Hikuli, Peyotillo, or False Peyote. They primarily contain the substance mescaline and other psychoactive alkaloids.
Above left: Ariocarpus retusus
Above right: Astrophyton asterias
Below left: Aztekium riterii
Below right: Ariocarpus fissuratus

Left: The earliest known botanical illustration of *Lophophora williamsii,* published in 1847. It has been found in archaeological sites more than seven thousand years of age. It was probably the first and most spectacular vision-inducing plant encountered by the Spanish conquerors of Mexico.

> "You see how it is when we walk for the Peyote.
> How we go, not eating, not drinking, with much will.
> All of one heart. How one goes being Huichol.
> That is our unity. That is what we must defend."
> —Ramón Medina Silva

Left: In Huichol geography, Wirikuta, the place of the ancestor-gods, is the locality of the origin of the sacred life of the tribe. Peyote grows here and is collected on the annual pilgrimages made by small groups of devout Huichols. The trip to Wirikuta is long and arduous, with the pilgrims traveling as Ancient Ones. Like the gods, they refrain from food, sex, and sleep during this extraordinary trip. When they first enter the domain of their Paradise, the *mara'akame* Ramón Medina Silva gestures toward Kaukayari (power spots) that once were the living forms of the gods.

However, no anthropologist ever participated in or observed a Peyote hunt until the 1960s, when anthropologists and a Mexican writer were permitted by Huichols to accompany several pilgrimages. Once a year, the Huichols make a sacred trip to gather Hikuri, as the sacred cactus is called. The trek is led by an experienced *mara'akame* or shaman, who is in contact with Tatewari (Our grandfather-fire). Tatewari is the oldest Huichol god, also known as Hikuri, the Peyote-god. He is personified with Peyote plants on his hands and feet, and he interprets all the deities to the modern shamans, often through visions, sometimes indirectly through

food taken for the stay in Wirikuta is corn tortillas. The pilgrims, however, eat Peyote while in Wirikuta. They must travel great distances. Today, much of the trek is done by car, but formerly the Indians walked some two hundred miles.

The preparation for gathering Peyote involves ritual confession and purification. Public recitation of all sexual encounters must be made, but no show of shame, resentment, or jealousy, nor any expression of hostility, occurs. For each offense, the shaman makes a knot in a string that, at the end of the ritual, is burned. Following the confession, the group, preparing to set out for Wirikuta—

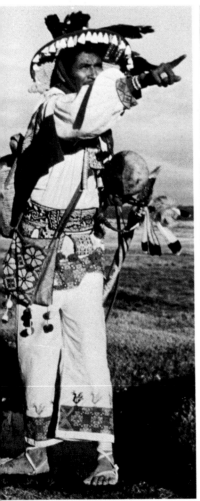

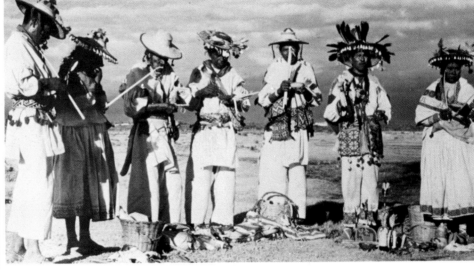

Kauyumari (the Sacred Deer Person and culture hero). Tatewari led the first Peyote pilgrimage far from the present area inhabited by the nine thousand Huichols into Wirikuta, an ancestral region where Peyote abounds. Guided by the shaman, the participants, usually ten to fifteen in number, take on the identity of deified ancestors as they follow Tatewari "to find their life."

The Peyote hunt is literally a hunt. Pilgrims carry Tobacco gourds, a necessity for the journey's ritual. Water gourds are often taken to transport water back home from Wirikuta. Often the only

an area located in San Luís Potosí—must be cleansed before journeying to paradise.

Upon arriving within sight of the sacred mountains of Wirikuta, the pilgrims are ritually washed and pray for rain and fertility. Amid the praying and chanting of the shaman, the dangerous crossing into the Otherworld begins. This passage has two stages: first, the Gateway of the Clashing Clouds, and second, the opening of the Clouds. These do not represent actual localities but exist only in the "geography of the mind"; to the participants the passing

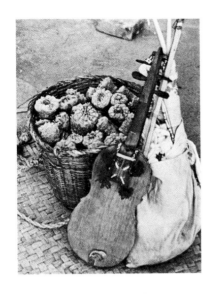

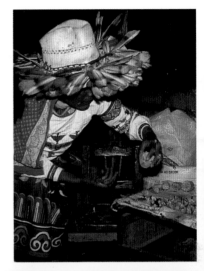

Right: A Peyote hunter spreads out his harvest at home.

Left: The baskets carried to Wirikuta contain only a few personal and ceremonial objects. On the return trip they are filled with the Peyote buttons collected on the pilgrimage. The Huichol say that Peyote is "very delicate," so the heavily laden baskets are carefully transported back to the Sierras in order to avoid bruising the cactus. Leaning against the basket is a Huichol violin, used to provide music for the Peyote dancing.

Below right: Huichol Indians returning from a pilgrimage.

Below left: A Peyote hunter with a basketful of Peyote cacti.

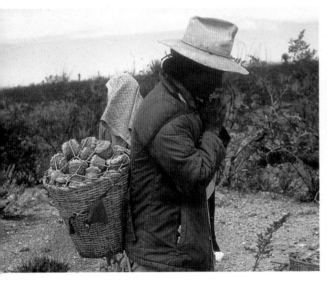

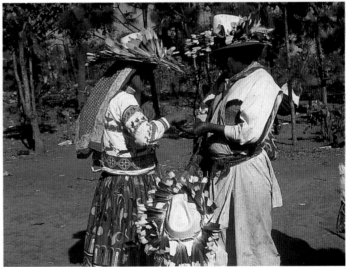

from one to the other is an event filled with emotion.

Upon arrival at the place where the Peyote is to be hunted, the shaman begins ceremonial practices, telling stories from the ancient Peyote tradition and invoking protection for the events to come. Those on their first pilgrimage are blindfolded, and the participants are led by the shaman to the "cosmic threshold," which only he can see. All celebrants stop, light candles, and murmur prayers, while the shaman, imbued with supernatural forces, chants.

Finally, Peyote is found. The shaman has seen the deer tracks. He draws his arrow and shoots the cactus. The pilgrims make offerings to this first Hikuri. More Peyote is sought, basketfuls of the plant eventually being collected. On the following day, more Peyote is collected, some of which is to be shared with those who remain at home. The rest is to be sold to the Cora and Tarahumara Indians, who use Peyote but do not have a quest.

The ceremony of distributing Tobacco is then carried out. Arrows are placed pointing to the four points of the compass; at midnight a fire is built.

Page 148 right: Each pilgrim has brought offerings to Peyote. After these gifts are carefully displayed, the pilgrims raise candles in the direction of the ascending sun. They weep and pray that the gods accept their offering, while Ramón (second from right) fervently chants.

Right: A Huichol sacrificial bowl decorated with Peyote designs.

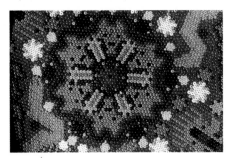

According to the Huichol, Tobacco belongs to fire.

The shaman prays, placing the offering of Tobacco before the fire, touching it with feathers, then distributing it to each pilgrim, who puts it into his gourd, symbolizing the birth of Tobacco.

The Huichol Peyote hunt is seen as a return to Wirikuta or Paradise, the archetypal beginning and end of a mythical

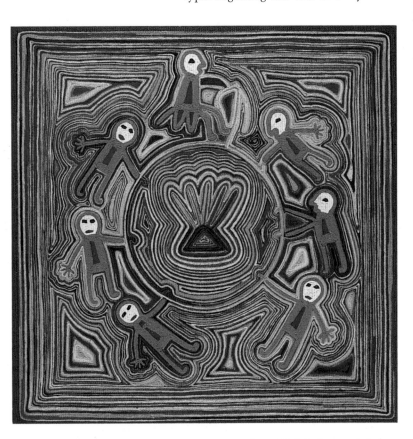

Above: "It is one, it is a unity; it is ourselves." These words of Huichol *mara'akame* Ramón Medina Silva describe the mystical rapport unfolding among communicants in the Peyote ceremonies that is such an important dimension in the lives of these people. In this yarn painting, six *peyoteros* and the shaman (on top) achieve that unity in a field of fire. In the center of the *peyoteros* is Tatewari, the First Shaman, as a five-plumed fire.

past. A modern Huichol *mara'akame* expressed it as follows: "One day all will be as you have seen it there, in Wirikuta. The First People will come back. The fields will be pure and crystalline, all this is not clear to me, but in five more years I will know it, through more revelations. The world will end, and the unity will be here again. But only for pure Huichol."

Among the Tarahumara, the Peyote

cult is less important. Many buy their supplies of the cactus, usually from Huichol. Although the two tribes live several hundred miles apart and are not closely related, they share the same name for Peyote—Hikuri—and the two cults have many points of resemblance.

The Tarahumara Peyote dance may be held at any time during the year for health, tribal prosperity, or for simple worship. It is sometimes incorporated into other established festivals. The principal part of the ceremony consists of dances and prayers followed by a day of feasting. It is held in a cleared area, neatly swept. Oak and pine logs are dragged in for a fire and oriented in an east-west direction. The Tarahumara name for the dance means "moving about the fire," and except for Peyote itself, the fire is the most important element.

The leader has several women assistants who prepare the Hikuri plants for use, grinding the fresh cacti on a metate, being careful not to lose one drop of the resulting liquid. An assistant catches all liquid in a gourd, even the water used to wash the metate. The leader sits west of the fire, and a cross may be erected opposite him. In front of the leader, a small hole is dug into which he may spit. A Peyote may be set before him on its side or inserted into a root-shaped hole bored in the ground. He inverts half a gourd over the Peyote, turning it to scratch a circle in the earth around the cactus. Removing the gourd temporarily, he draws a cross in the dust to represent the world, thereupon replacing the gourd. This apparatus serves as a resonator for the rasping stick: Peyote is set under the resonator, since it enjoys the sound.

Incense from burning copal is then offered to the cross. After facing east, kneeling, and crossing themselves, the leader's assistants are given deer-hoof rattles or bells to shake during the dance.

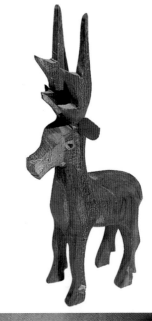

The ground-up Peyote is kept in a pot or crock near the cross and is served in a gourd by an assistant: he makes three rounds of the fire if carrying the gourd to the leader, one if carrying it to an ordinary participant. All the songs praise Peyote for its protection of the tribe and for its "beautiful intoxication."

Healing ceremonies are often carried out like the Huichol's.

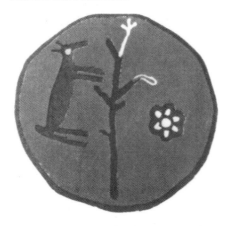

The Tarahumara leader cures at daybreak. The first terminates dancing by giving three raps. He rises, accompanied by a young assistant, and, circling the patio, he touches every forehead with water. He touches the patient thrice, and placing his stick to the patient's head, he raps three times. The dust produced by the rapping, even though infinitesimal, is a powerful health- and life-giver and is saved for medicinal use.

The final ritual sends Peyote home. The leader reaches toward the rising sun and raps thrice. "In the early morning, Hikuli had come from San Ignacio and from Satapolio riding on beautiful green doves, to feast with the Tarahumara at the end of the dance when the people sacrifice food and eat and drink. Having bestowed his blessings, Hikuli forms himself into a ball and flies to his shelter at the time."

Peyote is employed as a religious sacrament among more than forty American Indian tribes in many parts of the United States and western Canada. Because of its wide use, Peyote early attracted the attention of scientists and legislators and engendered heated and, unfortunately, often irresponsible opposition to its free use in American Indian ceremonies.

It was the Kiowa and Comanche Indians, apparently, who in visits to a native group in northern Mexico first learned of this sacred American plant. Indians in the United States had been restricted to reservations by the last half

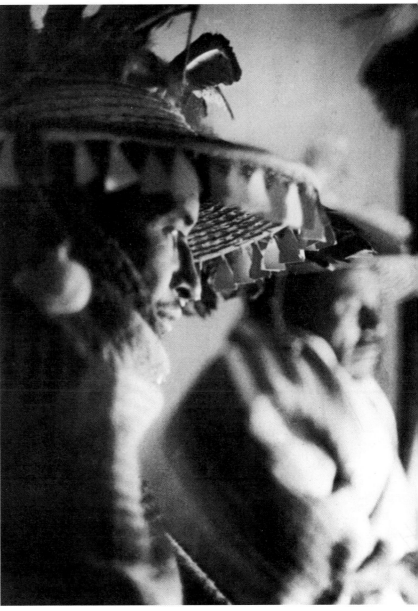

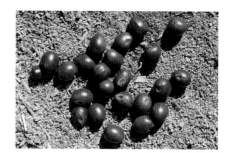

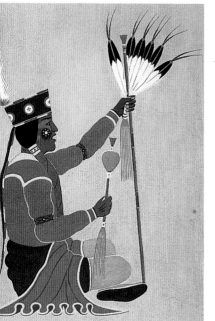

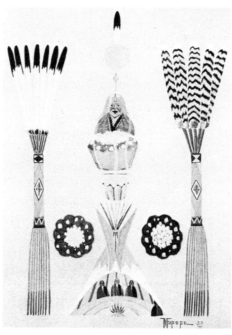

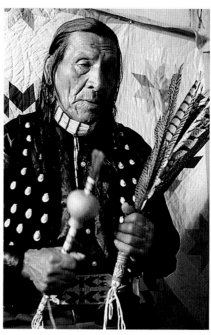

Above left: The roadman in the Native American Church officiates at the Peyote meeting as a representative of the Great Spirit. It is his duty to show the "Peyote road" to the participants. The roadman in Stephen Mopope's painting holds traditional ceremonial objects associated with the religion: the fan, staff, and rattle. On his cheek is painted the crown of a Peyote plant. In the center picture, also by Mopope, chanting participants sit inside the sacred tepee, in the middle of which is Father Fire and the crescent moon altar. Above the tepee is the Peyote water drum. The photograph on the far right depicts the Sioux medicine man Henry Crow Dog chanting at a Peyote meeting on the Rosebud Reservation.

Above middle: Also by Mopope. This shows the participant who sits singing in the interior of his sacred tipi. In the middle is Father Fire and the sickle shaped altar. Above the tipi is the water container.

Above right: Sioux Medicine Man Henry Crow Dog at a Peyote Gathering on the Rosebud reservation.

of the nineteenth century, and much of their cultural heritage was disintegrating and disappearing. Faced with this disastrous inevitability, a number of Indian leaders, especially from tribes relocated in Oklahoma, began actively to spread a new kind of Peyote cult adapted to the needs of the more advanced Indian groups of the United States.

The Kiowa and Comanche were apparently the most active proponents of the new religion. Today it is the Kiowa-Comanche type of Peyote ceremony that, with slight modifications, prevails north of the Mexican border. This ceremony, to judge from the rapid spread of the new Peyote religion, must have appealed strongly to the Plains tribes and later to other groups.

Success in spreading the new Peyote cult resulted in strong opposition to its practice from missionary and local governmental groups. The ferocity of this opposition often led local governments to enact repressive legislation, in spite of overwhelming scientific opinion that Indians should be permitted to use Peyote in religious practices. In an attempt to protect their rights to free reli-

gious activity, American Indians organized the Peyote cult into a legally recognized religious group, the Native American Church. This religious movement, unknown in the United States before 1885, numbered 13,300 members in 1922. In 1993 there were at least 300,000 members among seventy different tribes.

Indians of the United States, living far from the natural area of Peyote, must use the dried top of the cactus, the so-called mescal button, legally acquired by either collection or purchase and distribution through the U.S. postal services. Some American Indians still send pilgrims to gather the cactus in the fields, following the custom of Mexican Indians, but most tribal groups in the United States must procure their supplies by purchase and mail.

A member may hold a meeting in gratitude for the recovery of health, the safe return from a voyage, or the success of a Peyote pilgrimage; it may be held to celebrate the birth of a baby, to name a child, on the first four birthdays of a child, for doctoring, or even for general thanksgiving.

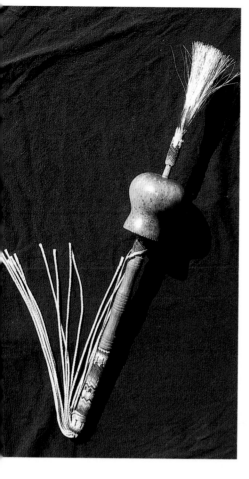

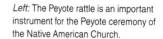

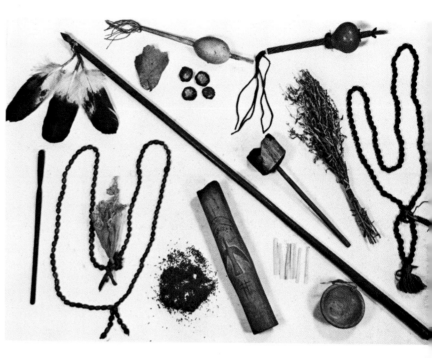

The Kickapoo hold a Peyote service for the dead, and the body of the deceased is brought into the ceremonial tepee. The Kiowa may have five services at Easter, four at Christmas and Thanksgiving, six at the New Year. Especially among the Kiowa, meetings are held only on Saturday night. Anyone who is a member of the Peyote cult may be a leader or "roadman." There are certain taboos that the roadman, and sometimes all participants, must observe. The older men refrain from eating salt the day before and after a meeting, and they may not bathe for several days following a Peyote service. There seem to be no sexual taboos, as in the Mexican tribes, and the ceremony is free of licentiousness. Women are admitted to meetings to eat Peyote and to pray, but they do not usually participate in the singing and drumming. After the age of ten, children may attend meetings, but do not take part until they are adults.

Peyote ceremonies differ from tribe to tribe. The typical Plains Indian service takes place usually in a tepee erected over a carefully made altar of earth or clay; the tepee is taken down as soon as the all-night ceremony is over. Some tribes hold the ceremony in a wooden round-house with a permanent altar of cement inside, and the Osage and Quapaw Indians often have electrically lighted round-houses.

The Father Peyote (a large "mescal button" or dried top of the Peyote plant) is placed on a cross or rosette of sage leaves at the center of the altar. This crescent-shaped altar, symbol of the spirit of Peyote, is never taken from the altar during the ceremony. As soon as the Father Peyote has been put in place, all talking stops, and all eyes are directed toward the altar.

Tobacco and corn shucks or blackjack oak leaves are passed around the circle of worshipers, each making a cigarette for use during the leader's opening prayer.

The next procedure involves purification of the bag of mescal buttons in cedar incense. Following this blessing, the roadman takes four mescal buttons from the bag, which is then passed around in a clockwise direction, each worshiper taking four. More Peyote

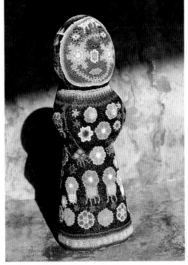

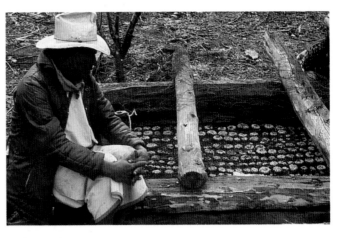

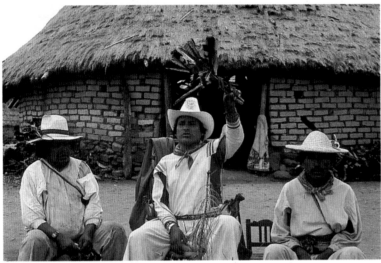

Above: A Huichol shaman *(mara'akame)* sings with his assistants in front of the temple in which the Peyote ceremony will take place.

Page 155 top: The ground Peyote is mixed with water and given to the participants at the intoxicating ceremony.

may be called for at any time during the ceremony, the amount consumed being left to personal discretion. Some peyotists eat up to thirty-six buttons a night, and some boast of having ingested upwards of fifty. An average amount is probably about twelve.

Singing starts with the roadman, the initial song always being the same, sung or chanted in a high nasal tone. Translated, the song means: "May the gods bless me, help me, and give me power and understanding."

Sometimes, the roadman may be asked to treat a patient. This procedure varies in form. The curing ritual is almost always simple, consisting of praying and frequent use of the sign of the cross.

Peyote eaten in ceremony has assumed the role of a sacrament in part because of its biological activity: the sense of well-being that it induces and the psychological effects (the chief of which is the kaleidoscopic play of richly colored visions) often experienced by those who indulge in its use. Peyote is considered sacred by Native Americans, a divine "messenger" enabling the individual to communicate with God without the medium of a priest. It is an earthly representative of God to many peyotists. "God told the Delawares to do good even before He sent Christ to the whites who killed Him . . .," an Indian explained to an anthropologist. "God made Peyote. It is His power. It is the power of Jesus. Jesus came afterwards on this earth, after Peyote . . . God (through Peyote) told the Delawares the same things that Jesus told the whites."

Correlated with its use as a religious sacrament is its presumed value as a medicine. Some Indians claim that if Peyote is used correctly, all other medicines are superfluous. Its supposed curative properties are responsible probably more than any other attribute for the rapid diffusion of the Peyote cult in the United States.

The Peyote religion is a medico-religious cult. In considering Native American medicines, one must always

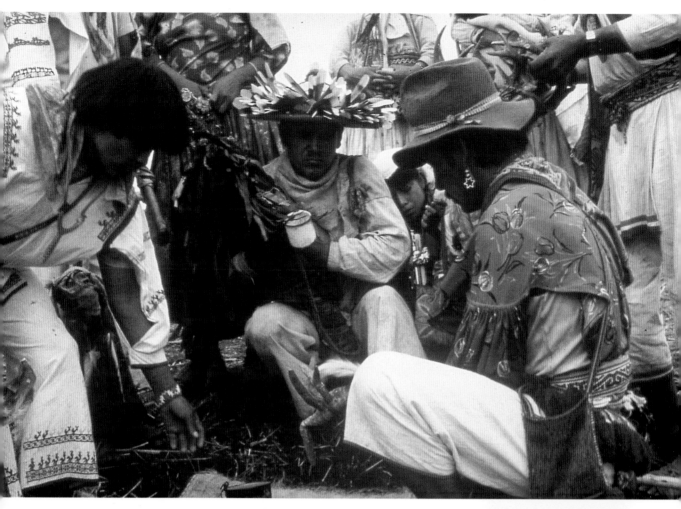

bear in mind the difference between the aboriginal concept of a medicinal agent and that of our modern Western medicine. Indigenous societies, in general, cannot conceive of natural death or illness but believe that they are due to supernatural interference. There are two types of "medicines": those with purely physical effects (that is, to relieve toothache or digestive upsets); and the medicines, *par excellence,* that put the medicine man into communication, through a variety of visions, with the malevolent spirits that cause illness and death.

The factors responsible for the rapid growth and tenacity of the Peyote religion in the United States are many and interrelated. Among the most obvious, however, and those most often cited, are: the ease of legally obtaining supplies of the hallucinogen; lack of federal restraint; cessation of intertribal warfare; reservation life with consequent intermarriage and peaceful exchange of social and religious ideas; ease of transportation and postal communication; and the general attitude of resignation toward encroaching Western culture.

In the year 1995 the use of peyote by members of the Native American Church was made legal by Bill Clinton!

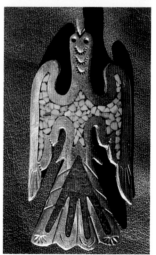

Above: A modern Peyote bird of the Navajo.

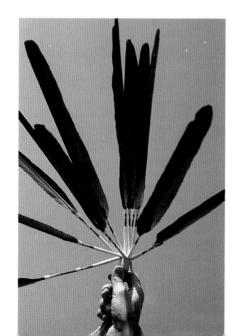

Left: A Peyote fan (Navajo) made from peacock feathers is used by the Indians to induce visions.

LITTLE FLOWERS OF THE GODS

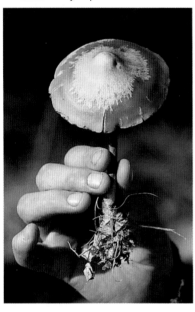

Above: One of the largest fruiting bodies of *Psilocybe azurescens* ever found.

"There is a world beyond ours, a world that is far away, nearby, and invisible. And there is where God lives, where the dead live, the spirits and the saints, a world where everything has already happened and everything is known. That world talks. It has a language of its own. I report what it says. The sacred mushroom takes me by the hand and brings me to the world where everything is known. It is they, the sacred mushrooms, that speak in a way I can understand. I ask them and they answer me. When I return from the trip that I have taken with them, I tell what they have told me and what they have shown me."

Thus does the famous Mazatec shaman María Sabina reverently describe the god-given powers of the intoxicating mushrooms that she uses in her ceremony, which has come down from ages past.

Few plants of the gods have ever been held in greater reverence than the sacred mushrooms of Mexico. So hallowed were these fungi that the Aztecs called them Teonanácatl ("divine flesh") and used them only in the most holy of their ceremonies. Even though, as fungi, mushrooms do not blossom, the Aztecs referred to them as "flower," and the Indians who still use them in religious rituals have endearing terms for them, such as "little flowers."

When the Spaniards conquered Mexico, they were aghast to find the natives worshiping their deities with the help of inebriating plants: Peyotl, Ololiuqui, Teonanácatl. The mushrooms were es-pecially offensive to the European ecclesiastical authorities, and they set out to eradicate their use in religious practices.

"They possessed another method of intoxication, which sharpened their cruelty; for if they used certain small toadstools ... they would see a thousand visions and especially snakes ... They called these mushrooms in their language *teunamacatlth,* which means 'God's flesh,' or of the Devil whom they worshiped, and in this wise with that bitter victual by their cruel God were they houseled."

In 1656, a guide for missionaries argued against Indian idolatries, including mushroom ingestion, and recommended their extirpation. Not only do reports condemn Teonanácatl, but actual illustrations also denounce it. One depicts the devil enticing an Indian to eat the fungus; another has the devil performing a dance upon a mushroom.

"But before explaining this [idolatry]," one of the clerics said, "I wish to explain the nature of the said mushrooms [that] were small and yellowish, and to collect them the priests and old men, appointed as ministers for these impostures, went to the hills and remained almost the whole night in sermonizing and in superstitious praying. At dawn, when a certain little breeze which they know begins to blow, they would gather them, attributing to them deity. When they are eaten or drunk, they intoxicate, depriving those who partake of them of their senses and making them believe a thousand absurdities."

1. *Psilocybe mexicana*
2. *Psilocybe semperviva*
3. *Psilocybe yungensis*
4. *Psilocybe caerulescens* var. *mazatecorum*
5. *Psilocybe caerulescens* var. *nigripes*

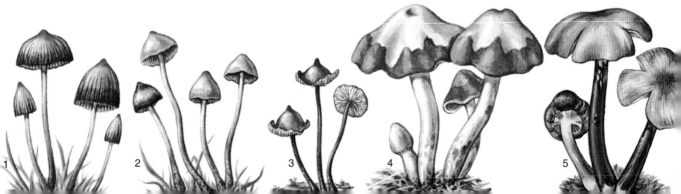

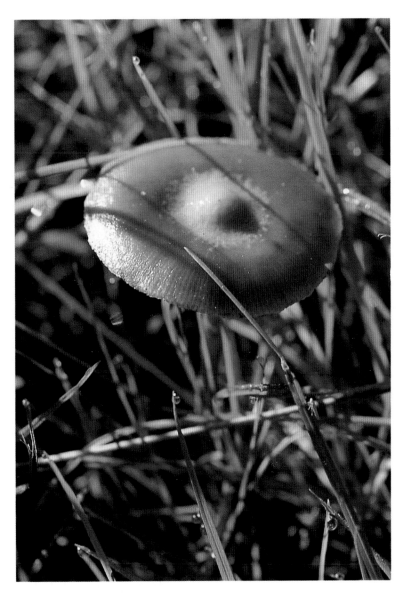

Dr. Francisco Hernández, personal physician to the king of Spain, wrote that three kinds of intoxicating mushrooms were worshiped. After describing a lethal species, he stated that "others when eaten cause not death but madness that on occasion is lasting, of which the symptom is a kind of uncontrolled laughter. Usually called *teyhuintli*, these are deep yellow, acrid and of a not displeasing freshness. There are others again which, without inducing laughter, bring before the eyes all kinds of visions, such as wars and the likeness of demons. Yet others are there not less desired by princes for their fiestas and banquets, of great price. With night-long vigils are they sought, awesome and terrifying. This kind is tawny and somewhat acrid."

For four centuries nothing was known of the mushroom cult; and it was even doubted that mushrooms were used hallucinogenically in ceremony. The Church fathers had done such a successful job of driving the cult into hiding through persecution that no anthropologist or botanist had ever uncovered the religious use of these mushrooms until this century.

In 1916 an American botanist finally proposed a "solution" to the identification of Teonanácatl, concluding that Teonanácatl and the Peyote were the same drug. Motivated by distrust of the chroniclers and Indians, he intimated that the natives, to protect Peyote, were indicating mushrooms to the authorities. He argued that the dried, brownish, disklike crown of Peyote resembles a

6. *Psilocybe cubensis*
7. *Psilocybe wassonii*
8. *Psilocybe hoogshagenii*
9. *Psilocybe siligineoides*
10. *Panaeolus sphinctrinus*

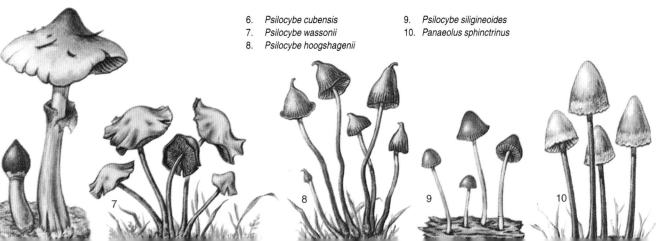

Below: In Europe and North America there are countless modern artifacts that reflect the contemporary mushroom cult.

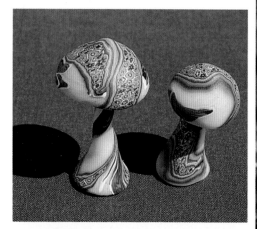

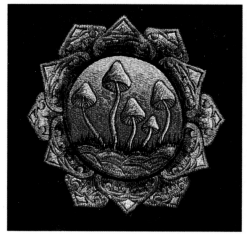

Above: Mushrooms with psychoactive properties are found around the world. In many places T-shirts with mushroom motifs are available for the traveling mushroom lover. Embroidery from Kathmandu, Nepal.

Above right: The *Psilocybe pelliculosa* is a relatively weak moderately active mushroom from the Pacific North West.

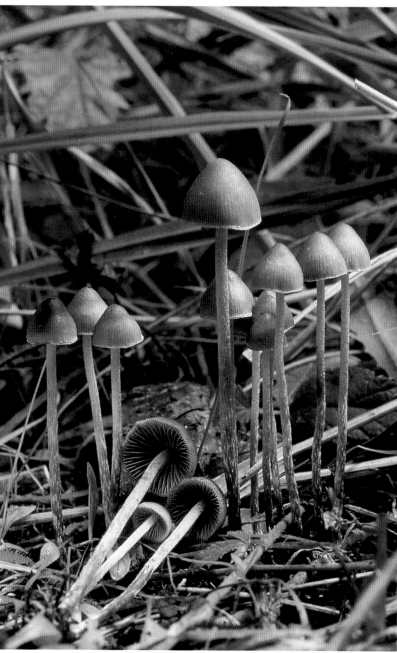

dried mushroom—so remarkably that it will even deceive a mycologist. It was not until the 1930s that an understanding of the role of hallucinogenic mushrooms in Mexico and a knowledge of their botanical identification and chemical composition started to become available. In the late 1930s the first two of the many species of sacred Mexican mushrooms were collected and associated with a modern mushroom ceremony. Subsequent field research has resulted in the discovery of some two dozen species. The most important belong to the genus *Psilocybe,* twelve of which have been reported, not including *Stropharia cubensis,* sometimes considered a *Psilocybe.* The most important species appear to be *Psilocybe mexicana, P. cubensis,* and *P. caerulescens.*

These various mushrooms are now known to be employed in divinatory and religious rites among the Mazatec, Chinantec, Chatino, Mixe, Zapotec, and Mixtec of Oaxaca; the Nahua and possibly the Otomi of Puebla; and the Tarascans of Michoacan. The present center of intensive use of the sacred mushrooms is among the Mazatec.

Mushrooms vary in abundance from year to year and at different seasons. There may be years when one or more species are rare or absent—they vary in their distribution and are not ubi-

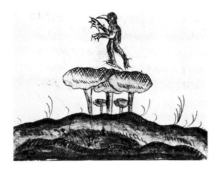

quitous. Furthermore, each shaman has his own favorite mushrooms and may forgo others; María Sabina, for example, will not use *Psilocybe cubensis.* And certain mushrooms are used for specific purposes. This means that each ethnobotanical expedition may not expect to find the same assortment of species employed at one time, even in the same locality and by the same people.

Chemical studies have indicated that psilocybine and, to a lesser extent, psilocine are present in many of the species of the several genera associated with the Mexican ceremony. In fact, these compounds have been isolated from many species of *Psilocybe* and other genera in widely separated parts of the world, although the evidence available suggests that only in Mexico are psilocybine-containing mushrooms at present utilized in native ceremonies.

The modern mushroom ceremony is an all-night seance that may include a curing ritual. Chants accompany the main part of the ceremony. The intoxication is characterized by fantastically colored visions in kaleidoscopic movement and sometimes by auditory hallucinations, and the partaker loses himself in unearthly flights of fancy.

The mushrooms are collected in the forests at the time of the new moon by a virgin girl, then taken to a church to remain briefly on the altar. They are never sold in the marketplace. The Mazatec call the mushrooms Nti-si-tho, in which "Nti" is a particle of reverence and endearment; the rest of the name means "that which springs forth." A Mazatec explained this thought poetically: "The little mushroom comes of itself, no one knows whence, like the wind that comes we know not whence nor why."

The male or female shaman chants for hours, with frequent clapping or percussive slaps on the thighs in rhythm with the chant. María Sabina's chanting, which has been recorded, studied, and translated, in great part proclaims humbly her qualifications to cure and to interpret divine power through the mush-

The Chemistry of Teonanácatl

Teonanácatl, the sacred mushrooms of Mexico, owe their hallucinogenic effects to two alkaloids known as psilocybine and psilocine.

The main component, psilocybine, is the phosphoric acid ester of psilocine, which occurs usually only in trace elements. Psilocybine and psilocine, being tryptamine derivatives, belong to the class of indole alkaloids. Their crystals are shown on page 23; their chemical structure on page 186. The chemical relationship of these hallucinogens to the physiological compound serotonine is especially significant. Serotonine, the molecular model of which is shown on page 187, is a neurotransmitter and, therefore, important in the biochemistry of psychic functions. Both psilocybine and psilocine can be produced synthetically. The active dose in man is 6–12 mg. Twenty to 30 mg induce strong visions.

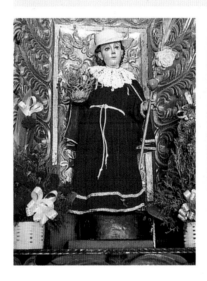

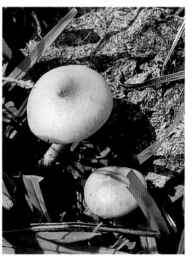

rooms. Excerpts from her chant, all in the beautiful tonal Mazatec language, give an idea of her many "qualifications."

"Woman who thunders am I, woman who sounds am I.
Spiderwoman am I, hummingbird woman am I . . .
Eagle woman am I, important eagle woman am I.
Whirling woman of the whirlwind am I, woman of a sacred, enchanted place am I,
Woman of the shooting stars am I."

R. Gordon Wasson, the first non-Indian fully to witness the Mazatec

Above left: In Mexico an unusual saint named El Niño is worshiped in the Catholic Church. The Mexican Indians understand him as an embodiment of the sacred mushroom, which they also call Niño. (Altar in San Cristóbal de Las Casas, Chiapas)

Above right: The tropical Magic Mushroom *Psilocybe cubensis (Stropharia cubensis)* was first gathered in Cuba and mycologically ascertained. It grows in all tropical zones, preferring cow manure.

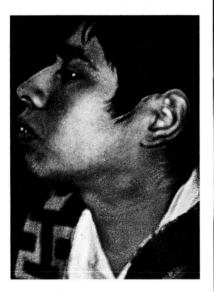

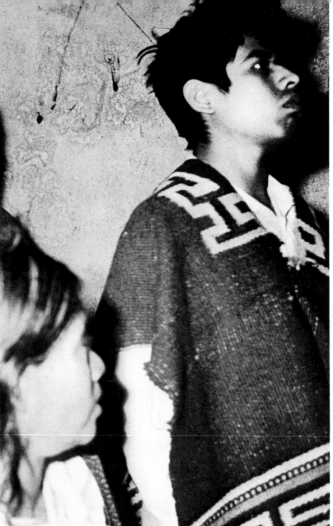

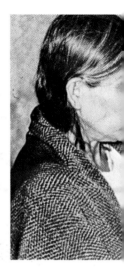

In 1958, the famous Mazatec shaman María Sabina performed a *Velada* (night vigil) on behalf of a seventeen-year-old youth, Pefecto José Garcia, who was seriously ill.

Left to right: Pefecto awaits the commencement of the *Velada*.

Pefecto stands up at the beginning of the ceremony, and María Sabina turns her head to gaze at him.

The shaman has incensed pairs of sacred mushrooms and hands Pefecto the intoxicating plant for ingestion.

Pefecto has heard the unfavorable diagnosis, which María Sabina has learned through the help of the mushrooms—that there is no hope for his recovery. He collapses in terror and despair.

The shaman and her daughter, adverse diagnosis notwithstanding, continue to chant, hoping for more insight—even though she has learned that Pefecto's soul has been irrevocably lost.

ceremony, wrote the following understanding thoughts about this use of the mushrooms:

"Here let me say a word about the nature of the psychic disturbance that the eating of the mushroom causes. This disturbance is wholly different from the effect of alcohol, as different as night from day. We are entering upon a discussion in which the vocabulary of the English language, of any European language, is seriously deficient.

"There are no apt words in it to characterize one's state when one is, shall we say, 'bemushroomed.' For hundreds, even thousands, of years, we have thought about these things in terms of alcohol, and we now have to break the bounds imposed on us by our alcoholic obsession. We are all, willy-nilly, confined within the prison walls of our everyday vocabulary. With skill in our choice of words, we may stretch accepted meanings to cover slightly new feelings and thoughts, but when a state of mind is utterly distinct, wholly novel, then all our old words fail. How do you

tell a man who has been born blind what seeing is like? In the present case this is an especially apt analogy, because superficially the bemushroomed man shows a few of the objective symptoms of one who is intoxicated, drunk. Now virtually all the words describing the state of drunkenness, from 'intoxicated' (which literally means 'poisoned') through the scores of current vulgarisms, are contemptuous, belittling, pejorative. How curious it is that modern civilized man finds surcease from care in a drug for which he seems to have no respect! If we use by analogy the terms suitable for alcohol, we prejudice the mushroom, and since there are few among us who have been bemushroomed, there is danger that the experience will not be fairly judged. What we need is a vocabulary to describe all the modalities of a divine inebriant . . ."

Upon receiving six pairs of mushrooms in the ceremony, Wasson ate them. He experienced the sensation of his soul being removed from his body and floating in space. He saw "geometric

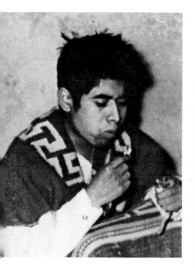
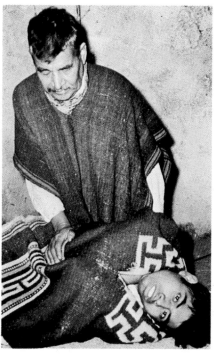
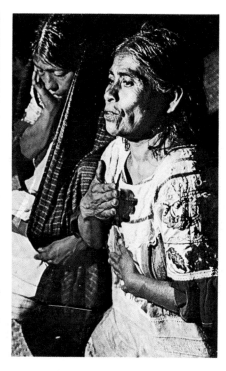

patterns, angular, in richest colors, which grew into architectural structures, the stonework in brilliant colors, gold and onyx and ebony, extending beyond the reach of sight, in vistas measureless to man. The architectural visions seemed to be oriented, seemed to belong to the ... architecture described by the visionaries of the Bible." In the faint moonlight, "the bouquet on the table assumed the dimensions and shape of an imperial conveyance, a triumphant car, drawn by ... creatures known only to mythology."

Mushrooms have apparently been ceremonially employed in Mesoamerica for many centuries. Several early sources have suggested that Mayan languages in Guatemala had mushrooms named for the underworld. Miniature mushroom stones, 2,200 years of age, have been found in archaeological sites near Guatemala City, and it has been postulated that stone mushroom effigies buried with a Mayan dignitary suggested a connection with the Nine Lords of the Xibalba, described in the sacred book

Popol Vuh. Actually, more than two hundred mushroom stone effigies have been discovered, the oldest dating from the first millennium B.C. Although the majority are Guatemalan, some have been unearthed in El Salvador and Honduras and others as far north as Veracruz and Guerrero in Mexico. It is now clear that whatever the use of these "mushroom stones," they indicate the great antiquity of a sophisticated sacred use of hallucinogenic mushrooms.

A superb statue of Xochipilli, Aztec Prince of Flowers, from the early sixteenth century, was recently discovered on the slopes of the volcano Mt. Popocatepetl (see illustration, p. 62). His face is in ecstasy, as though seeing visions in an intoxication; his head is slightly tilted, as though hearing voices. His body is engraved with stylized flowers that have been identified as sacred, most of them inebriating, plants. The pedestal on which he sits is decorated with a design representing cross-sections of the caps of *Psilocybe aztecorum*, a hallucinogenic mushroom known only from

"The *niños santos (Psilocybe mexicana)* heal. They lower fevers, cure colds, and give freedom from toothaches. They pull the evil spirits out of the body or free the spirit of the sick."

—María Sabina

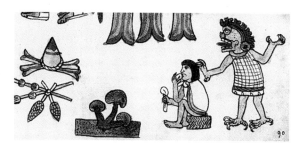

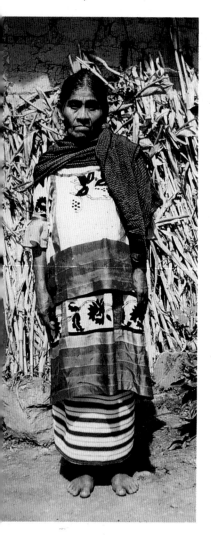

Above: Albert Hofmann visited the shaman María Sabina in 1962 and took many portraits of her.

Page 163: The sincerity and absolute faith in the revelatory power of the mushrooms is evident in these photographs of María Sabina, who, during the nightlong chanting and clapping ceremony, feels herself fully in contact with the other world, which the mushrooms have allowed her to visit.

this volcano. Thus Xochipilli undoubtedly represents not simply the Prince of Flowers but more specifically the Prince of Inebriating Flowers, including the mushrooms that, in Nahuatl poetry, were called "flowers" and "flowers that intoxicate."

Have psilocybine-containing mushrooms ever been employed as magicoreligious hallucinogens in the New World? The answer is probably yes.

A species of *Psilocybe* and possibly also *Panaeolus* are used today near the classic Maya ceremonial center of Palenque, and hallucinogenic mushrooms have been reported in use along the border between Chiapas in Mexico and Guatemala. Whether these modern mushroom practices in the Maya region represent vestiges of former use or have been recently introduced from Oaxaca it is not possible as yet to say.

Nevertheless, evidence is now accumulating to indicate that a mushroom cult flourished in prehistoric times—from 100 B.C. to about A.D. 300–400 in northwestern Mexico: in Colima, Jalisco, and Nayarit. Funerary effigies, with two "horns" protruding from the head, are believed to represent male and female "deities" or priests associated with mushrooms. Traditions among contemporary Huichol Indians in Jalisco also suggest the former religious use of these fungi "in ancient times."

What about South America, where these psychoactive mushrooms abound? There is no evidence of such use today, but indications of their apparent former employment are many. The Yurimagua Indians of the Peruvian Amazon were reported in the late seventeenth and early eighteenth centuries to be drinking a potently inebriating beverage made from a "tree fungus." The Jesuit report stated that the Indians "mix mushrooms that grow on fallen trees with a kind of reddish film that is found usually attached to rotting trunks. This film is very hot to the taste. No person who drinks this brew fails to fall under its effects after three draughts of it, since it is so strong, or more correctly, so toxic." It has been suggested that the tree mushroom might have been the psychoactive *Psilocybe yungensis,* which occurs in this region.

In Colombia, many anthropomorphic gold pectorals with two domelike ornaments on the head have been found. They are in the so-called Darien style, and the majority of them have been unearthed in the Sinú area of northwestern Colombia and in the Calima region on the Pacific coast. For lack of a better term, they have been called "telephone-bell gods," since the hollow semispherical ornaments resemble the bells of old-fashioned telephones. It has been suggested that they represent mushroom effigies. The discovery of similar artifacts in Panama and Costa Rica and one in Yucatán might be interpreted to suggest a prehistoric continuum of a sacred mushroom cult from Mexico to South America.

Farther to the south in South America, there is archaeological evidence that may suggest the religious importance of mushrooms. Moche effigy stirrup vessels from Peru, for example, have mushroomlike cephalic ornaments.

While the archaeological evidence is convincing, the almost complete lack of reference in colonial literature to such use of mushrooms, and the absence of any known modern hallucinogenic use of mushrooms among aboriginal groups of South America, gives cause for caution in the interpretation of what otherwise might easily be interpreted as ancient mushroom effigies from south of Panama. If, however, it becomes evident that the various archaeological artifacts from South America mentioned above do represent hallucinogenic mushrooms, then the area for their significance in America will be greatly amplified.

"I take the 'little one who springs up out of the earth'
(Psilocybe caerulescens) and I see God.
I see him springing up
out of the earth."
—María Sabina

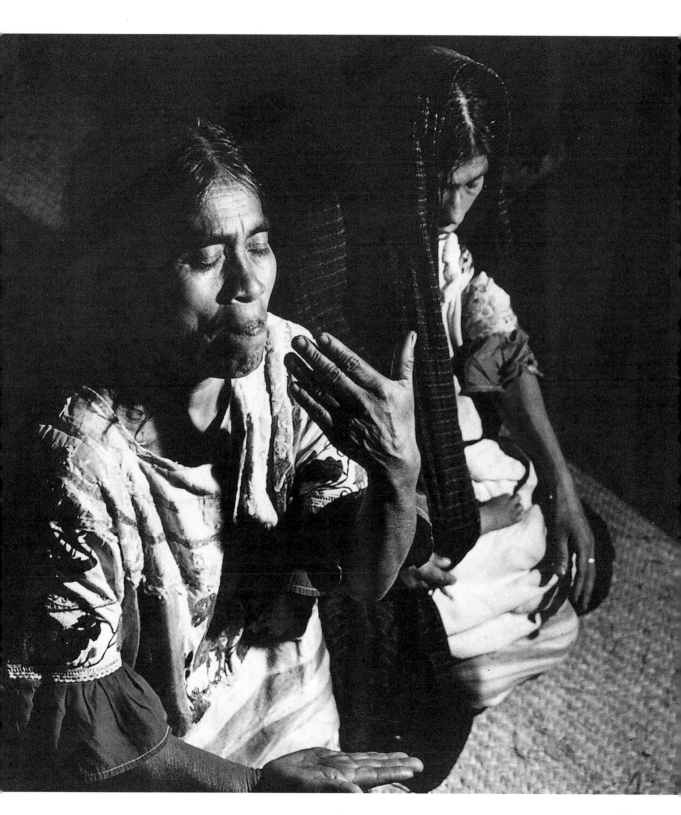

DIVINER'S SAGE

Right: Salvia divinorum is easy to recognize by its square stem.

Below: A paste made of the fresh leaves of Salvia divinorum is chewed slowly.

Closely associated with the Indian mushroom cults is the use of another psychoactive plant, Hierba de la Pastora *(Salvia divinorum)*. It is not entirely clear if it was used in the pre-Spanish times. It is possible that it was the Pipiltzintzintli of the Aztecs.

The male or female shamans of the Mazatecs of Oaxaca use *Salvia divinorum,* which is also known as *hoja de la*

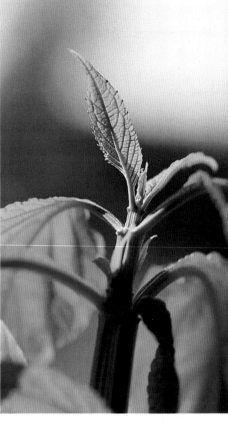

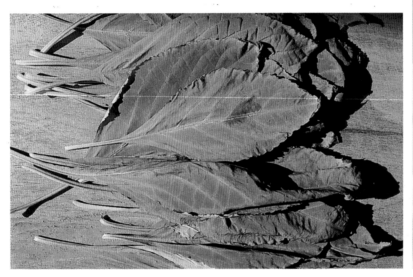

Page 165 top left: Painted nettle is used by the Mazatecs as a replacement for Salvia divinorum.

Page 165 top right: Coleus pumilus is considered by the Mazatecs to be related to Salvia divinorum.

Page 165 middle: Salvia divinorum in the Mexican rain forest.

pastora (leaf of the shepherd) or *pastora,* in rituals associated with divination or healing, generally as a substitute for the otherwise preferred psychoactive mushrooms. María Sabina remarked: "When I am in the time that there are no mushrooms and want to heal someone who is sick, then I must fall back on the leaves of *pastora.* When you grind them up and eat them, they work just like the *niños.* But, of course, *pastora* has nowhere near as much power as the mushrooms."

The ritual use is remarkably similar to the use of mushrooms. *Salvinia divinorum* rituals take place at night in complete darkness and stillness. Either the healer is alone with the patient or there are also other patients and possibly some healthy participants present. Before the shaman chews and sucks on the leaves, they are held over some

burning Copal incense, and some prayers are said to consecrate the leaves. After chewing the leaves, the participants lie down and remain as still and silent as possible. Salvia rituals last barely longer than one to two hours, as the effects of the leaves last a significantly shorter time than those of mushrooms. If the visions are strong enough, the healer finds the cause of the illness, or some other problem. He or she gives the patient appropriate advice and ends the meeting.

Salvia divinorum, which is also known as Aztec sage, is native to the Mazatec areas of the Sierra Madre Oriental in the Mexican state of Oaxaca. It grows naturally in tropical rain forests in an altitude of three hundred to eighteen hundred meters. *Salvia divinorum,* because of its limited geographic habitat, belongs to the rarest of psychoactive

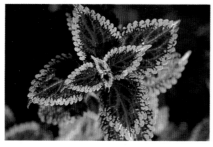

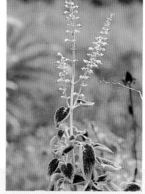

plants, but is cultivated by plant lovers all over the world. This reproduction is achieved with cuttings.

The Mazatecs take thirteen pairs of fresh leaves (twenty-six leaves altogether) and twist them into a kind of cigar or chaw, which is put into the mouth and sucked or chewed. The juice is not swallowed, but the active ingredients are absorbed through the mucous membranes in the side of the mouth. For one of these cigars, it takes at least six fresh leaves, but one can use eight or ten leaves for a stronger effect. The effects with the chewing method begin in almost exactly ten minutes and last approximately forty-five minutes.

The dried leaves can also be smoked. With this method, half of a fairly large leaf (two or three deep inhalations) induces a strong psychoactive reaction. Generally, one or two leaves are smoked.

Most people who have smoked, chewed, or taken a tincture of *Salvia divinorum* report very bizarre, unusual psychoactive effects, which are not very comparable with euphoric or psychedelic substances. There is often perceived to be a "bending" of space; and a feeling of swaying or out-of-body experiences is also typical.

In the traditional taxonomy of the Mazatecs, *Salvia divinorum* is related to two forms of labiates. Salvia is known as the "mother" *(la hembra), Coleus pumilus* is considered to be the "father" *(el macho),* and *Coleus blumei* is known as *el nene* (the child) and *el ahiajado,* the godchild. The fresh leaves are used just as those of *Salvia divinorum*—that is, they are chewed like chewing tobacco. This connection gives the Coleus the reputation of being psychoactive plants.

What Was Pipiltzintzintli?

The ancient Aztecs knew and used a plant called *Pipiltzintzintli* (the purest little prince) very similarly to the use of *Psilocybe mexicana* in entheogenic rituals. There are masculine and feminine forms of this plant, *macho* and *hembra*. In the National Archives in Mexico City, there are Inquisition files from the years 1696, 1698, and 1706 that mention Pipiltzintzin and hint at its intoxicating effects. Various authors have taken this to be *Salvia divinorum*.

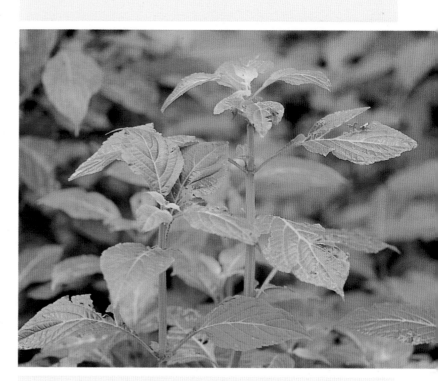

The Chemistry of *Salvia divinorum*

The leaves contain the neocerodan-diterpenes salvinorin A and salvinorin B (also known as divinorin A and divinorin B), as well as two other, similar substances that have not yet been precisely identified. The main ingredient is salvinorin A (chemical formula: $C_{23}H_{28}O_8$), which has extreme consciousness-altering effects with amounts as small as 150–500mg. Salvinorin is not an alkaloid. It was first described by Ortega et al. by the name of salvinorin (1982). Later, Valdes et al. described it under the name of divinorin A (1984). The neurochemistry of salvinorin is still an unsolved puzzle. The ingredients have not bound to any receptors in any receptor tests (the NovaScreen method). The plant also contains loliolid.

CACTUS OF THE FOUR WINDS

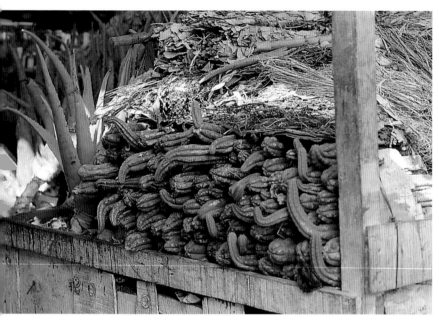

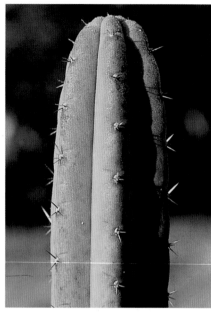

Above left: Pieces of San Pedro piled up for sale in the "witches' market" in Chiclayo in northern Peru.

Above right: The fast-growing San Pedro cactus develops few, if any, thorns when cultivated.

"San Pedro has a special symbolism in *curanderismo* [folk healing] for a reason: San Pedro is always in tune with . . . the powers of animals, of strong personages or beings, of serious beings, of beings that have supernatural power. . ."

The San Pedro cactus, *Trichocereus pachanoi,* represents undoubtedly one of the most ancient of the magic plants of South America. The oldest archaeological evidence, a Chavín stone carving in a temple in northern Peru, goes back to 1300 B.C. Almost equally old textiles from Chavín depict the cactus with jaguar and hummingbird figures. Peruvian ceramics made between 1000 and 700 B.C. show the plant in association with the deer; and others, several hundred years later, have the cactus with the jaguar and stylized spirals illustrating the hallucinogenic experiences induced by the plant. On the southern coast of Peru, large ceramic urns of the Nazca culture, dated 100 B.C.–A.D. 500, depict San Pedro.

The use of *Trichocereus* was widespread in Peru when the Spanish arrived. One ecclesiastical report said that shamans "drink a beverage they call Achuma which is a water they make from the sap of some thick and smooth cacti . . ." and "as it is very strong, after they drink it they remain without judgment and deprived of their senses, and they see visions that the devil represents to them . . ." As with Peyote in Mexico, the Roman Church fought against the San Pedro cactus: "This is the plant with which the devil deceived the Indians . . . in their paganism, using it for their lies and superstitions . . . those who drink lose consciousness and remain as if dead; and it has even been seen that some have died because of the great frigidity to the brain. Transported by the drink, the Indians dreamed a thousand absurdities and believed them as if they were true . . ."

The modern use of the San Pedro cactus, along the coastal regions of Peru and in the Andes of Peru and Bolivia, has been greatly affected by Christian influence—influences even in the name applied to the plant, originating possibly in the Christian belief that St. Peter holds the keys to heaven. But the overall context of the moon-oriented ritual surrounding its use indicates that it is truly an amalgan of pagan and Christian elements.

San Pedro is now employed to cure sickness, including alcoholism and in-

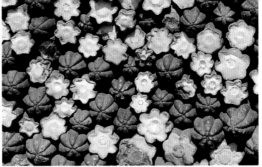

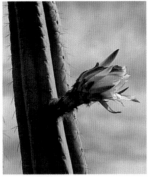

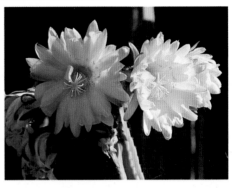

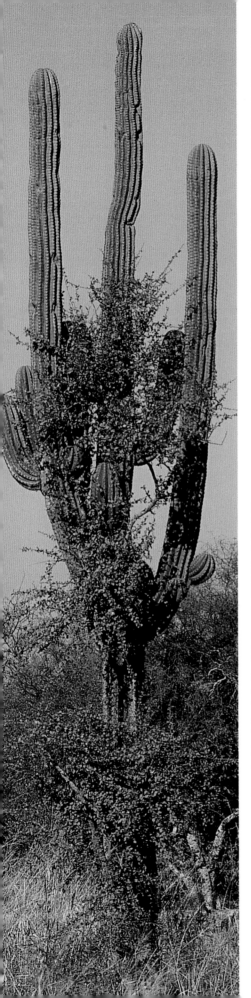

The Chemistry of San Pedro

Trichocereus contains as its main alkaloid mescaline, responsible for the visual hallucinogenic effects. From dried specimens of San Pedro, 2 percent mescaline has been isolated. In addition, hordenine has also been detected.

sanity, for divination, to undo love witchcraft, to counter all kinds of sorcery, and to ensure success in personal ventures. It is only one—but the principal one—of many "magical" plants known to and used by shamans and collected near sacred lagoons high in the Andes.

At these lagoons, shamans go annually for purification and to visit special individuals, experts in sorcery and "owners" of divine plants capable of awaking, with San Pedro, supernatural spiritual powers. Even the sick exert themselves to make pilgrimages to these remote holy places. It is thought that the penitent may undergo a metamorphosis in these lagoons and that the plants, especially San Pedro, from these areas possess extraordinarily powerful properties to cure illness and to influence witchcraft.

Shamans specify four "kinds" of the cactus, distinguished by the number of ribs: those with four ribs are rare and considered to be the most potent, with very special supernatural powers, since the four ribs represent the "four winds" and the "four roads."

The cactus is known in northern coastal Peru as San Pedro, in the northern

Top: The San Pedro cactus (*Trichocereus pachanoi*).

Above left: The flowers of San Pedro remain closed during the daytime.

Above right: In the early evening the large flowers of the San Pedro blossom in sumptuous splendor.

Far left: A species from the *Trichocereus* genus that has not yet been botanically categorized. It grows in northwestern Argentina, where it is also called San Pedro and used psycho-actively.

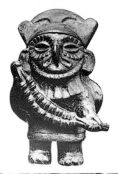

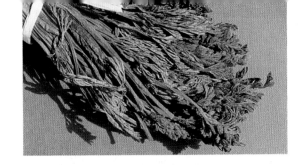

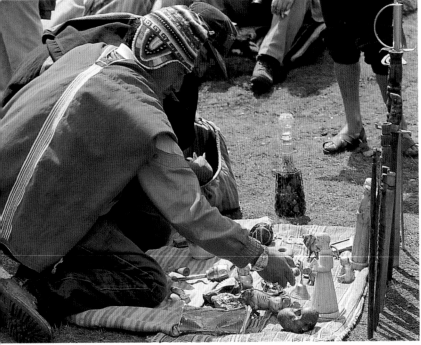

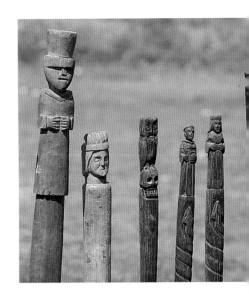

Top left: A ceramic pot from the Chimú culture, A.D. 1200. The owl-faced female depicted on this vessel is probably an herbalist and shaman; she holds Huachuma *(Trichocereus)*. Even today in native markets, the women who sell the hallucinogenic cactus are usually both herbalists and shamans, and according to native beliefs, the owl is associated with these women.

Top right: There are many herbs called "conduro" that belong to different genera (for example, *Lycopodium*) and are traditionally used as ingredients in the San Pedro drink.

Middle: A north Peruvian *curandero* (healer) sets up his "mesa" for the San Pedro ritual on the banks of Shimbe Lake.

Below right: The mesa is surrounded by magical staves. They are either from pre-Columbian graves or modern replicas made from the Amazonian Chonta Palm.

Andean area as Huachuma, and in Bolivia as Achuma; the Bolivian term *chumarse* ("to get drunk") is derived from Achuma. Aguacolla and Gigantón are its Ecuadorean names.

The stems of the cactus, normally purchased in the market, are sliced like bread and boiled for up to seven hours in water. After the drinking of San Pedro, other medicinal herbs, the help of which is frequently sought, begin to talk to the shaman, activating his own "inner power." San Pedro may be taken alone, but often other plants, separately boiled, are added and the drink is then called Cimora. Among the numerous plant additives employed are the Andean cactus *Neoraimondia macrostibas*, a species of the amaranthaceous *Iresine*, the euphorbiaceous *Pedilanthus tithymaloides*, and *Isotoma longiflora* of the Campanulaceae. All of these plants, except *Iresine*, may have biodynamic principles. *Iresine* has the reputation of curing "insanity." *Brugmansia aurea* and *B. sanguinea*, two potent hallucinogens in their own right, are frequently added.

Only in recent years has San Pedro been correctly identified. In early chemical and psychiatric studies in Peru, the cactus was misidentified as *Opuntia cylindrica*. Only recently have studies indicated the great significance of the vegetal additives, an investigation that deserves more attention. On occasion, magic demands that other additives be employed; powdered bones and cemetery dust are commonly used to ensure the effectiveness of the brew. As one observer has stated: San Pedro is "the catalyst that activates all the complex forces at work in a folk healing session, especially the visionary and divinatory powers" of the shaman, who can make himself the owner of another man's identity. But the magic of San Pedro goes far beyond curing and divination, for it is believed to guard houses like a dog, whistling in an unearthly fashion and forcing intruders to flee in terror.

The principal effects of *Trichocereus pachanoi* have been described by a shaman: "... the drug first produces ... drowsiness or a dreamy state and a feeling of lethargy ... a slight dizziness ... then a great 'vision,' a clearing of all the faculties ... It produces a light numb-

168

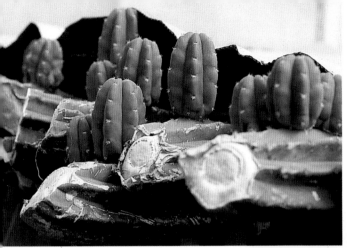

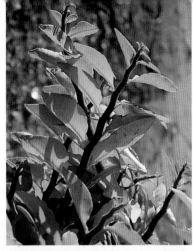

ness in the body and afterward a tranquillity. And then comes detachment, a type of visual force ... inclusive of all the senses ... including the sixth sense, the telepathic sense of transmitting oneself across time and matter ... like a kind of removal of one's thought to a distant dimension."

"Four-ribbed cacti ... are considered to be very rare and very lucky ... to have special properties
because they correspond
to the 'four winds' and the 'four roads,'
supernatural powers associated with the cardinal points ..."
—Douglas Sharon

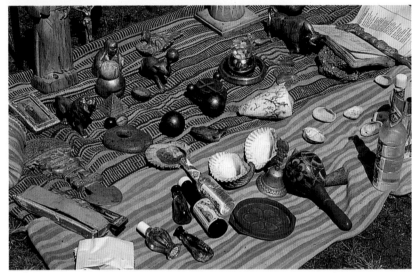

During the ritual, participants are "set free from matter" and engage in flight through cosmic regions. It was probably shamans who used the San Pedro cactus that a Spanish officer in Cuzco, Peru, described in the sixteenth century: "Among the Indians, there was another class of wizards, permitted by the Incas to a certain degree, who are like sorcerers. They take the form they want and go a long distance through the air in a short time; and they see what is happening, they speak with the devil, who answers them in certain stones or in other things that they venerate ..." Ecstatic magical flight is still characteristic of the contemporary San Pedro ceremony: "San Pedro is an aid which one uses to render the spirit more pleasant, more manageable ... One is transported across time, matter, and distance in a rapid and safe fashion ..."

The shaman may take the drug himself or give it only to the patient, or both may take it. The aim of this shamanic curing ritual is to make the patient "bloom" during the night ceremony, to make his subconscious "open like a flower," even like the night-blooming *Trichocereus* itself. Patients sometimes are contemplative and calm, sometimes break into dancing or even throw themselves writhing on the ground.

As with so many other hallucinogens, here is a plant given by the gods to man to help him experience an ecstasy—separation of the soul from the body—"in a very tenuous, simple fashion and almost instantaneously." This ecstasy provides preparations for the sacred flight that enables man to experience mediation between his mortal existence and the supernatural forces—an activity establishing direct contact through this plant of the gods.

Top left: Harvested and stored pieces of San Pedro continue living and often begin growing again after months, even years.

Top right: The Wolf's Milk plant *(Pedilanthus tithymaloides)* is sometimes added to the San Pedro drink in order to strengthen its effects. Sometimes is has been said that *Pedilanthus* is hallucinogenic, but this has not been proved.

Above: The view of the mesa gives a clear impression of the syncretic cosmology of the modern healer. Gods and deities from different cultures lay next to snail shells, archaeological objects, and perfume bottles.

VINES OF THE SERPENT

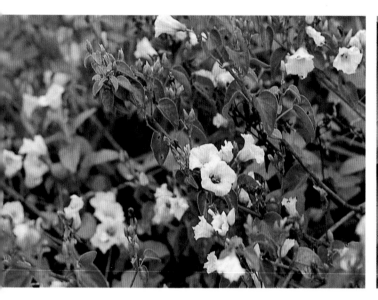

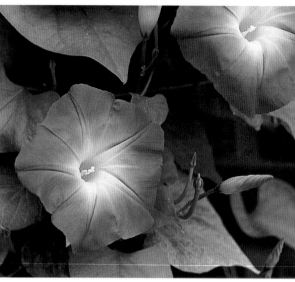

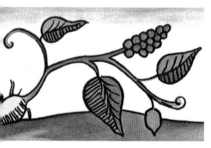

Top left: The Ololiuqui vine *Turbina corymbosa.*

Top right: Flying Saucers are a favorite cultivated strain of the enchanting Morning Glory, *Ipomoea violacea.*

Above: An early painting of Ololiuqui from Sahagún's *Historia de las Cosas de Nueva España,* written in the second half of the sixteenth century, clearly depicts the plant as a Morning Glory.

Four centuries ago, a Spanish missionary in Mexico wrote: "Ololiuqui . . . deprives all who use it of their reason . . . The natives communicate in this way with the devil, for they usually talk when they become intoxicated with Ololiuqui, and they are deceived by various hallucinations which they attribute to the deity which they say resides in the seeds . . ."

A recent report indicates that Ololiuqui has not lost its association with the deity in Oaxaca: "Throughout these references we see two cultures in a duel to death [the Spanish and the Indians] [with] the tenacity and wiles of the Indians defending their cherished Ololiuqui. The Indians seem to have won out. Today in almost all the villages of Oaxaca one finds the seeds still serving the natives as an ever present help in time of trouble." As with the sacred mushrooms, the use of the hallucinogenic Morning Glories, so significant in the life of pre-Hispanic Mexico, hid in the hinterlands until the present century.

A Spanish report written shortly after the Conquest stated that the Aztecs have "an herb called *coatl-xoxo uhqui* [green snake], and it bears a seed called *Ololiuqui.*" An early drawing depicts it as a Morning Glory with congested fruits, cordate leaves, a tuberous root, and a twining habit. In 1651, the physician of the king of Spain, Francisco Hernández, identified Ololiuqui as a Morning Glory and professionally reported: "Ololiuqui, which some call Coaxihuitl or snake plant, is a twining herb with thin, green, cordate leaves; slender, green, terete stems; and long, white flowers. The seed is round and very much like coriander, whence the name [in Nahuatl, the term *Ololiuqui* means 'round thing'] of the plant. The roots are fibrous and slender. The plant is hot in the fourth degree. It cures syphilis and mitigates pain which is caused by chills. It relieves flatulency and removes tumors. If mixed with a little resin, it banishes chills and stimulates and aids in a remarkable degree in cases of dislocations, fractures, and pelvic troubles in women. The seed has some medicinal use. If pulverized or taken in a decoction or used as a poultice on the head or forehead with milk and chili, it is said to cure eye troubles. When drunk, it acts as an aphrodisiac. It has a sharp taste and is very hot. Formerly, when the priests wanted to commune with their gods and to receive a message from them, they ate this plant to induce a delirium. A thousand visions and satanic hallucinations appeared to them. In its manner of action, this plant can be compared with *Solanum maniacum* of

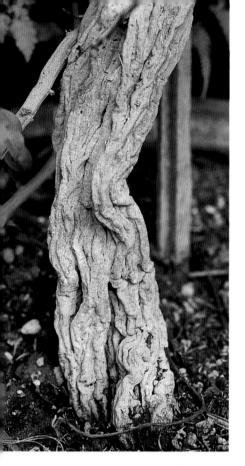

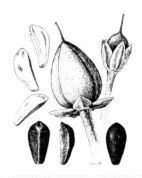

The Chemistry of the Ololiuqui

Lysergic acid alkaloids are the hallucinogenic compounds of Ololiuqui. They are indole alkaloids that have also been isolated from Ergot. Lysergic acid amide, also known as ergine, and lysergic acid hydroxyethylamide are the main components of the alkaloid mixture in Ololiuqui. Their molecular arrangement is shown on page 187. The tryptamine radical in the ring structure of lysergic acid establishes its relationship with these ergoline alkaloids as well as with the active principles of *Psilocybe* and of the brain hormone serotonine.

LSD, lysergic acid diethylamide, a semi-synthetic compound, is the most potent hallucinogen known today. It differs from lysergic acid amide only by replacement of two hydrogen atoms for two ethyl groups (p. 187). The active principle of Ololiuqui (hallucinogenic dose 2–5 mg), however, is about 100 times less potent than LSD (hallucinogenic dose 0.05 mg).

Dioscorides. It grows in warm places in the fields."

Other early references stated that "Ololiuqui is a kind of seed like the lentil . . . produced by a species of ivy . . .; when it is drunk, this seed deprives of his senses him who has taken it, for it is very powerful" and that "it will not be wrong to refrain from telling where it groes, for it matters little that this plant be here described or the Spaniards be made acquainted with it." Another writer marveled: "It is remarkable how much faith these natives have in the seed, for . . . they consult it as an oracle to learn many things . . . especially those . . . beyond the power of the human mind to penetrate . . . They consult it through one of their deceiving doctors, some of whom practice Ololiuqui drinking as a profession . . . If a doctor who does not drink Ololiuqui wishes to free a patient of some trouble, he advises the patient himself to partake . . . The doctor appoints the day and hour when the drink must be taken and establishes the reason for the patient's drinking it. Finally, the one drinking Ololiuqui . . . must seclude himself in his room . . . No one must enter during his divination . . . He . . . believes the Ololiuqui . . . is revealing what he wants to know. When the delirium is passed, the doctor comes out of seclusion reciting a thousand

Above left: The very woody trunk of the Ololiuqui vine.

Above right: The capsules and seeds of *Ipomoea violacea* are characteristic.

Below: The European bindweed *Convolvulus tricolor* also contains psychoactive alkaloids, although there is no knowledge of any traditional use.

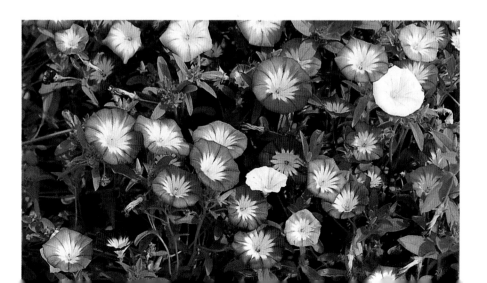

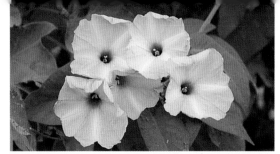

Right: In South America the bindweed *Ipomoea carnea* is used as an inebriant. It also has the psychoactive alkaloid ergotine.

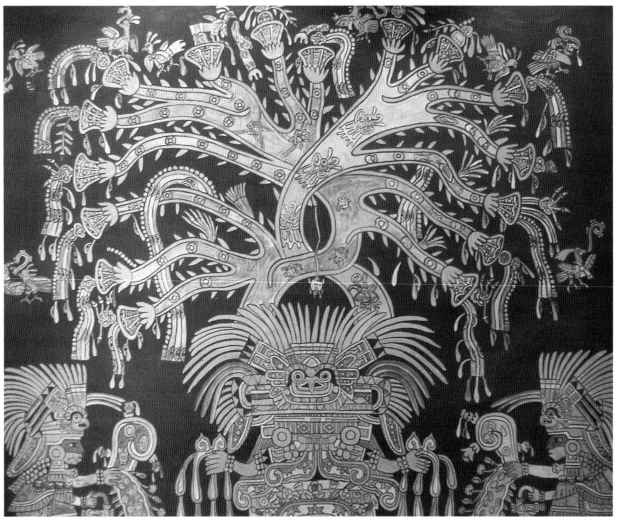

Above: An ancient Indian Mother Goddess and her priestly attendants with a highly stylized vine of Ololiuqui, in one of the murals from Teotihuacán, Mexico, dated about A. D. 500. Hallucinogenic nectar appears to flow from the blossoms of the plant, and "disembodied eyes" and birds are other stylistic features associated with hallucinogenic intoxication.

fabrications . . . thus keeping the patient deceived." The confession of an Aztec penitent illustrates the Ololiuqui association with witchcraft: "I have believed in dreams, in magic herbs, in Peyote, in Ololiuqui, in the owl . . ."

The Aztecs prepared a salve that they employed in making sacrifices: "They took poisonous insects . . . burned them and beat the ashes together with the foot of the *ocotl,* Tobacco, Ololiuqui and some live insects. They presented this diabolical mixture to their gods and rubbed their bodies with it. When thus anointed, they became fearless to every danger." Another reference asserted that "they place the mixture be-

fore their gods, saying that it is the food of the gods . . . and with it they become witch-doctors and commune with the devil."

In 1916, an American botanist suspected erroneously that Ololiuqui was a species of *Datura.* His reasons were several: *Datura;* was a well-known intoxicant; its flower resembled a Morning Glory; no psychoactive principle was known from the Morning Glory family; the symptoms of Ololiuqui intoxication resembled those caused by *Datura;* and "a knowledge of botany has been attributed to the Aztecs which they were far from possessing . . . The botanical knowledge of the early Span-

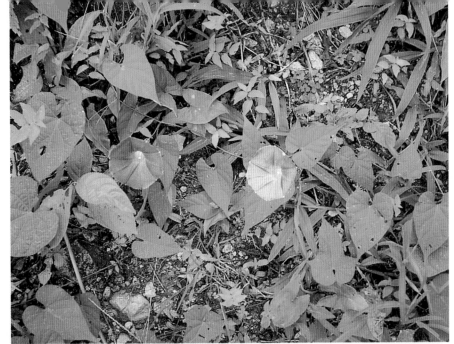

Left: The Morning Glory *Ipomoea violacea* as a wildflower in southern Mexico.

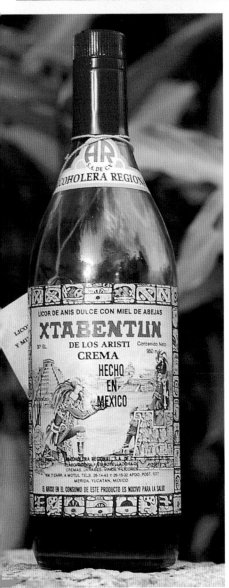

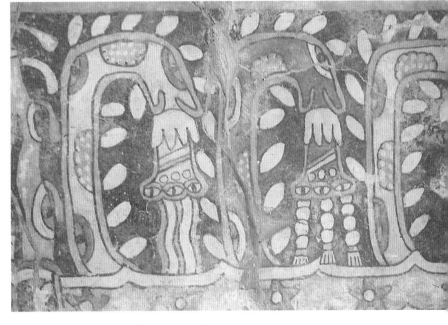

ish writers ... was perhaps not much more extensive." This misidentification was widely accepted.

Only in 1939 was identifiable material of *Turbina corymbosa* collected among the Chinantec and Zapotec of Oaxaca, where it was cultivated for hallucinogenic use. The Chinantec name *A-mu-kia* means "medicine for divination." Thirteen seeds are usually ground up and drunk with water or in an alcoholic beverage. Intoxication rapidly begins and leads to visual hallucinations. There may be an intervening stage of giddiness, followed by lassitude, euphoria, and drowsiness and a somnambulistic narcosis. The Indian may be

Above: Depiction of Morning Glories and visionary eyes on an ancient Indian wall painting in Tepantitla (Teotihuacán).

Left: Xtabentun, "the Jewel Cordial" as it is called, is made out of honey from the Ololiuqui flower.

173

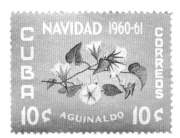

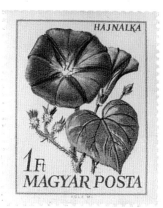

Below: A Zapotec shaman in San Bartolo Yautepec, Mexico, preparing an infusion of seeds of *Ipomoea violacea*.

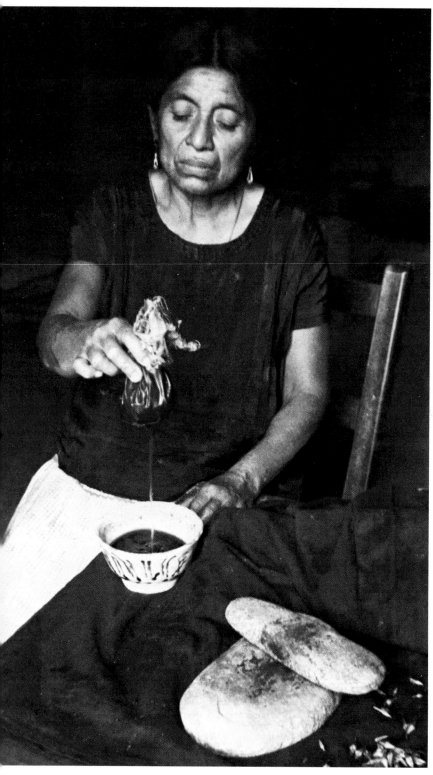

dimly aware of what is going on and is susceptible to suggestions. The visions are often grotesque, portraying people or events. The natives say that the intoxication lasts three hours and seldom has unpleasant aftereffects. Ololiuqui is taken at night and, in contrast to Peyote and the mushrooms, is administered to a single individual alone in a quiet, secluded place.

The use of seeds of *Turbina corymbosa* has been recorded for the Chinantec, Mazatec, and others in Oaxaca. They are known in Oaxaca as Piule, although each tribe has its own name for the seeds.

The name *Ololiuqui* seems to have been applied to several plants by the Aztecs, but only one was psychoactive. Of one, an early report states: "There is an herb called Ololiuqui or Xixicamatic which has leaves like miltomate [*Physalis* sp.] and thin, yellow flowers. The root is round and as large as a cabbage." This plant could not be *Turbina corymbosa*, but its identity remains a mystery. The third Ololiuqui, also called *Hueyytzontecon*, was used medicinally as a purgative, a characteristic suggesting the Morning Glory family, but the plant is not convolvulaceous.

Another Morning Glory, *Ipomoea violacea*, was valued as a sacred hallucinogen among the Aztecs, who called the seeds Tlitliltzin, from the Nahuatl term for "black" with a reverential suffix. The seeds of this Morning Glory are elongate, angular, and black, whereas those of *Turbina corymbosa* are round and brown. One ancient report mentions both, asserting that Peyote, Ololiuqui, and Tlitliltzin are all psychoactive. *Ipomoea violacea* is used especially in the Zapotec and Chatin area of Oaxaca, where it is known as Badoh Negro or, in Zapotec, Badungás. In some Zapotec villages both *Turbina corymbosa* and *Ipomoea violacea* are known; in others, only the latter is used. The black seeds are often

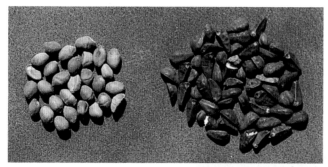

called *macho* ("male") and men take them; the brown seeds, called *hembra* ("female"), are ingested by women. The black seeds are more potent than the brown, according to the Indians, an assertion borne out by chemical studies. The dose is frequently seven or a multiple of seven; at other times, the familiar thirteen is the dose.

As with *Turbina*, Badoh Negro seeds are ground and placed in a gourd with water. The solid particles are strained out, and the liquid is drunk. Revelations of the cause of illness or divinations are provided during the intoxication by "intermediaries"—the fantastical *baduwin*, or two little girls in white who appear during the séance.

A recent report of the use of seeds of *Ipomoea violacea* among the Zapotec indicates that Badoh Negro is indeed a significant element in the life of these Indians: ". . . Divination about recovery in sickness is also practiced by means of a plant which is described as a narcotic. This plant . . . grows in the yard . . . of a family who sells its leaves and seeds . . . to administer to patients . . . The patient, who must be alone with the curer if not in a solitary place where he cannot hear even a cock's crow, falls into a sleep during which the little ones, male and female, the plant children *[bador]*, come and talk. These plant spirits will also give information about lost objects." The modern ritual with Morning Glory seeds now has incorporated Christian elements. Some of the names—Semilla de la Virgen ("seed of the Virgin") and Hierba María ("Mary's herb")—show union of the Christian with the pagan, and clearly an indication that *Turbina corymbosa* and *Ipomoea violacea* are considered gifts from the gods.

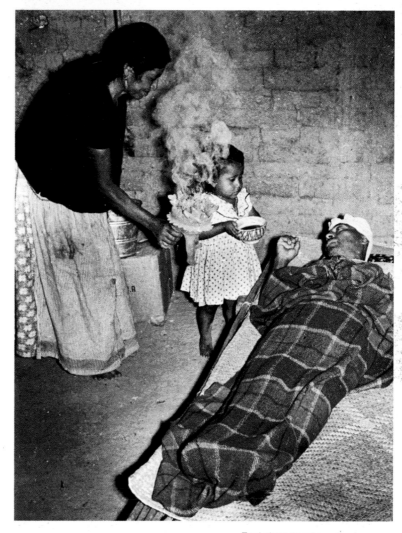

Top: Left are the ocher-colored, somewhat round seeds of *Turbina corymbosa*. On the right are the black, angular seeds of the *Ipomoea violacea*.

Above: The shaman administers the infusion to a patient, assisted by a young girl. The brew must be taken at night in a secluded and quiet place. The patient's problems will be diagnosed by the shaman from interpretation of what he says while under the influence of the plants.

175

SEMEN OF THE SUN

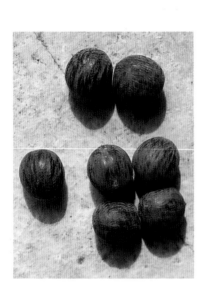

Above: The seeds of *Virola surinamensis,* called Ucuba, are used ethnomedicinally.

Below right: The most important species of *Virola* in hallucinogenic preparations is *V. theiodora,* of the northwestern Amazon. *Virola* is an American genus related to the Old World genus of the Nutmeg. The tiny flowers of *Virola* have a highly pungent fragrance.

At the beginning of time, Father Sun practiced incest with his daughter, who acquired Viho by scratching her father's penis. Thus the Tukano received this sacred snuff from the sun's semen, and since it is still hallowed, it is kept in containers called *muhipu-nuri,* or "penis of the sun." This hallucinogen enables the Tukano to consult the spirit world, especially Viho-mahse, the "snuff-person," who, from his dwelling in the Milky Way, tends all human affairs. Shamans may not contact other spiritual forces directly but only through the good graces of Viho-mahse. Consequently, the snuff represents one of the most important tools of the *payé* or shamans.

Although the sixty species of *Virola* are spread throughout tropical forests of the New World and psychoactive principles have been found in at least a dozen species, it is only in the western Amazon and adjacent parts of the Orinoco basin that this genus has been used as the source of a sacred inebriant.

The species most important as sources of the intoxicating snuff are *V. calophylla, V. calophylloidea, V. elongata,* and *V. theiodora,* the last being without doubt the most frequently employed. Yet locally, *V. rufula, V. cuspidata,* and other species may supply the drug. There are Indians—the primitive nomadic Makú of the Rio Piraparaná of Colombia, for example—who ingest the red "bark-resin" directly, with no preparation, using *V. elongata.* Other tribes, especially the Bora and Witoto, swallow pellets made from the paste of the "resin," valuing for this purpose *V. peruviana, V. surinamensis, V. theiodora,* and possibly *V. loretensia.* There is vague evidence that shamans in Venezuela may smoke the bark of *V. sebifera* "at dances when curing fevers" or that they may boil the bark and drink the liquor "to drive away evil spirits."

"Sometimes when they travel or go hunting, they say:
'I must carry my Epená against those spirits,
so that they do not persecute us.'
They take Epená in the night if they hear the noises of those spirits of the forest.
They inhale it to drive them away . . ."
—Ettore Biocca

Although the mythological significance and magico-religious use of Epená snuff is indicative of a great age, the drug was not known until very recently. Perspicacious plant-explorer though he was, Spruce failed to discover this fundamental psychoactive use of *Virola,* notwithstanding his special study of the group that resulted in the discovery of a number of species new to science. The earliest reference to this hallucinogen dates from the beginning of this century, when a German ethnologist reported on the Yekwana of the upper Orinoco area.

It was not, however, until 1938 and 1939 that the botanical association of *Virola* with the snuff was made. The Brazilian botanist Ducke reported that the leaves of *V. theiodora* and *V. cuspidata* represented the source. The leaves, of course, are never used, but this report first focused attention on *Virola,* which, until then, had never been suspected as a hallucinogen.

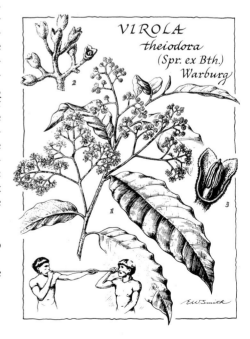

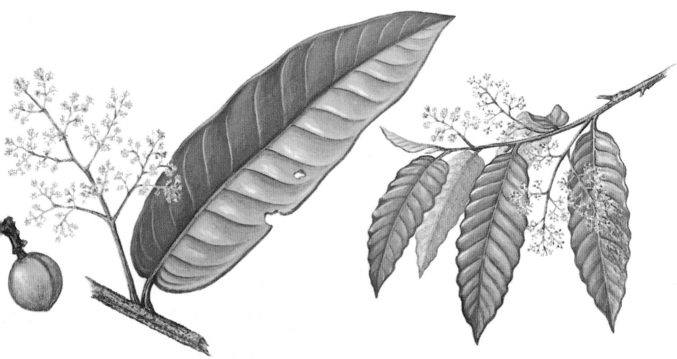

The first detailed description and specific identification of the drug, however, was published in 1954 when its preparation and use among medicine men of Colombian Indians was described. Taken mainly by shamans among the Barasana, Makuna, Tukano, Kabuyaré, Kuripako, Puinave, and other tribes in eastern Colombia, the drug was employed ritualistically for diagnosis and treatment of disease, prophecy, divination, and other magico-religious purposes. At that time, *V. calophylla* and *V. calophylloidea* were indicated as the species most valued, but later work in Brazil and elsewhere has established the primacy of *V. theiodora*.

Recent field studies have shown that the psychoactive snuff is used among many Indian groups in Amazonian Colombia, the uppermost Orinoco basin of Colombia and Venezuela, the Rio Negro, and other areas of the western Amazon of Brazil. The southernmost locality of its known use is among the Paumaré Indians of the Rio Purús in the southwestern Amazon of Brazil.

The snuff is apparently most highly prized and most deeply involved in aboriginal life among the sundry Indian tribes collectively called Waiká in the upper Orinoco of Venezuela and the northern affluents of the Rio Negro of Brazil. These groups are variously named, but are most commonly known to anthropologists as the Kirishaná, Shiriana, Karauetaré, Karimé, Parahuré, Surará, Pakidái, and Yanomamo. They generally refer to the snuff as Epená,

Ebena, Nyakwana, or some variant of these terms. In northwestern Brazil, this snuff and others are often generically known as Paricá.

Unlike the Colombian Indians, among whom the use of the snuff is usually restricted to shamans, these tribes may often take the drug in daily life. All male members of the group above the ages of thirteen or fourteen may participate. The hallucinogen is often snuffed in frighteningly excessive amounts and, in at least one annual ceremony, constantly over a two- or three-day period.

The powder is prepared in a variety of ways. Among the Colombian Indians, the bark is stripped from the trees in the early morning and the soft inner layers are scraped. The shavings are kneaded in cold water for twenty minutes. The brownish liquid is then filtered and boiled down to a thick syrup that, when dried, is pulverized and mixed with ashes of the bark of a wild cacao tree.

The various groups of Waiká have several other methods of preparation. Those living in the Orinoco area frequently rasp the cambial layer of the bark and trunk and gently dry the shavings over a fire so that they may be stored for future use. When a supply of the drug is needed, the shavings are wetted and boiled for half an hour or more, the resulting liquid being reduced to a syrup that, after drying, is ground to a powder and finely sifted. This dust is then mixed with equal amounts of a powder prepared from the dried, aromatic leaves of

Above left: Leaf, flowers, and young fruit of the rain forest tree *Virola calophylla.*

Above right: A branch of *Virola theiodora* with flowers.

177

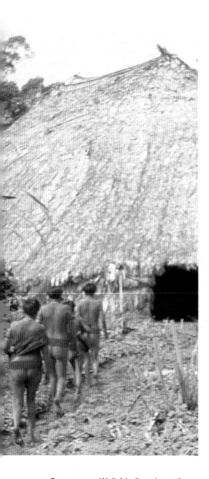

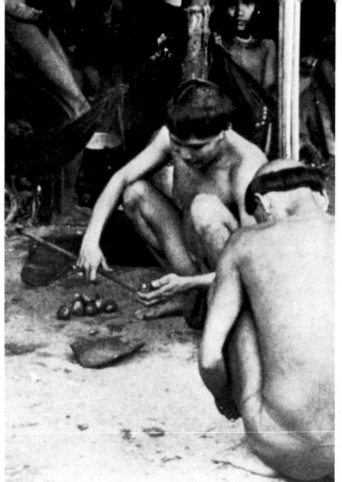

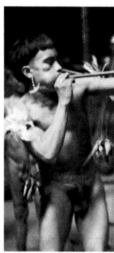

Once a year, Waiká Indians in north-eastern Brazil come together from miles around for an endocannibalistic cere-mony for which a huge quantity of *Virola* snuff is made and consumed. The ceremony held in typical round houses commemorates the dead of the previous year.

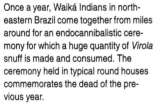

a small plant, *Justicia pectoralis* var. *ste-nophylla,* cultivated for this purpose. Fi-nally, a third ingredient is added: the ashes of the bark of an Ama or Amasita, a beautiful and rare leguminous tree, *Eli-zabetha princeps.* The hard outer bark, cut into small pieces, is placed in glowing embers, then removed and allowed to smolder to ashes.

In more eastern areas of Waiká coun-try in Brazil, the preparation of the snuff takes place mainly in the forest. Trees are felled and long strips of bark are peeled from the trunk. A copious flow of liquid that rapidly turns a blood red accumulates on the inner surface of the bark. After gently heating the strips, the shaman gathers the "resin" into an earthenware pot that is set on the fire. When the pot of red liquid is reduced to a thick syrup, it is sun-dried, crystal-lizing into a beautiful amber-red solid that is meticulously ground to an extre-mely fine dustlike consistency. This powder—Nyakwana snuff—may be employed directly, but usually the pul-verized leaves of *Justicia* are added "to make it smell better."

The Bora, Muinane, and Witoto In-dians of Amazonian Colombia and ad-jacent Peru use *Virola* not as a snuff, but by oral administration. They ingest small pellets or pills made from the re-sin to induce an intoxication during which the medicine men communicate with the "little people." These Indians utilize several species: *V. theiodora, V. pavonis,* and *V. elongata,* as well as possibly *V. surinamensis* and *V. loreten-sis.* The Bora of Peru indicate that they have used a related myristicaceous ge-nus, *Iryanthera macrophylla,* as the source of a narcotic paste for making the pellets.

The Witoto of Colombia completely decorticate the trunk of a *Virola* tree. The ·shiny cambial layer on the inner surface of the bark and adhering to the bare trunk is rasped off with the back of a machete, and the raspings are care-fully collected in a gourd. This material gradually darkens to a brownish red. The still moist raspings are kneaded, squeezed repeatedly, and pressed over a wicker sieve. The liquid that oozes through, primarily of cambial sap, has a light "coffee and milk" hue. Without further preparation, this liquid is quickly boiled, possibly to inactivate enzymes that might destroy the active

Waiká Indians consume incredible amounts of *Virola* powder, using large snuffing tubes made of the stems of maranthaceous plants. The tubes are filled with three to six teaspoonfuls of snuff for each inhalation.

After a stage of hyperactivity and stimulation during which the participants who have inhaled the snuff engage the *hekula* spirits, a period of disturbed somnolescence sets in during which nightmarish visual hallucinations continue *(left)*.

Waiká shamans frequently employ *Virola* snuff or Epená in ritual curing *(below left)*. The intricate relationship between magico-religious and "medicinal" practices of these peoples makes it difficult to distinguish the boundaries of the supernatural and the pragmatic. In fact, the Indian himself does not make a distinction between these two areas.

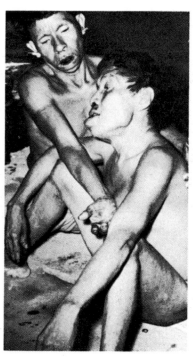

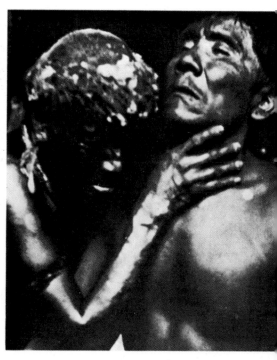

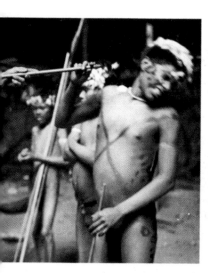

Application of the snuff is a vigorous process, the powder being blown far into the nostrils and sinuses. It causes an immediate lacrimation and excessive discharge of mucus from the nose.

principles, and is then allowed to simmer, with frequent stirring, until its volume is reduced. When the liquid finally becomes pasty, the vessel is taken from the fire, and the paste is rolled into pellets for immediate use. These pellets may keep their potency, according to the natives, for about two months.

When the pellets are not for immediate consumption, they are usually coated with a "salt," as the natives say, prepared from any of numerous plants. The "salt" is always made by the same process. The plant material is first burned and the ashes are placed in a crude funnel made of leaves or bark. Water seeps slowly through the ashes, dripping out through a hole at the bottom to be collected beneath. The filtrate is then boiled down until a gray-white residue or "salt" remains. The pellets of sticky resin are rolled in this powder. There is apparently a large assortment of plants employed for this "salt," which the Witoto call Le-sa. The lecythidaceous *Gustavia poeppigiana* is a common source of the ashes for the filtration. In the same family, the bark of the huge tree *Eschweilera itayensis* is va-

lued. An unidentified tree of this family, known to the natives as Cha-pe-na, is used. The woody stump of a species of *Carludovica* or *Sphaeradenia* of the Cyclanthaceae is reduced to ashes for this purpose. The leaves and fragrant inflorescence of the aroid *Spathiphyllum cannaefolium* give an ash that leaches out a high-quality "salt." The bark of a wild species of *Theobroma*, or several small palms, probably species of *Geonoma* and *Bactris,* are similarly used.

The Bora of Peru strip pieces of bark, only from the lower four to eight ft (1.5–2.5 m) of the trunk. The

A Mahekototen shaman *(above)* struggling against death, an ever-present threat. The Waiká believe that communication with the spirit world occurring during *Virola* intoxication enables the shaman to stave off death, which they explain as the result of the activity of malevolent spirits.

The Chemistry of Epená

The chemical analysis of various *Virola* snuffs revealed about a half-dozen closely related indole alkaloids belonging to the simple, open-chained or closed-ring tryptamine derivatives with a tetrahydro-β-carboline system. The main constituents of these snuffs are 5-methoxy-*N,N*-dimethyltryptamine and Dimethyltryptamine. 6-methoxy-*N,N*-dimethyltryptamine, monomethyltryptamine, and 2-methyl- and 1,2-dimethyl-6-methoxy-tetrahydro-β-carboline usually occur only in trace amounts. The alkaloid mixtures are almost identical to those isolated from the *Anadenanthera* snuff powders.

179

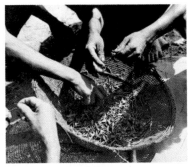

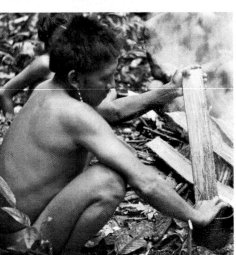

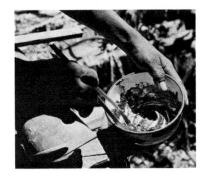

"This is a magical snuff . . . prepared from the bark of a certain tree . . .
the sorcerer blows a little . . . through a reed . . . into the air.
Next he snuffs, whilst . . . he absorbs the powder
into each nostril successively . . .
immediately the witch doctor begins singing and yelling wildly,
all the while pitching the upper part of his body
backwards and forwards."
—Theodor Koch-Grünberg (1923)

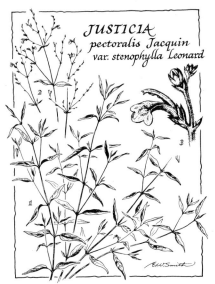

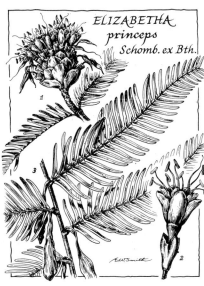

hard, brittle outer layer of bark is chipped off, leaving only the softer inner phloem. This layer quickly turns brown from congealed oxidized "resin" and is vigorously pounded on a log with a mallet until it is shredded. These shredded sections are soaked in water with occasional kneading for half an hour or more, when the pot is brought to a vigorous boil for another half hour. The bark material, squeezed dry, is then removed, and the remaining liquid is boiled with constant stirring until only a thick paste remains. Small pellets for ingestion are then made from this paste.

Fewer plants are used by the Bora for preparing the "salt" for coating the pellets: the leaves and stump of a species of *Carludovica* and of a palm of the genus *Scheelea*.

The hallucinogenic principles appear to be present mainly in the almost colorless exudate from the inner surface of the bark, which appears as soon as the bark is stripped from the tree. This resinlike substance quickly turns reddish in a typical oxidase-type reaction and then darkens, drying to a hard, glossy mass. In specimens dried for chemical study, it appears as a sticky, dark reddish brown gummy material. This material in many species contains tryptamines and other indolic hallucinogens. Observation of the process indicates that the reason for scraping the surface of the bark is to obtain all traces of the cambial layer that adhere to it. The drug is prepared from the cambial sap, which is quickly boiled, causing coagulation of protein and possibly polysaccharides, and then simmered slowly to reduce the volume to near dryness.

The whole process resembles that

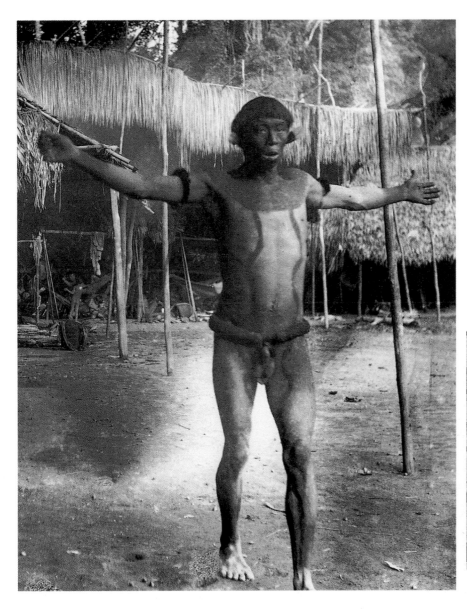

Page 180 left, top to bottom: The Waiká carefully pick over the leaves of *Justicia* before drying them as an additive to the *Virola* snuff.

One method of preparing *Virola* snuff starts with the accumulation of the red, resinlike liquid on the inner bark and its solidification by heat (as shown in the photograph of a Waiká Indian).

A Witoto Indian beats the syrup left after boiling down *Virola* resin.

Page 180 middle and right: Justicia leaves are highly aromatic when dried and are, on occasion, added to *Virola* snuff. They may, however, also be the source of a hallucinogenic snuff.

Among the Waiká, the invariable ashes mixed with *Virola* powder come from the burning of the bark of a beautiful but rare tree, *Elizabetha princeps.*

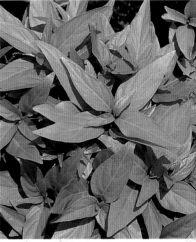

used for isolation of natural products from the cambium of other trees, coniferine from gymnosperms, for example, except that ethyl alcohol or acetone is now used, rather than heat, to destroy enzyme activity, which might otherwise act adversely on the desired product.

The "resin" of *Virola* plays an important role in everyday native medicine: several species are valued as antifungal medicines. The resin is spread over infected areas of the skin to cure ringworm and similar dermatological problems of fungal origin that are so prevalent in the humid tropical rain forests. Only certain species are chosen for this therapeutic use—and the choice seems not to have any relationship to the hallucinogenic properties of the species.

Indians who are familiar with *Virola* trees from the point of view of their hallucinogenic potency exhibit uncanny knowledge of different "kinds"—which to a botanist appear to be indistinguishable as to species. Before stripping the bark from a trunk, they are able to predict how long the exudate will take to turn red, whether it will be mild or peppery to the tongue when tasted, how long it will retain its potency when made into snuff, and many other hidden characteristics. Whether these subtle differences are due to age of the tree, season of the year, ecological situations, conditions of flowering or fruiting, or other environmental or physiological factors it is at present impossible to say—but there is no doubt about the Indian's expertness in recognizing these differences, for which he often has a terminology, so significant in his hallucinogenic and medicinal use of the trees.

Above left: Indians under *Virola* intoxication characteristically have faraway, dreamlike expressions that are, of course, due to the active principles of the drug, but which the natives believe are associated with the temporary absence of the shamans' souls as they travel to distant places. The chants during the incessant dancing performed by shamans may at times reflect conversations with spirit forces. This transportation of the soul to other realms represents to the Waiká one of the most significant values of the effects of this hallucinogen.

Above right: The leaves of *Justicia pectoralis* var. *stenophylla* are an important ingredient in the snuff that is made from the *Virola.*

GATEWAY TO DREAMTIME

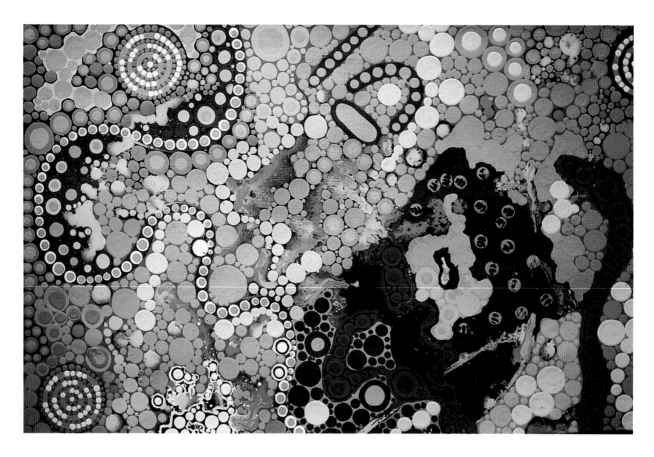

Above: Pituri bushes are represented by the gray dots on this painting by Aboriginal artist Walangari Karntawarra Jakamarra (detail from oil painting, 1994).

The psychoactive use of Pituri is probably the longest continuous use of a psychoactive substance in the history of humanity. The Australian Aborigines have the longest continuous culture of the world. The ancestors of today's Aborigines chewed Pituri 40,000 to 60,000 years ago.

Pituri refers in the broadest sense to all plants or plant materials with additional ingredients that are used for hedonistic or magical purposes by the Australian Aborigines. Generally, the term *Pituri* refers to a plant from the nightshade family, *Duboisia hopwoodii*.

Usually, the Pituri leaves are mixed with alkaline plant ashes and chewed like chewing tobacco. Pituri removes hunger and thirst and induces intense dreams, which is probably why the Aborigines use Pituri as a magic substance. In the Aboriginal magic, entering the dream state, the transcendent

Below: The trunk of the Pituri bush.

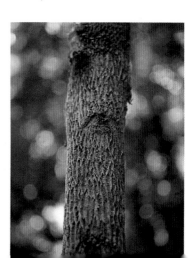

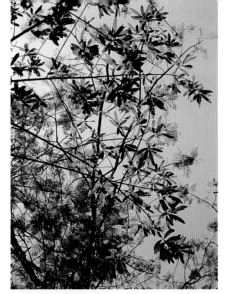

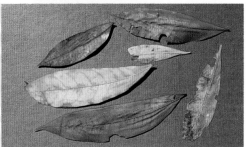

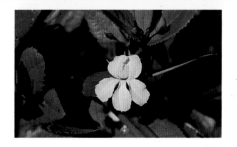

The Chemistry of Pituri

Duboisia hopwoodii contains various strongly stimulating but also toxic alkaloids (piturin, D-nor-nicotine and nicotine). D-nor-nicotine seems to be the main active substance, and myosimin, *N*-formylnornicotine, cotinin, *N*-acetylnornicotine, anabasine, anabatin, anatalline, and bipyridyl are also present.

The hallucinogenic tropanalkaloid hyoscyamine has been discovered in the roots, as well as traces of scopalamine, nicotine, nornicotine, metanicotine, myosmine, and *N*-formylnornicotine. *Duboisia myoporoides* contains large quantities of scopolamine.

Plants Whose Ashes Are Added to Pituri

Protaceae
    Grevillea striata R. BR. (Ijinyja)
Mimosaceae (Leguminosae)
    Acacia aneura F. Muell. ex Benth. (Mulga)
    Acacia coriacea DC. (Awintha)
    Acacia kempeana F. Muell. (Witchitty bush)
    Acacia lingulata A. Cunn. ex. Benth.
    Acacia pruinocarpa
    Acacia salicina Lindley
Caesalpiniaceae (Leguminosae)
    Cassia spp.
Rhamnaceae
    Ventilago viminalis Hook. (Atnyira)
Myrtaceae
    Eucalyptus microtheca F. Muell. (Angkirra)
    Eucalyptus spp. (Gums)
    Eucalyptus sp. (Red gum)
    Melaleuca sp.

primal condition of being is an essential concept. This dream state is an altered state of consciousness.

In this dream state, all magical processes and acts affect the "normal consciousness." It seems as if there are various types of Pituri for various uses and each of these varieties is linked with various songs, totems, and appropriate "dream songs" or "songlines." There are some songlines that are sung as "Pituri-songs." Pituri has a connection to the place that it grows. There is even a Pituri clan. Pituri carries with it the "dream of the place" where it grows and can instill it into humans.

The Pituri bush *(Duboisia hopwoodii)* was described by the German-Australian botanist Ferdinand J. H. von Müller (1825–1896). The plants, as well as the dried or fermented leaves, play a significant role in the domestic economy as a valuable good for barter. Although *Duboisia hopwoodii* is widespread in Australia, some areas are better for collection and harvesting than others. The leaves are filled with the power of the land in which they grow. Before the Aborigines had contact with Europeans, there was a far-reaching trading system in the central desert, which gave rise to the so-called Pituri roads and paths.

Various additives are mixed with the dried or fermented leaves and chewed. One will use plant ashes, another uses animal hair to hold the material together: plant fibers, yellow ochre, eucalyptus resin, and, most recently, sugar. The effects of the various Pituri preparations differ markedly. Some are arousing, while others are weak stimulants; some are euphoric, while others can induce visions.

Top: The Pituri bush.

Middle: The fermented Pituri leaves.

Bottom: The *Goodenia* is a Pituri replacement for the leaves of *Duboisia hopwoodii.* Plants of the genus *Goodenia* are ethnobotanically significant medicinal and nutritional plants for the Aborigines.

183

CHEMICAL STRUCTURES OF HALLUCINOGENS

Chemical determination of the molecular structure of the hallucinogenic principles in sacred plants has led to remarkable results.

Almost all plant hallucinogens contain the element nitrogen and therefore belong to the large class of chemical compounds known as alkaloids.

divinorum are the most significant examples that do not contain nitrogen. The main active principle of *Cannabis* is tetrahydrocannabinol (THC), while the main active principle of *Salvia divinorum* is salvinorin.

The principal plant hallucinogens are closely

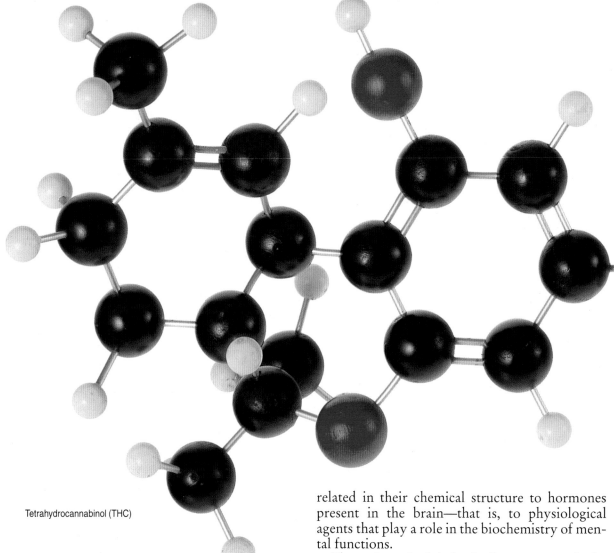

Tetrahydrocannabinol (THC)

related in their chemical structure to hormones present in the brain—that is, to physiological agents that play a role in the biochemistry of mental functions.

The active principle in the Peyote cactus is the alkaloid mescaline, a compound closely related to the brain-hormone norepinephrine (noradrenaline). Norepinephrine belongs to the group of physiological agents known as neurotransmitters because they function in the chemical transmission of impulses between neurons (nerve

The term *alkaloid* is used by chemists for the nitrogenous metabolic products of plants that have alkaline properties and are therefore "alkali-like" (alkaloid). Among the more important plants with psychoactive properties, only Hemp and *Salvia*

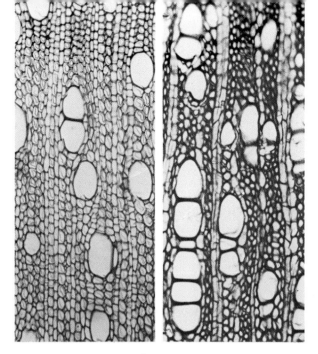

Recent studies show differences in the internal structure of wood between *Cannabis sativa (far left)* and *C. indica.* As shown in these microscopic cross-sections, one of the most significant differences is the usually single conducive vessels in the former species as contrasted with the consistently grouped vessels in the latter.

THC, found only in *Cannabis,* is concentrated in the resin and is absent from the woody tissue, which for this reason is specifically exempted from control in American *Cannabis* legislation.

lanine, which is widely distributed in the human organism.

The models of mescaline and noradrenaline molecules on page 186 clearly show the close relationship in chemical structure of these two agents.

Psilocybine and psilocine, the active principles of Teonanácatl, the hallucinogenic Mexican mushrooms, are derived from the same basic compound as the brain hormone serotonine: tryptamine. Tryptamine also is the basic compound of an essential amino acid, which is tryptophane. The relationship can be clearly seen in the molecular models shown on page 186.

There is another Mexican sacred plant, Ololiuqui (Morning Glory), the hallucinogenic principles of which are derivatives of tryptamine. In this case, tryptamine is incorporated in a complex ring structure that has been called ergolin. The molecular models on page 187 show the structural relationship between lysergic acid amide and lysergic acid hydroxyethylamide (the two principal active constituents of Ololiuqui), the neurotransmitter serotonine, and psilocybine and psilocine.

That the important plant hallucinogens and the brain hormones serotonine and noradrenaline have the same basic structure cannot be due to mere chance. This astounding relationship may explain the psychotropic potency of these hallucinogens. Having the same basic structure, these hallucinogens may act at the same sites in the nervous system as the above-mentioned brain hormones, like similar keys fitting the same lock. As a result, the psychophysiological functions associated with those brain sites are altered, suppressed, stimulated, or otherwise modified.

The ability of hallucinogens to produce changes in brain function is due not only to their having a particular chemical composition, but also to the peculiar spatial arrangement of the atoms in their molecules. This can be seen very clearly in the case of the most powerful hallucinogen known today, lysergic acid diethylamide. LSD may be regarded as a chemically modified form of an active principle in Ololiuqui. The only difference between the semi-synthetic drug lysergic acid diethylamide and the natural Ololiuqui hallucinogen lysergic acid amide is that two hydrogen atoms of the

The molecular models of hallucinogens on pages 186–87 show the chemical elements of which these substances consist and the manner in which the atoms of these elements are related to one another in the molecules. The black balls mean carbon atoms, the white hydrogen, the red oxygen, the green nitrogen, and the yellow ball in the psilocybine molecule indicates a phosphoric atom. There is, in fact, no space between atoms connected with each other; they touch. Moreover, atoms of various elements are of different sizes. Only the especially small size of the hydrogen atoms has been indicated in these models.

It is hardly possible to imagine the real dimension of atoms and molecules: 0.1 mg (a tenth of a thousandth of a gram) of a hallucinogen, barely visible, consists of about 2×10^{17} ($= 200,000,000,000,000,000$) molecules.

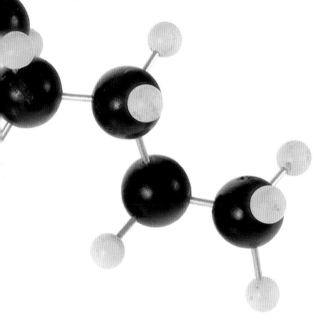

cells). Mescaline and norepinephrine have the same basic chemical structure. Both are derivatives of a substance known to chemists as phenylethylamine. Another derivative of phenylethylamine is the essential amino acid phenyla-

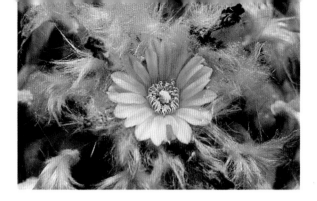

Peyotl *(Lophophora williamsii)*

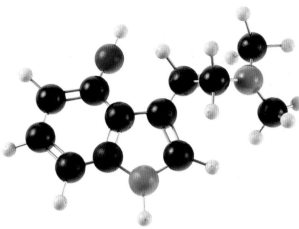

Psilocine
(hallucinogenic principle of Teonanácatl)

amide have been replaced in the diethylamide by two ethyl groups. With LSD, a dose of 0.05 milligram will produce a deep hallucinogenic intoxication of some hours' duration. With iso-LSD, which differs from LSD only in the spatial arrangement of the atoms, ten times that dose has no effect whatsoever.

The molecular models of LSD and iso-LSD on page 187 show that, while the atoms are linked to each other in the same way, their spatial arrangement is different.

Molecules differing only in spatial arrangement are known as stereoisomers. Stereoisomers can exist only with molecules that are asymmetrical in structure, and one of the theoretically possible spatial arrangements is in general more active.

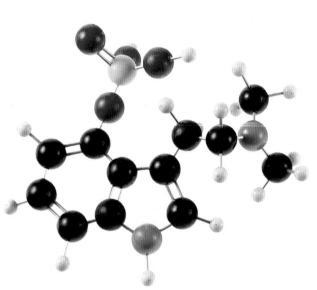

Psilocybine
(hallucinogenic principle of Teonanácatl)

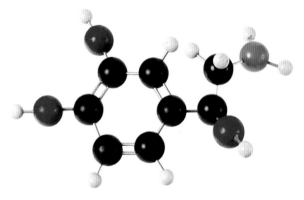

Noradrenaline
(a brain hormone)

Next to chemical composition, spatial configuration plays the most crucial role in determining not only hallucinogenic but also general pharmacological activity.

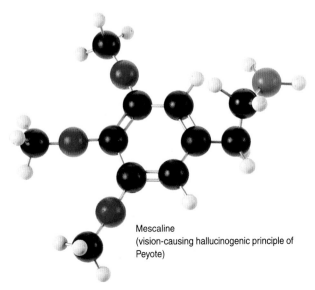

Mescaline
(vision-causing hallucinogenic principle of Peyote)

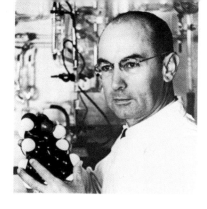

Dr. Albert Hofmann, born 1906, discoverer of LSD and the hallucinogenic principles of Teonanácatl and of Ololiuqui, is shown here with the molecular model of LSD in his pharmaceutic-chemical research laboratory, Sandoz, Basel, Switzerland, 1943.

Page 186: The comparison between Mescaline and Noradrenaline and between Psilocybine and Psilocine with Serotonine shows the relationship in the chemical structure between the hallucinogens and brain hormones.

The close chemical relationship between the active principles of Ololiuqui and LSD, the most potent hallucinogen known today, is evident when comparing the molecular models of Lysergic Acid Amide and Lysergic Acid Hydroxyethylamide with Lysergic Acid Diethylamide.

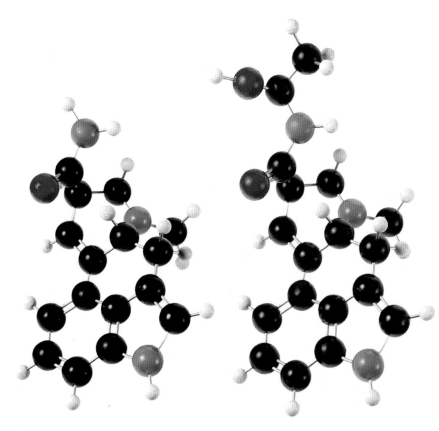

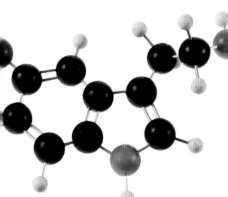

Lysergic acid amide
(hallucinogenic principle of
Ololiuqui)

Lysergic Acid Hydroxyethylamide
(hallucinogenic principle of
Ololiuqui)

LSD
(semi-synthetic hallucinogen)

iso-LSD
(semi-synthetic compound)

Serotonine
(a brain hormone)

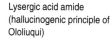

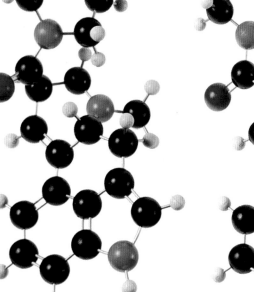

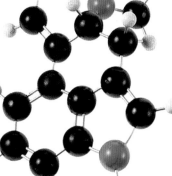

The active properties of hallucinogens are due not only to their composition with certain atoms; the spatial arrangement of the atoms in the molecule is equally important in determining the hallucinogenic effects. As an example, LSD and iso-LSD *(at right)* consist of the same elements, but they differ in the spatial arrangement of the diethylamide group. In comparison to LSD, iso-LSD is practically without hallucinogenic effect.

USES OF HALLUCINOGENS IN MEDICINE

The use of pure hallucinogenic compounds in medicine has the same basis as the use of the source plants in magico-religious ceremonies. The effects in both cases consist of profound psychic alterations in the experience of reality. Not only is perception of the outside world affected,

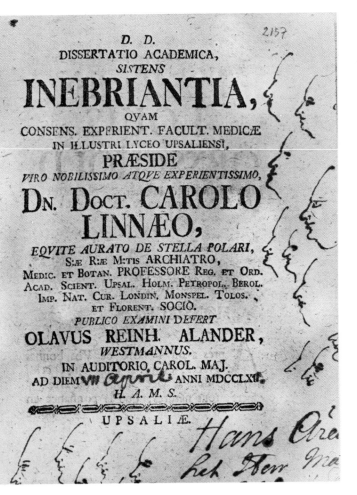

but perception of the subject's own personality is also transformed. The changes in sensory experience of the outside world are due to a shift in sensitivity of the sense organs. Sensory perception, particularly with regard to vision and hearing, is stimulated by hallucinogens. These changes in self-awareness indicate the profound influence of the drugs, which affect the very core of our being: consciousness.

Our experience of reality is incomprehensible without a subject, an ego, that perceives this reality. The subjective experience of so-called objective reality is the result of interactions between external sensory signals, mediated by the sense organs, and the ego, which brings this information to the level of conscious awareness. In this situation, one can think of the external world as a sender of information or signals and the deep self as a receiver. The translator in this case is the ego. In the absence of one of these—either the sender or the receiver—reality does not exist. There is no music on the radio, and the screen is blank. If we adhere to this concept of reality as the product of the interaction between sender and receiver, the perception of a different reality under the influence of hallucinogens may be explained by the fact that the brain, which is the site of consciousness, undergoes dramatic biochemical changes. The receiver is thus set for wavelengths other than those associated with normal, everyday reality. From this perspective, the subjective experience of reality is infinite, depending on the capacity of the receiver, which can be greatly changed through biochemical modification of the brain field.

In general, we experience life from a rather limited point of view. This is the so-called normal state. However, through hallucinogens the perception of reality can be strongly changed and expanded. These different aspects or levels of one and the same reality are not mutually exclusive. They form an all-encompassing, timeless, transcendental reality.

The possibility of changing the wavelength setting on the "ego receiver," and, with this, to produce changes in the awareness of reality, constitutes the real significance of hallucinogens. This ability to create new and different images of the world is why hallucinogenic plants were, and still are, regarded as sacred.

What is the essential, characteristic difference between everyday reality and the images seen during hallucinogenic inebriation? In normal states of consciousness—in everyday reality—ego and outside world are separated; one stands face to face with the outside world; it has become an object. Under the influence of hallucinogens, the borderline between the experiencing ego and the outside world disappears or becomes blurred,

Page 188: The first treatise on inebriants is apparently the doctoral thesis of Alander, a student of Linnaeus, who is the father of modern botany. This thesis, defended in 1762 at Uppsala, was a mixture of scientific and pseudo-scientific information. An observer present at the thesis defense may have doodled these profiles, possibly depicting the academic examiners.

Below: Visionary experiences produced by hallucinogens are a source of inspiration for painters. These two watercolors by Christian Rätsch emerged after taking LSD and show the mystical character of the experience.

depending on the degree of inebriation. A feedback mechanism is set up between receiver and sender. Part of the ego reaches out to the external world, into the objects around us; they begin to come to life, acquiring a deeper and different meaning. This may be a joyful experience or a

ecstasy known as the *unio mystica* or, in the experience of Eastern religious life, as *samadhi* or *satori*. In both of these states, a reality is experienced that is illuminated by that transcendental reality in which creation and ego, sender and receiver, are One.

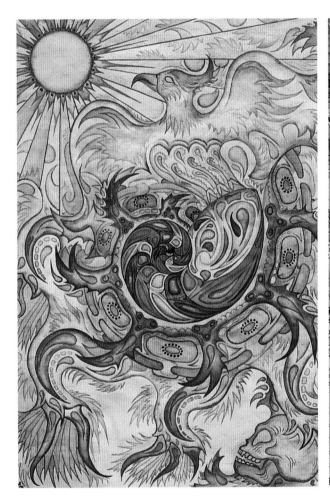

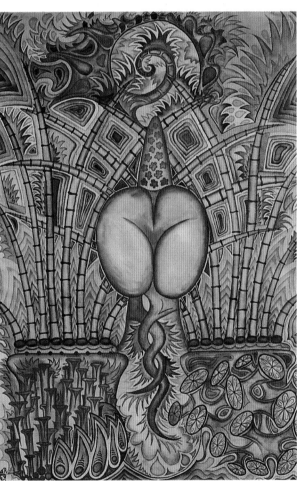

demonic one, involving the loss of the trusted ego. The new ego feels linked in bliss with outside objects in a special way and also with other human beings. The experience of deep communication with the outside world may even culminate in the sensation of being at one with the whole of creation.

This state of cosmic consciousness that under favorable circumstances may be attained with hallucinogens is related to the spontaneous religious

The changes in consciousness and perception that may be experimentally produced with hallucinogens have found a number of different applications in medicine. The pure substances most commonly used in this field are mescaline, psilocybine, and LSD. Recent research has been concerned mainly with the most powerful hallucinogen known so far, LSD, a substance that is a chemically modified form of the active principle in Ololiuqui.

In psychoanalysis, breaking the habitual experience of the world can help patients caught in an ego-centered problem cycle to escape from their fixation and isolation. With the I-Thou barrier relaxed or even removed under the influence of a hallucinogen, better contact may be established with the psychiatrist, and the patient may become more open to psychotherapeutic suggestion.

Hallucinogenic stimulation also often causes forgotten or repressed past experiences to be clearly recalled. It can be of crucial importance in psychotherapy to bring back to conscious awareness events that led to a psychological disturbance. Numerous reports have been published on how the influence of hallucinogens used during psychoanalysis revived memories of past events, even those from very early childhood. This is not the usual form of remembering, but involves actually going through the experience again: it is not *réminiscence* but *réviviscence,* as the French psychiatrist Jean Delay put it.

The hallucinogen does not in itself effect a cure but rather plays the role of a medicinal aid to be used in the total context of psychoanalysis or psychotherapy, to make these more effective and to reduce the period of treatment required. There are two different ways of using it for this purpose.

One method, developed in European hospitals, is known as psycholysis. It consists of giving medium doses of the hallucinogen on a number of

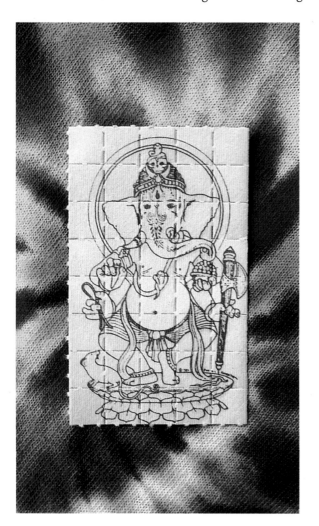

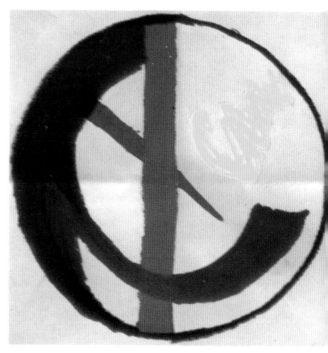

successive occasions at specific intervals. The patient's experiences under the influence of the hallucinogen are discussed in a group session that follows and are expressed through painting, drawing, and the like. The term *psycholysis* was invented by Ronald A. Sandison, an English psychotherapist of the Jungian school. The "-lysis" component indicates the dissolving of psychological tensions and conflicts.

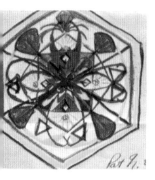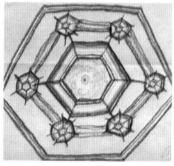

The second method is the one generally preferred in the United States. After intensive psychological preparation appropriate to each individual, the patient is given a single very high dose of the hallucinogen. This "psychedelic therapy" is intended to produce a mystic, religious state of ecstasy that should provide a starting point for restructuring the patient's personality. The term *psychedelic* means "mind manifesting." It was coined by the psychiatrist Humphrey Osmond.

The use of hallucinogens as an aid to psychoanalysis and psychotherapy is based on effects

analysis and psychotherapy, are still the subject of dispute in medical circles. However, this applies also to other techniques, such as electroshock, insulin treatment, and psychosurgery, all of which carry far greater danger than the use of hallucinogens, which, in expert hands, may be regarded as virtually without risk.

Some psychiatrists hold the view that the faster retrieval of forgotten or repressed traumatic experiences frequently seen with these drugs and the shorter period of treatment are not advantageous. They believe that this method does not allow sufficient time for the full psychotherapeutic utilization and integration of the material made conscious, and that the beneficial effects are of shorter duration than if traumatic experiences are

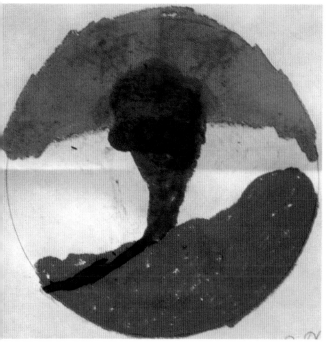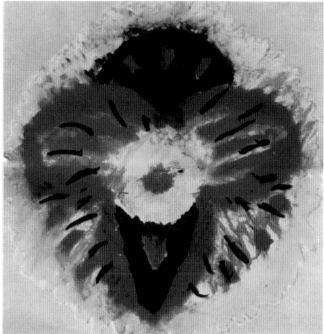

that are the opposite of those psychotropic drugs known as tranquilizers. These drugs tend rather to suppress the patient's problems and conflicts, making them appear less serious and no longer so important, whereas the hallucinogens bring conflicts to the surface and make them more intense, so that they may be more clearly recognizable and open to psychotherapy.

Hallucinogenic drugs, as an adjunct to psycho-

brought back to conscious awareness more gradually and dealt with in stages.

Psycholysis and psychedelic therapy both require very careful preparation of the patient before the hallucinogen is given. If there is to be a really positive gain from the experience, patients must not be frightened by the unusual effects produced by the drug. Careful selection of patients to be treated is also important, for not

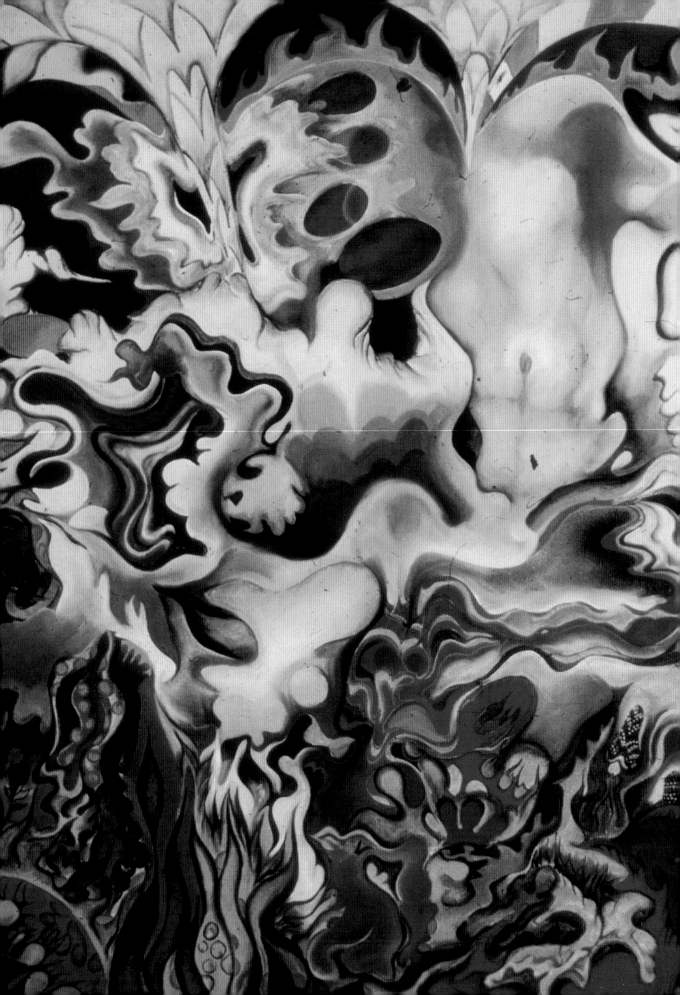

Page 192: In the 1960s, many artists in the United States and Europe experimented with hallucinogens in order to enhance the creative process. The painting on the left is an example of this genre.

Below: Only a few artists are capable of expressing the visionary realms while directly under the influence of hallucinogens. The two paintings by Fred Weidmann were executed while under the influence of *Psilocybe cyanescens*. Both are acrylic on marbled paper.

Left: *Slipping and Sliding 1* (There exists another painting from the same day.)

Right: *The Garden of Pan*

every type of psychic disorder responds equally well to this form of therapy. To be successful, therefore, hallucinogen-assisted psychoanalysis or psychotherapy requires special knowledge and experience.

One of the most important aspects of the clinical training of a psychotherapist working with

could be considered a "model of psychosis," but major differences have in fact been found between psychotic states and hallucinogenic inebriation. However, hallucinogenic intoxication can serve as a model for studying the biochemical and electrophysiological changes that occur with abnormal mental states.

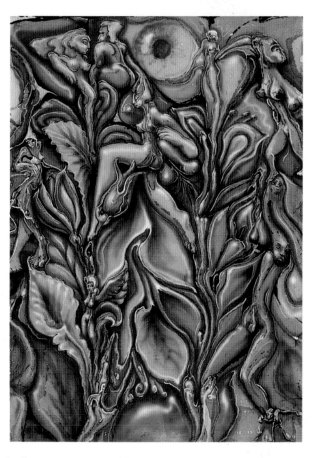

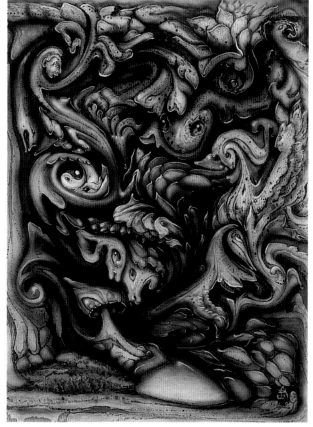

hallucinogens is self-experimentation with these substances. Through these experiences, therapists can gain direct knowledge of the worlds that their patients enter and, thereby, have much greater understanding of the dynamics of the unconscious.

Hallucinogens may also be used in experimental studies to determine the nature of mental disorders. Certain abnormal mental states produced by hallucinogens in normal subjects are, in some respects, similar to the symptoms of schizophrenia and other mental diseases. At one time it was even thought that hallucinogenic intoxication

One area where the medical use of hallucinogens, and particularly LSD, touches on serious ethical questions is in the care of the dying. Doctors in American hospitals observed that the very severe pain suffered by cancer patients, which no longer responded to conventional painkillers, could be partly or completely relieved by LSD. This action is probably not analgesic in the usual sense. What is thought to happen is that the perception of pain disappears; under the influence of the drug, the patient's mind becomes separated from his body to such an extent that physical pain

Below: During visionary experiences, many people see spirals, whirlpools, and milky ways. The artist Nana Nauwald depicted such an experience in her painting *The Middle Is Everywhere*.

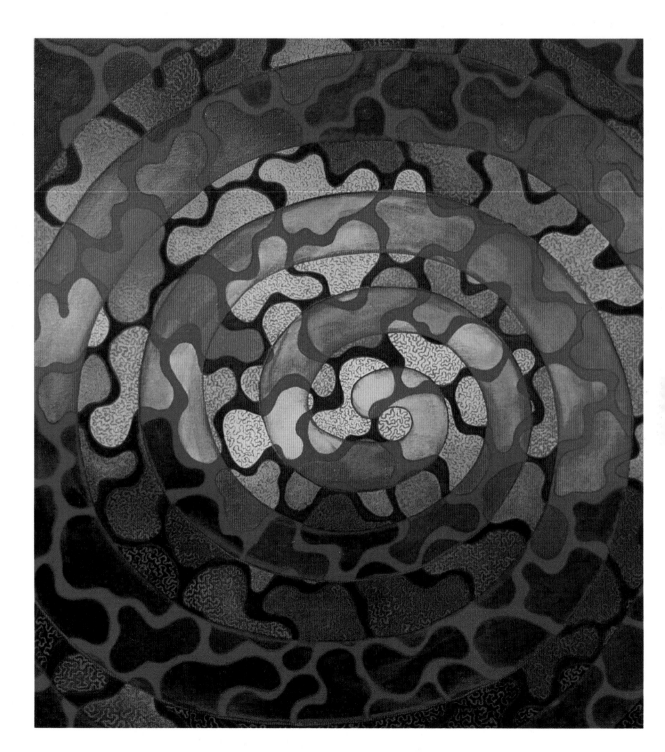

no longer reaches it. If the use of hallucinogens in this type of case is to be effective, it is again absolutely necessary to prepare the patient mentally and to explain the kind of experience and the changes that he may undergo. Great benefit derives also from guiding the patient's thoughts

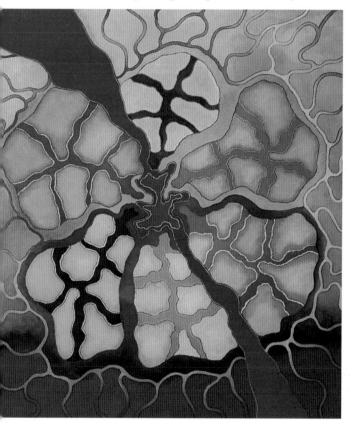

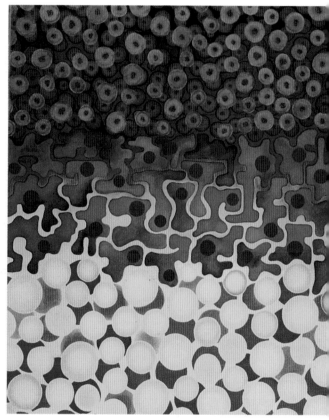

Below left: The painting *Spirit and Matter Are Indivisible* documents a recurring hallucinogen-influenced experience.

Below right: Many people recognize the *Will to Live* when they have tasted the plants of the gods. Nana Nauwald expresses this artistically.

toward religious aspects, which can be done by a clergyman or by a psychotherapist. There have been numerous reports of how dying individuals, free from pain in LSD ecstasy, have come to perceive the meaning of life and death, and have died in peace, reconciled to their fate and free from fear.

The medical use of hallucinogenic drugs differs from the shamanistic use of hallucinogenic sacred plants by medicine men and healer-priests in that the latter usually themselves eat the plant, or drink a decoction made from it; whereas in conventional medicine, the hallucinogenic substance is given only to the patient. In both instances, however, the same psychological effects are utilized, for the same drug actions that serve as an aid to psychoanalysis and psychotherapy also give the shaman unusual powers of divination and healing. They consist of the loosening or even dissolution of the I-Thou barrier, with the result that objective everyday consciousness dissolves into the mystic experience of One-ness.

EPILOGUE

One of the leading lights of the interdisciplinary investigations of hallucinogens was Louis Lewin, the famous Berlin toxicologist. More than a half a century ago, he captured the all-pervading significance of hallucinogens to the cultural evolution of the human race when he wrote in his book *Phantastica:*

"From the beginning of our knowledge of man, we find him consuming substances of no nutritive value but taken for the sole purpose of producing for a certain time a feeling of contentment, ease, and comfort . . .

"Their potential energy has covered the whole earth and established communication between various races, in spite of dividing mountains and sundering seas. These substances have formed a bond of union between men of opposite hemispheres, the uncivilized and the civilized; they have forced passages which, once open, proved of use for other purposes: they produced in ancient races characteristics which have endured to the present day, evidencing the marvelous degree of intercourse that existed between different people just as certainly and as exactly as a chemist can judge the relations of two substances by their reactions. Hundreds or thousands of years were necessary to establish contact between whole nations by these means . . .

"The motives for the occasional or habitual use of these drugs are of greater interest than collection of facts concerning them. Here all kinds of human contrasts meet: barbarism and civilization, with all their various degrees of material possessions, social status, knowledge, belief, age and gifts of body, mind, and soul.

"On this plane meet artisan and sybarite, ruler and subject; the savage from some distant island or from the Kalahari Desert associates with poet, philosophers, scientists, misanthropes, and philanthropists; the man of peace rubs shoulders with the man of war, the devotee with the atheist.

"The physical impulses which bring under their spell such diverse classes of mankind must be extraordinary and far-reaching. Many have expressed opinions about them, but have probed and understood their intrinsic properties, and fewer still perceived the inner-most significance and the motives for the use of substances in which such energies are stored."

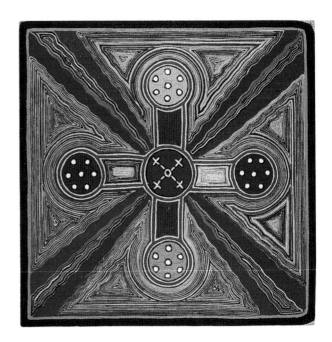

Above: In Huichol, the term *nierika* refers to a portway between so-called ordinary and non-ordinary realities. It is a passageway and, at the same time, a barrier between worlds. *Nierika,* a decorated ceremonial disk, is also said to mean "mirror" as well as "face of the deity." This *nierika* shows the four cardinal directions and the sacred center. The coordinating axis is placed in a field of fire.

Several early scientific investigators can be credited with beginning the interdisciplinary research on hallucinogenic plants and psychoactive substances. In 1855, Ernst Freiherr von Bibra published *Die narkotischen Genussmittel und der Mensch,* in which he considered some seventeen psychoactive plants. He urged chemists to study diligently an area so promising and so full of enigmas. Mordecai Cooke, a British mycologist, published a number of specialized papers on fungi. His only popular, nontechnical publication, *The Seven Sisters of Sleep,* was an interdisciplinary study of psychoactive plants, published in 1860.

Half a century after von Bibra's work and undoubtedly sparked by it, another outstanding book appeared. Carl Hartwich's extensive *Die menschlichen Genussmittel,* published in 1911, considered at length and with an interdisciplinary emphasis about thirty psychoactive plants, and he mentioned a number of others in passing. Pointing out that von Bibra's pioneering book was dated, that chemical and botanical research on these curiously active plants had scarcely begun in 1855, he optimistically maintained that by 1911, such studies were either well under way or had already been completed.

Thirteen years later, in 1924, perhaps the most influential figure in psychopharmacology, Louis Lewin, published his *Phantastica,* a book of extraordinary interdisciplinary depth. It presented a total story of some twenty-eight plants and a few synthetic compounds that are used around the world for their stimulating or inebriating effects, emphasizing their importance to scientific research, especially in the fields of botany, ethnobotany, chemistry, pharmacology, medicine, psychology, and psychiatry, as well as to ethnology, history, and sociology. Lewin wrote that "the contents of this book will provide a starting point from which original research in the above-mentioned departments of science maybe pursued."

From the 1930s to today, interdisciplinary activity in psychopharmacology, botany, and anthropology began uninterruptedly to increase. Many amplifications and clarifications of older knowledge have been made and new discoveries in sundry fields have followed one another in close succession. In spite of the pharmaceutical, phytochemical, and ethnobotanical advances that have been made in the past 150 years, there still remains a tremendous amount of work to be done on these "plants of the gods."

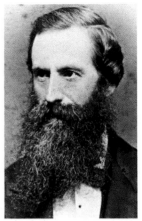

ERNST FREIHERR VON BIBRA
1806–1878

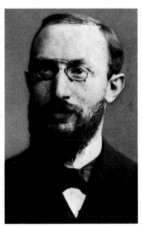

MORDECAI COOKE
1825–1913

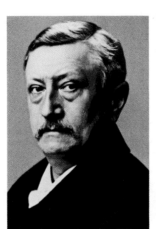

CARL HARTWICH
1851–1917

LOUIS LEWIN
1850–1929

PHOTO CREDITS

Arnau, F., *Rauschgift,* Lucerne 1967: 101 below right

A-Z Botanical Coll., London: 17 above left

Biblioteca Apostolica Vaticana, Vatican City (Codex Barberini Lat. 241 fol. 29r): 111 left

Biblioteca Medicea Laurenziana, Florence: 159 above (Photo: Dr. G. B. Pineider)

Biblioteca Nazionale Centrale di Firenze, Florence: 162 above (Photo: G. Sansoni)

Biedermann, H., *Lexikon der Felsbildkunst,* Graz 1976: 83 above

Bildarchiv Bucher, Lucerne: 17 below right

Biocca, E., Yanoàma, Bari 1965 (Photo: Padre L. Cocco): 178 middle, 178/179, 179 middle, right, 181 left

Black Star, New York: 96 middle, left and right (Photo C. Henning)

Bouvier, N., Cologny-Genève: 82

Brill, D., College Park, Georgia: 168 above left

Carroll, L., *Alice's Adventures in Wonderland,* New York 1946: 101 below left

Coleman Collection, Uxbridge: 17 above, center left

Curtis Botanical Magazine, vol. III, third series, London 1847: 147 below

Editions Delcourt, Paris: 89 above left

EMB Archives, Lucerne: 5. 13 above, centerright, 28/29, 36 (9, 10), 38 (14,15), 40 (22, 25 below), 43 (35), 44 (38, 39), 46 (46) and below, 48 (52, 53) and below, 49 (55, 56), 53 (70, 72) and below, 56 (84) and below, 58 (89, 90), 59 (93), 60 (96), 62, 88, 118, 119, 122 above, 132, 133 right, 145 above, 177, 187 above

Emboden, W., California State University, Northridge: 95 right

Erdoes, R., New York and Santa Fe: 152 right

ETH-Bibliothek, Zurich: 197 center left

Forman, W., Archive, London: 62 right

Fröhlich, A., Lucerne: 186 above

Fuchs, L., *New Kreuterbuch,* Basel 1543: 31 left

Furst, P. T., New York State University, Albany, New York: 172 below

Goodman, Mill Valley, California: 96 center left

Halifax Collection, Ojai, California: 150 below, 190/191 middle, 191 above, 196

Harvard Botanical Museum, Cambridge, Mass.: 31 center left, 98 above, 152 left, 153 above right, 170 below, 185 above, 197 above

Hernández de Alba, G., Nuestra Gente Namuy Misag, Bogotá: 143 left

Hofmann, Dr. A., Burg i. L.: 23, 162 left

Holford, M., Loughton: 105 below

Holmstedt, B., Karolinska Institute, Stockholm: 197 below

Hunt Institute for Botanical Documentation, Carnegie-Mellon University, Pittsburgh: 188

Kaufmann, P. B., Department of Botany, University of Michigan, Ann Arbor: 99

Kobel, H., Sandoz Research Laboratories, Basel: 103 below right

Koch-Grünberg, T., *Zwei Jahre unter den Indianern,* Berlin, 1910: 127 left

Köhler, *Medizinal-Pflanzenatlas,* vol. I, Gera-Untermhaus 1887: 21 below, 31 center left

Krippner, S., San Francisco: 192

Leuenberger, H., Yverdon: 111 right

Lyckner, K.-Ch., Hamburg: 110 above left

Moreau de Tours, J., *Du Hachisch et de l'alimentation Mentale,* Paris 1845: 100 below

Museo del Oro, Bogotá: 64

Museum of Fine Arts, Boston, Gift of Mrs. W. Scott Fritz: 108 left

Museum of the American Indian, Heye Foundation, New York: 152 middle

Museum Rietberg, Zurich: 2 (Photo: Kammerer/Wolfsberger), 10/11 Sammlung von der Heydt (Photo: Wettstein & Kauf)

Myerhoff, B., Los Angeles: 148, 149 above left, 151 below

Nauwald, N., Südergellersen: 194, 195

Negrin, J., Mexico: 63 (Photo: L. P. Baker))

New Yorker, New York: 100 top

Österreichische Nationalbibliothek, Vienna (Codex Vindobonensis S. N. 2644—*Tacuinum Sanitatis in Medicina*—Folio 40): 87 below

Ott, J., Xalapa: 56 (82)

Parker, A.: Yale University, New Haven: 97 below left

Pelt, J. M., *Drogues et plantes magiques,* Paris 1971: 151 above left

Perret, J., Lucerne: 184–187 (models by Dr. A. Hofmann)

Petersen, W.: Mecki bei den 7 Zwergen, Köln (© for the Mecki-character: Diehl-Film, Munich): 84 center right

Photoarchiv Emil Schulthess Erben, Zurich: 24

Radio Times Hulton Picture Library, London: 4

Rätsch, C., Hamburg: 7, 8, 13 center, right, 17 below, center left, 18, 19, 21 above, 22, 24/25, 27, 30, 34, 35, 36, 37 (8), 38 (16, 17), 39, 40, (23, 24), 42, 43 (34, 36, 37), 44 (40, 41), 45, 46 (45, 47, 48), 47, 48 (53), 49 (57), 50, 51, 52, 53, (69, 71), 54, 55 (77, 78, 80), 56 (81, 83), 57, 58 (91), 59 (92, 94), 60 (95, 97), 83 below, 84 above, center left, below, 85 above right, below, 86, 97 above left, above right, 89 below, 90 below, 91, 92, 93, 94, 95 above, 96 above, below, 97, above left, above right, 101 above, 102, 103 above right, below right, 104, 105 right, 106, 107 above, below left, below right, 108 above right, below, 109, 110 below left, right, 112, 113 above below left, 114 above, 115 above, 117

left, above left, 120, 121, 122 below, 123, 124, 125, 128, 129, 130, 131, 134, 135, 136, 137, 138, 139, 140, 141, 142 right, 144, 145 below, 146, 147 above, 150 above, 151 above right, 152 above, 153 above left, 154 above left, 155 below, 156 above, 157 above, 158, 159 below, 164, 165, 166, 167, 168 above right, middle, below, 169, 170 above left, below, 172 above, 173, 175 above, 176 left, 181 right, 182, 189, 190 left

Rauh, Prof., Dr. W., Institut für Systematische Botanik und Pflanzengeographie der Universität Heidelberg: 16 above right, middle, below, 17 middle, 60

Roger Viollet, Paris: 116 right

Royal Botanical Gardens, Kew. 117 below right, 126 left, 197 center right

Sahagún, B. de, *Historia General de las Cosas de Nueva España,* Mexico 1829: 107 below middle

Salzman, E.: Denver, Colorado: 85 above left

Samorini, G.: Dozza: 112 right, 113 below right, 114 below, 115 below

Scala, Florence: 105 left

Schaefer, S. B.: McAllen, Texas: 6, 149 above right, middle, 154 above right, below, 155 above

Schmid, X.: Wetzikon: 55 (79)

Schultes, R. E., Harvard Botanical Museum, Cambridge, Mass.: 98 below, 117 above right, 126 middle, right, 127 right, 133 left, 142, 178

Schuster, M., Basel: 118 above left, 119 above middle

Science Photo Library, London (Long Ashton Research Station, University of Bristol): 31 right

Sharma, G., University of Tennessee, Martin: 98 center right

Sinsemilla: *Marijuana Flowers* © Copyright 1976, Richardson, Woods and Bogart. Permission granted by: And/Or Press, Inc., PO Box 2246, Berkeley, CA 94702: 97 below right

Smith, E. W., Cambridge, Mass.: 156/157 below, 171 above right, 176 right

Starnets, P. Olympia: 158 right

Tobler, R., Lucerne: 16 above left, 81

Topham, J., Picture Library, Edenbridge: 17 above right, 90 above

Valentini, M. B., *Viridarium reformatum, seu regnum vegetabile,* Frankfurt a. Main 1719: 80

Wasson, R. G., Harvard Botanical Museum, Cambridge, Mass.: 14, 15 (Photo A. B. Richardson), 174 below, 175 below (Photo: C. Bartolo)

Weidmann, F., Munich: 193

Zentralbibliothek Zurich (Ms. F23, p. 399): 89 above right

Zerries, O., Munich: 118 below right, 118/119, 119 above right

ACKNOWLEDGMENTS

Should this book succeed in giving its readers a better understanding of the role of hallucinogenic plants in the cultural development of man through the centuries, we must thank the patience and friendliness of shamans and other native peoples with whom we have had the happy opportunity of working.

The debt that we owe for the faithful cooperation and encouragement of our many professional colleagues over the years can be neither easily nor adequately put into words, but nonetheless it is deeply appreciated.

To the sundry scientific institutions and many libraries that have freely and fully helped us in so many ways, both before and during the preparation of the book, we express our heartfelt thanks. Without this support, the book never could have been born in its present form.

The generosity of the many individuals and institutions that have made available, often at great expense of time and research, the extensive illustrative material for this volume—much of it hitherto unpublished—has heartened us during the frequent frustrations that we have met in our efforts to produce a book conceived with a fresh and forward-looking overview of one of the fundamental elements of human culture—the hallucinogens.

Christian Rätsch thanks Claudia Müller-Ebeling, Nana Nauwald, Stacy Schaefer, Arno Adelaars, Felix Hasler, Jonathan Ott, Giorgio Samorini, and Paul Stamets for comments on the revision.

BIBLIOGRAPHY

Aaronson, Bernard & Humphrey Osmond (ed.)
1970 *Psychedelics*. New York: Anchor Books.

Adovasio, J. M. & G. F. Fry
1976 "Prehistoric Psychotropic Drug Use in Northeastern Mexico and Trans-Pecos Texas" *Economic Botany* 30: 94–96.

Agurell, S.
1969 "Cactaceae Alkaloids. I." *Lloydia* 32: 206–216.

Aiston, Georg
1937 "The Aboriginal Narcotic Pitcheri" *Oceania* 7(3): 372–377.

Aliotta, Giovanni, Danielle Piomelli, & Antonio Pollio
1994 "Le piante narcotiche e psicotrope in Plinio e Dioscoride" *Annali dei Musei Civici di Revereto* 9(1993): 99–114.

Alvear, Silvio Luis Haro
1971 *Shamanismo y farmacopea en el reino de Quito*. Quito, Instituto Ecuatoriana de Ciencias Naturales (Contribución 75).

Andritzky, Walter
1989 *Schamanismus und rituelles Heilen im Alten Peru* (2 volumes). Berlin: Clemens Zerling.
1989 "Ethnopsychologische Betrachtung des Heilrituals mit Ayahuasca *(Banisteriopsis caapi)* unter besonderer Berücksichtigung der Piros (Ostperu)" *Anthropos* 84: 177–201.
1989 "Sociopsychotherapeutic Functions of Ayahuasca Healing in Amazonia" *Journal of Psychoactive Drugs* 21(1): 77–89.
1995 "Sakrale Heilpflanze, Kreativität und Kultur: indigene Malerei, Gold- und Keramikkunst in Peru und Kolumbien" *Curare* 18(2): 373–393.

Arenas, Pastor
1992 "El 'cebil' o el 'árbol de la ciencia del bien y del mal'" *Parodiana* 7(1–2): 101–114.

Arévalo Valera, Guillermo
1994 *Medicina indígena Shipibo-Conibo: Las plantas medicinales y su beneficio en la salud*. Lima: Edición Aidesep.

Baer, Gerhard
1969 "Eine Ayahuasca-Sitzung unter den Piro (Ost-Peru)" *Bulletin de la Société Suisse des Americanistes* 33: 5–8.
1987 "Peruanische ayahuasca-Sitzungen" in: A. Dittrich & Ch. Scharfetter (ed.), *Ethnopsychotherapie*, S. 70–80, Stuttgart: Enke.

Barrau, Jacques
1958 "Nouvelles observations au sujet des plantes hallucinôgenes d'usage autochtone en Nouvelle-Guinée" *Journal d'Agriculture Tropicale et de Botanique Appliquée* 5: 377–378.
1962 "Observations et travaux récents sur les vé-gétaux hallucinogènes de la Nouvelle-Guinée" *Journal d'Agriculture Tropicale et de Botanique Appliquée* 9: 245–249.

Bauer, Wolfgang, Edzard Klapp & Alexandra Rosenbohm
1991 *Der Fliegenpilz: Ein kulturhistorisches Museum*. Cologne: Wienand-Verlag.

Beringer, Kurt
1927 *Der Meskalinrausch*. Berlin: Springer (reprint 1969).

Bianchi, Antonio & Giorgio Samorini
1993 "Plants in Association with Ayahuasca" *Jahrbuch für Ethnomedizin und Bewußtseinsforschung* 2: 21–42, Berlin: VWB.

Bibra, Baron Ernst von
1995 *Plant Intoxicants: A Classic Text on the Use of Mind-Altering Plants*. Technical notes by Jonathan Ott. Healing Arts Press: Rochester, VT. Originally published as *Die Narcotische Genußmittel und der Mensch*. Verlag von Wilhelm Schmid, 1885.

Bisset, N. G.
1985a "Phytochemistry and Pharmacology of *Voacanga* Species" *Agricultural University Wageningen Papers* 85(3): 81–114.
1985b "Uses of *Voacanga* Species" *Agricultural University Wageningen Papers* 85(3): 115–122.

Blätter, Andrea
1995 "Die Funktionen des Drogengebrauchs und ihre kulturspezifische Nutzung" *Curare* 18(2): 279–290.
1996 "Drogen im präkolumbischen Nordamerika" *Jahrbuch für Ethnomedizin und Bewußtseinsforschung* 4 (1995): 163–183.

Bogers, Hans, Stephen Snelders & Hans Plomp
1994 *De Psychedelische (R)evolutie*. Amsterdam: Bres.

Bové, Frank James
1970 *The Story of Ergot*. Basel, New York: S. Karger.

Boyd, Carolyn E. & J. Philip Dering
1996 "Medicinal and Hallucinogenic Plants Identified in the Sediments and Pictographs of the Lower Pecos, Texas Archaic" *Antiquity* 70 (268): 256–275

Braga, D. L. & J. L. McLaughlin
1969 "Cactus Alkaloids. V: Isolation of Hordenine and *N*-Methyltyramine from *Ariocarpus retusus*" *Planta Medica* 17: 87.

Brau, Jean-Louis
1969 *Vom Haschisch zum LSD*. Frankfurt/M.: Insel.

Bunge, A.
1847 "Beiträge zur Kenntnis der Flora Rußlands und der Steppen Zentral-Asiens" *Mem. Sav. Etr. Petersb.* 7: 438.

Bye, Robert A.
1979 "Hallucinogenic Plants of the Tarahumara" *Journal of Ethnopharmacology* 1: 23–48.

Callaway, James
1995 "Some Chemistry and Pharmacology of Ayahuasca" *Jahrbuch für Ethnomedizin und Bewußtseinsforschung* 3(1994): 295–298, Berlin: VWB.
1995 "Pharmahuasca and Contemporary Ethnopharmacology" *Curare* 18(2): 395–398.

Campbell, T. N.
1958 "Origin of the Mescal Bean Cult" *American Anthropologist* 60: 156–160.

Camporesi, Piero
1990 *Das Brot der Träume*. Frankfurt/New York: Campus.

Carstairs, G. M.
1954 "Daru and Bhang: Cultural Factors in the Choice of Intoxicants" *Quarterly Journal for the Study of Alcohol* 15: 220–237.

Chao, Jew-Ming & Ara H. Der Marderosian
1973 "Ergoline Alkaloidal Constituents of Hawaiian Baby Wood Rose, *Argyreia nervosa* (Burm.f.) Bojer" *Journal of Pharmaceutical Sciences* 62(4): 588–591.

Cooke, Mordecai C.
1989 *The Seven Sisters of Sleep*. Lincoln, MA: Quarterman Publ. (reprint 1860).

Cooper, J. M.
1949 "Stimulants and Narcotics" in: J. H. Stewart (ed.), *Handbook of South American Indians*, Bur. Am. Ethnol. Bull. 143(5): 525–558.

Cordy-Collins, Alana
1982 "Psychoactive Painted Peruvian Plants: The Shamanism Textile" *Journal of Ethnobiology* 2(2): 144–153.

Davis, Wade
1996 *One River: Explorations and Discoveries in the Amazon Rain Forest*. New York: Simon & Schuster.

De Smet, Peter A. G. M. & Laurent Rivier
1987 "Intoxicating Paricá Seeds of the Brazilian Maué Indians" *Economic Botany* 41(1): 12–16.

DeKorne, Jim
1995 *Psychedelischer Neo-Schamanismus*. Löhrbach: Werner Pieper's MedienXperimente (Edition Rauschkunde).

Deltgen, Florian
1993 *Gelenkte Ekstase: Die halluzinogene Droge Cají der Yebámasa-Indianer*. Stuttgart: Franz Steiner Verlag (Acta Humboldtiana 14).

Descola, Philippe
1996 *The Spears of Twilight: Life and Death in the Amazon Jungle.* London: HarperCollins.

Devereux, Paul
1992 *Shamanism and the Mystery Lines: Ley Lines, Spirit Paths, Shape-Shifting & Out-of-Body Travel.* London, New York, Toronto, Sydney: Quantum.
1997 *The Long Trip: A Prehistory of Psychedelia.* New York: Penguin/Arkana.

Diaz, José Luis
1979 "Ethnopharmacology and Taxonomy of Mexican Psychodysleptic Plants" *Journal of Psychedelic Drugs* 11(1–2): 71–101.

Dieckhöfer, K., Th. Vogel, & J. Meyer-Lindenberg
1971 "*Datura Stramonium* als Rauschmittel" *Der Nervenarzt* 42(8): 431–437.

Dittrich, Adolf
1996 *Ätiologie-unabhängige Strukturen veränderter Wachbewußtseinszustände.* Second edition, Berlin: VWB.

Dobkin de Rios, Marlene
1972 *Visionary Vine: Hallucinogenic Healing in the Peruvian Amazon.* San Francisco: Chandler.
1984 *Hallucinogens: Cross-Cultural Perspectives.* Albuquerque: University of New Mexico Press.
1992 *Amazon Healer: The Life and Times of an Urban Shaman.* Bridport, Dorset: Prism Press.

Drury, Nevill
1989 *Vision Quest.* Bridport, Dorset: Prism Press.
1991 *The Visionary Human.* Shaftesbury, Dorset: Element Books.
1996 *Shamanism.* Shaftesbury, Dorset: Element.

Duke, James A. & Rodolfo Vasquez
1994 *Amazonian Ethnobotanical Dictionary.* Boca Raton, FL: CRC Press.

DuToit, Brian M.
1977 *Drugs, Rituals and Altered States of Consciousness.* Rotterdam: Balkema.

Efron, Daniel H., Bo Holmstedt, & Nathan S. Kline (ed.)
1967 *Ethnopharmacologic Search for Psychoactive Drugs.* Washington, DC: U.S. Department of Health, Education, and Welfare.

Emboden, William A.
1976 "Plant Hypnotics Among the North American Indians" in: Wayland D. Hand (ed.), *American Folk Medicine: A Symposium,* S. 159–167, Berkeley: University of California Press.
1979 *Narcotic Plants* (revised edition). New York: Macmillan.

Escohotado, Antonio
1990 *Historia de las drogas* (3 vols.). Madrid: Alianza Editorial.

Eugster, Conrad Hans
1967 *Über den Fliegenpilz.* Zürich: Naturforschende Gesellschaft (Neujahrsblatt).
1968 "Wirkstoffe aus dem Fliegenpilz" *Die Naturwissenschaften* 55(7): 305–313.

Fadiman, James
1965 "*Genista canariensis*: A Minor Psychedelic" *Economic Botany* 19: 383–384.

Farnsworth, Norman R.
1968 "Hallucinogenic Plants" *Science* 162: 1086–1092.
1972 "Psychotomimetic and Related Higher Plants" *Journal of Psychedelic Drugs* 5(1): 67–74.
1974 "Psychotomimetic Plants. II" *Journal of Psychedelic Drugs* 6(1): 83–84.

Fericgla, Josep M.
1994 (ed.), *Plantas, Chamanismo y Estados de Consciencia.* Barcelona: Los Libros de la Liebre de Marzo (Collección Cogniciones).

Fernández Distel, Alicia A.
1980 "Hallazgo de pipas en complejos precerámicos del borde de la Puna Jujeña (Republica Argentina) y el empleo de alucinógenos por parte de las mismas cultura" *Estudios Arqueológicos* 5: 55–79, Universidad de Chile.

Festi, Francesco
1985 *Funghi allucinogeni: Aspetti psicofisiologici e storici.* Rovereto: Musei Civici di Rovereto (LXXXVI Pubblicazione).
1995 "Le erbe del diavolo. 2: Botanica, chimica e farmacologia" *Altrove* 2: 117–145.
1996 "*Scopolia carniolica* Jacq." *Eleusis* 5: 34–45.

Festi, Franceso & Giovanni Aliotta
1990 "Piante psicotrope spontanee o coltivate in Italia" *Annali dei Musei Civici di Rovereto* 5 (1989): 135–166.

Festi, Francesco & Giorgio Samorini
1994 "Alcaloidi indolici psicoattivi nei generi *Phalaris e Arundo (Graminaceae):* Una rassegna" *Annali dei Musei Civici di Rovereto* 9 (1993): 239–288.

Fields, F. Herbert
1968 "*Rivea corymbosa:* Notes on Some Zapotecan Customs" *Economic Botany* 23: 206–209.

Fitzgerald, J. S. & A. A. Sioumis
1965 "Alkaloids of the Australian Leguminosae V: The Occurrence of Methylated Tryptamines in *Acacia maidenii* F. Muell." *Australian Journal of Chemistry* 18: 433–434.

Flury, Lázaro
1958 "El Caá-pí y el Hataj, dos poderosos ilusiógenos indígenas" *América Indigena* 18(4): 293–298.

Forte, Robert (ed.)
1997 *Entheogens and the Future of Religion.* San Francisco: Council on Spiritual Practices/Promind Services (Sebastopol).

Friedberg, C.
1965 "Des Banisteriopsis utilisés comme drogue en Amerique du Sud" *Journal d'Agriculture Tropicale et de Botanique Appliquée* 12: 1–139.

Fühner, Hermann
1919 "Scopoliawurzel als Gift und Heilmittel bei Litauen und Letten" *Therapeutische Monatshefte* 33: 221–227.
1925 "Solanazeen als Berauschungsmittel: Eine historisch-ethnologische Studie" *Archiv für experimentelle Pathologie und Pharmakologie* 111: 281–294.
1943 *Medizinische Toxikologie.* Leipzig: Georg Thieme.

Furst, Peter T.
1971 "*Ariocarpus retusus*, the 'False Peyote' of Huichol Tradition" *Economic Botany* 25: 182–187.
1972 (ed.), *Flesh of the Gods.* New York: Praeger.
1974 "Hallucinogens in Pre-Columbian Art" in Mary Elizabeth King & Idris R. Traylor Jr. (ed.), *Art and Environment in Native America,* The Museum of Texas Tech, Texas Tech University (Lubbock), Special Publication no. 7.
1976 *Hallucinogens and Culture.* Novato, CA: Chandler & Sharp.
1986 *Mushrooms: Psychedelic Fungi.* New York: Chelsea House Publishers. [updated edition 1992]
1990 "Schamanische Ekstase und botanische Halluzinogene: Phantasie und Realität" in: G. Guntern (ed.), *Der Gesang des Schamanen,* S. 211–243, Brig: ISO-Stiftung.
1996 "Shamanism, Transformation, and Olmec Art" in: *The Olmec World: Ritual and Rulership,* S. 69–81, The Art Museum, Princeton University/New York: Harry N. Abrams.

Garcia, L. L., L. L. Cosme, H. R. Peralta, et al.
1973 "Phytochemical Investigation of *Coleus Blumei*. I. Preliminary Studies of the Leaves" *Philippine Journal of Science* 102: 1.

Gartz, Jochen
1986 "Quantitative Bestimmung der Indolderivate von *Psilocybe semilanceata* (Fr.) Kumm." *Biochem. Physiol. Pflanzen* 181: 117–124.
1989 "Analyse der Indolderivate in Fruchtkörpern und Mycelien von *Panaeolus subbalteatus* (Berk. & Br.) Sacc." *Biochemie und Physiologie der Pflanzen* 184: 171–178.
1993 *Narrenschwämme: Psychotrope Pilze in Europa.* Genf/Neu-Allschwil: Editions Heuwinkel.
1996 *Magic Mushrooms Around the World.* Los Angeles: Lis Publications.

Garza, Mercedes de la
1990 *Sueños y alucinación en el mundo náhuatl y maya.* México, D.F.: UNAM.

Gelpke, Rudolf
1995 *Vom Rausch im Orient und Okzident* (Second edition). With a new epilogue by Michael Klett. Stuttgart: Klett-Cotta.

Geschwinde, Thomas
1990 *Rauschdrogen: Marktformen und Wirkungsweisen.* Berlin etc.: Springer.

Giese, Claudius Cristobal
1989 "Curanderos": *Traditionelle Heiler in Nord Peru (Küste und Hochland).* Hohenschäftlarn: Klaus Renner Verlag.

Golowin, Sergius
1971 "Psychedelische Volkskunde" *Antaios* 12: 590–604.
1973 *Die Magie der verbotenen Märchen.* Gifkendorf: Merlin.

Gonçalves de Lima, Oswaldo
1946 "Observações sôbre o 'vinho da Jurema' utilizado pelos índios Pancurú de Tacaratú (Pernambuco)" *Arquivos do Instituto de Pesquisas Agronomicas* 4: 45–80.

Grinspoon, Lester & James B. Bakalar
1981 *Psychedelic Drugs Reconsidered.* New York: Basic Books.
1983 (eds.), *Psychedelic Reflections.* New York: Human Sciences Press.

Grob, Charles S. et al.
1996 "Human Psychopharmacology of Hoasca, a Plant Hallucinogen in Ritual Context in Brazil" *The Journal of Nervous and Mental Disease* 181(2): 86–94.

Grof, Stanislav
1975 *Realms of the Human Unconscious: Observations from LSD Research.* New York: Viking Press.

Grof, Stanislav and Joan Halifax.
1977 *The Human Encounter with Death.* New York: E. P. Dutton.

Guerra, Francisco
1967 "Mexican Phantastica: A Study of the Early Ethnobotanical Sources on Hallucinogenic Drugs" *British Journal of Addiction* 62: 171–187.
1971 *The Pre-Columbian Mind.* London: Seminar Press.

Guzmán, Gastón
1983 *The Genus Psilocybe.* Vaduz, Liechtenstein: Beihefte zur Nova Hedwigia, Nr. 74

Halifax, Joan
1979 *Shamanic Voices: A Survey of Visionary Narratives.* New York: E. P. Dutton
1981 *Die andere Wirklichkeit der Schamanen.* Bern, Munich: O. W. Barth/Scherz.

Hansen, Harold A.
1978 *The Witch's Garden.* Foreword by Richard Evans Schultes. Santa Cruz: Unity Press-Michael Kesend. Originally published as *Heksens Urtegard.* Laurens Bogtrykkeri, Tønder, Denmark, 1976.

Harner, Michael (ed.)
1973 *Hallucinogens and Shamanism.* London: Oxford University Press.

Hartwich, Carl
1911 *Die menschlichen Genußmittel.* Leipzig: Tauchnitz.

Heffern, Richard
1974 *Secrets of Mind-Altering Plants of Mexico.* New York: Pyramid.

Heim, Roger
1963 *Les champignons toxiques et hallucinogènes.* Paris: N. Boubée & Cie.
1966 (et al.) "Nouvelles investigations sur les champignons hallucinogènes" *Archives du Muséum National d'Histoire Naturelle,* (1965–1966).

Heim, Roger & R. Gordon Wasson
1958 "Les champignons hallucinogènes du Mexique" *Archives du Muséum National d'Histoire Naturelle,* Septième Série, Tome VI, Paris.

Heinrich, Clark
1998 *Die Magie der Pilze.* Munich: Diederichs.

Heiser, Charles B.
1987 *The Fascinating World of the Nightshades.* New York: Dover.

Höhle, Sigi, Claudia Müller-Ebeling, Christian Rätsch, & Ossi Urchs
1986 *Rausch und Erkenntnis.* Munich: Knaur.

Hoffer, Abraham & Humphry Osmond
1967 *The Hallucinogens.* New York and London: Academic Press.

Hofmann, Albert
1960 "Die psychotropen Wirkstoffe der mexikanischen Zauberpilze" *Chimia* 14: 309–318.
1961 "Die Wirkstoffe der mexikanischen Zauberdroge Ololiuqui" *Planta Medica* 9: 354–367.
1964 *Die Mutterkorn-Alkaloide.* Stuttgart: Enke.

1968 "Psychotomimetic Agents" in: A. Burger (ed.), *Chemical Constitution and Pharmacodynamic Action*, S. 169–235, New York: M. Dekker.
1980 *LSD, My Problem Child*. Translated by Jonathan Ott. New York: McGraw-Hill. Originally published as *LSD: mein Sorgenkind*. Stuttgart: Klett-Cotta, 1979.
1987 "Pilzliche Halluzinogene vom Mutterkorn bis zu den mexikanischen Zauberpilzen" *Der Champignon* 310: 22–28.
1989 *Insight, Outlook*. Atlanta: Humanics New Age. Originally published as *Einsichten/Ausblicken*. Basel: Sphinx Verlag, 1986.
1996 *Lob des Schauens*. Privately printed (limited edition of 150 copies).
Hofmann, Albert, Roger Heim, & Hans Tscherter
1963 "Présence de la psilocybine dans une espèce européenne d'Agaric, le *Psilocybe semilanceata* Fr. Note (*) de MM." in: *Comptes rendus des séances de l'Académie des Sciences* (Paris), t. 257: 10–12.
Huxley, Aldous
1954 *The Doors of Perception*. New York: Harper & Bros.
1956 *Heaven and Hell*. New York: Harper & Bros.
1999 *Moksha*. Preface by Albert Hofmann. Edited by Michael Horowitz and Cynthia Palmer. Introduction by Alexander Shulgin. Rochester, VT: Park Street Press.
Illius, Bruno
1991 *Ani Shinan: Schamanismus bei den Shipibo-Conibo (Ost-Peru)*. Münster, Hamburg: Lit Verlag (Ethnologische Studien Vol. 12).
Jain, S. K., V. Ranjan, E. L. S. Sikarwar, & A. Saklani
1994 "Botanical Distribution of Psychoactive Plants in India" *Ethnobotany* 6: 65–75.
Jansen, Karl L. R. & Colin J. Prast
1988 "Ethnopharmacology of Kratom and the *Mitragyna* Alkaloids" *Journal of Ethnopharmacology* 23: 115–119.
Johnston, James F.
1855 *The Chemistry of Common Life. Vol. II: The Narcotics We Indulge In*. New York: D. Appleton & Co.
1869 *Die Chemie des täglichen Lebens* (2 Bde.). Berlin.
Johnston, T. H. & J. B. Clelland
1933 "The History of the Aborigine Narcotic, Pituri" *Oceania* 4(2): 201–223, 268, 289.
Joralemon, Donald & Douglas Sharon
1993 *Sorcery and Shamanism: Curanderos and Clients in Northern Peru*. Salt Lake City: University of Utah Press.
Joyce, C. R. B. & S. H. Curry
1970 *The Botany and Chemistry of Cannabis*. London: Churchill.
Jünger, Ernst
1980 *Annäherungen-Drogen und Rausch*. Frankfurt/usw.: Ullstein.
Kalweit, Holger
1984 *Traumzeit und innerer Raum: Die Welt der Schamanen*. Bern etc.: Scherz.
Klüver, Heinrich
1969 *Mescal and Mechanisms of Hallucinations*. Chicago: The University of Chicago Press.
Koch-Grünberg, Theodor
1921 *Zwei Jahre bei den Indianern Nordwest-Brasiliens*. Stuttgart: Strecker & Schröder
1923 *Vom Roraima zum Orinoco*. Stuttgart:
Kotschenreuther, Hellmut
1978 *Das Reich der Drogen und Gifte*. Frankfurt/M. etc.: Ullstein.
Kraepelin, Emil
1882 *Über die Beeinflussung einfacher psychologischer Vorgänge durch einige Arzneimittel*. Jena.
La Barre, Weston
1970 "Old and New World Narcotics" *Economic Botany* 24(1): 73–80.
1979 "Shamanic Origins of Religion and Medicine" *Journal of Psychedelic Drugs* 11(1–2): 7–11.
1979 *The Peyote Cult* (5th edition). Norman: University of Oklahoma Press.
Langdon, E. Jean Matteson & Gerhard Baer (ed.)
1992 *Portals of Power: Shamanism in South America*. Albuquerque: University of New Mexico Press.

Larris, S.
1980 *Forbyde Hallucinogener? Forbyd Naturen at Gro!* Nimtoffe: Forlaget Indkøbstryk.
Leuenberger, Hans
1969 *Zauberdrogen: Reisen ins Weltall der Seele*. Stuttgart: Henry Goverts Verlag.
Leuner, Hanscarl
1981 *Halluzinogene*. Bern etc.: Huber.
1996 *Psychotherapie und religiöses Erleben*. Berlin: VWB.
Lewin, Louis
1997 *Banisteria caapi, ein neues Rauschgift und Heilmittel*. Berlin: VWB (reprint from 1929).
1998 *Phantastica: A Classic Survey on the Use and Abuse of Mind-Altering Plants*. Rochester, VT: Park Street Press. Originally published as *Phantastica-Die Betäubenden und erregenden Genußmittel. Für Ärtzte und Nichtärzte*. Berlin: Georg Stilke Verlag, 1924.
Lewis-Williams, J. D. & T. A. Dowson
1988 "The Signs of All Times: Entoptic Phenomena in Upper Paleolithic Art" *Current Anthropology* 29(2): 201–245.
1993 "On Vision and Power in the Neolithic: Evidence from the Decorated Monuments" *Current Anthropology* 34(1): 55–65.
Liggenstorfer, Roger & Christian Rätsch (eds.)
1996 *María Sabina-Botin der heiligen Pilze: Vom traditionellen Schamanentum zur weltweiten Pilzkultur*. Solothurn: Nachtschatten Verlag.
Li, Hui-Lin
1975 "Hallucinogenic Plants in Chinese Herbals" *Botanical Museum Leaflets* 25(6): 161–181.
Lin, Geraline C. & Richard A. Glennon (ed.)
1994 *Hallucinogens: An Update*. Rockville, MD: National Institute on Drug Abuse.
Lipp, Frank J.
1991 *The Mixe of Oaxaca: Religion, Ritual, and Healing*. Austin: University of Texas Press.
Lockwood, Tommie E.
1979 "The Ethnobotany of *Brugmansia*" *Journal of Ethnopharmacology* 1: 147–164.
Luna, Luis Eduardo
1984 "The Concept of Plants as Teachers Among Four Mestizo Shamans of Iquitos, Northeast Peru" *Journal of Ethnopharmacology* 11(2): 135–156.
1986 *Vegetalismo: Shamanism Among the Mestizo Population of the Peruvian Amazon*. Stockholm: Almqvist & Wiskell International (Acta Universitatis Stockholmiensis, Stockholm Studies in Comparative Religion 27).
1991 "Plant Spirits in Ayahuasca Visions by Peruvian Painter Pablo Amaringo: An Iconographic Analysis" *Integration* 1: 18–29.
Luna, Luis Eduardo & Pablo Amaringo
1991 *Ayahuasca Visions*. Berkeley: North Atlantic Books.
McKenna, Dennis J. & G. H. N. Towers
1985 "On the Comparative Ethnopharmacology of Malpighiaceous and Myristicaceous Hallucinogens" *Journal of Psychoactive Drugs* 17(1): 35–39.
McKenna, Dennis J., G. H. N. Towers, & F. Abbott
1994 "Monoamine Oxydase Inhibitors in South American Hallucinogenic Plants: Tryptamine and β-Carboline Constituents of Ayahuasca" *Journal of Ethnopharmacology* 10: 195–223 and 12: 179–211.
McKenna, Terence
1991 *The Archaic Revival*. San Francisco: Harper.
1992 "Tryptamine Hallucinogens and Consciousness" *Jahrbuch für Ethnomedizin und Bewußtseinsforschung* 1: 133–148, Berlin: VWB.
1992 *Food of the Gods: The Search for the Original Tree of Knowledge: A Radical History of Plants, Drugs and Human Evolution*. New York: Bantam Books.
1994 *True Hallucinations: Being an Account of the Author's Extraordinary Adventures in the Devil's Paradise*. London: Rider.
Mantegazza, Paolo
1871 *Quadri della natura umana: Feste ed ebbrezze* (2 volumes). Mailand: Brigola.
1887 *Le estasi umane*. Mailand: Dumolard.
Marzahn, Christian
1994 *Bene Tibi-Über Genuß und Geist*. Bremen: Edition Temmen.

Marzell, Heinrich
1964 *Zauberpflanzen-Hexentränke*. Stuttgart: Kosmos.
Mata, Rachel & Jerry L. McLaughlin
1982 "Cactus Alkaloids. 50: A Comprehensive Tabular Summary" *Revista Latinoamerica de Quimica* 12: 95–117.
Metzner, Ralph
1994 *The Well of Remembrance: Rediscovering the Earth Wisdom Myths of Northern Europe*. Appendix "The Mead of Inspiration and Magical Plants of the Ancient Germans" by Christian Rätsch. Boston: Shambhala.
Møller, Knud O.
1951 *Rauschgifte und Genußmittel*. Basel: Benno Schwabe.
Moreau de Tours, J. J.
1973 *Hashish and Mental Illness*. New York: Raven Press.
Müller, G. K. & Jochen Gartz
1986 "*Psilocybe cyanescens*-eine weitere halluzinogene Kahlkopfart in der DDR" *Mykologisches Mitteilungsblatt* 29: 33–35.
Müller-Eberling, Claudia & Christian Rätsch
1986 *Isoldens Liebestrank*. Munich: Kindler.
Müller-Ebeling, Claudia, Christian Rätsch, & Wolf-Dieter Storl
1998 *Hexenmedizin*. Aarau: AT Verlag.
Munizaga A., Carlos
1960 "Uso actual de *miyaya* (Datura stramonium) por los araucanos de Chiles" *Journal de la Société des Américanistes* 52: 4–43.
Myerhoff, Barbara G.
1974 *Peyote Hunt: The Sacred Journey of the Huichol Indians*. Ithaca: Cornell, University Press.
Nadler, Kurt H.
1991 *Drogen: Rauschgift und Medizin*. Munich: Quintessenz.
Naranjo, Plutarco
1969 "Etnofarmacología de las plantas psicotrópicas de América" *Terapia* 24: 5–63.
1983 *Ayahuasca: Etnomedicina y mitología*. Quito: Ediciones Libri Mundi.
Negrin, J.
1975 *The Huichol Creation of the World*. Sacramento, CA: Crocker Art Gallery.
Neuwinger, Hans Dieter
1994 *Afrikanische Arzneipflanzen und Jagdgifte*. Stuttgart: WVG.
Ortega, A., J. F. Blount, & P. S. Merchant
1982 "Salvinorin, a New Trans-Neoclerodane Diterpene from *Salvia divinorum* (Labiatae)" *J. Chem. Soc.*, Perkin Trans. I: 2505–2508.
Ortiz de Montellano, Bernard R.
1981 "Entheogens: The Interaction of Biology and Culture" *Reviews of Anthropology* 8(4): 339–365.
Osmond, Humphrey
1955 "Ololiuhqui: The Ancient Aztec Narcotic" *Journal of Mental Science* 101: 526–537.
Ott, Jonathan
1979 *Hallucinogenic Plants of North America*. (revised edition) Berkeley: Wingbow press.
1985 *Chocolate Addict*. Vashon, WA: Natural Products Co.
1993 *Pharmacotheon: Entheogenic Drugs, Their Plant Sources and History*. Kennewick, WA: Natural Products Co.
1995 *Ayahuasca Analogues: Pangoean Entheogens*. Kennewick, WA: Natural Products Co.
1995 "Ayahuasca and Ayahuasca Analogues: Pan-Gaean Entheogens for the New Millennium" *Jahrbuch für Ethnomedizin und Bewußtseinsforschung* 3(1994): 285–293.
1995 "Ayahuasca-Ethnobotany, Phytochemistry and Human Pharmacology" *Integration* 5: 73–97.
1995 "Ethnopharmacognosy and Human Pharmacology of *Salvia divinorum* and Salvinorin A" *Curare* 18(1): 103–129.
1995 *The Age of Entheogens & The Angels' Dictionary*. Kennewick, WA: Natural Products Co.
1996 "*Salvia divinorum* Epling et Játiva (Foglie della Pastora/Leaves of the Shepherdess)" *Eleusis* 4: 31–39.
1996 "Entheogens II: On Entheology and Entheobotany" *Journal of Psychoactive Drugs* 28(2): 205–209.

Ott, Jonathan & Jeremy Bigwood (ed.)
1978 *Teonanácatl: Hallucinogenic Mushrooms of North America.* Seattle: Madrona.

Pagani, Silvio
1993 *Funghetti.* Torino: Nautilus.

Pelletier, S. W.
1970 *Chemistry of Alkaloids.* New York: Van Nostrand Reinhold.

Pelt, Jean-Marie
1983 *Drogues et plantes magiques.* Paris: Fayard.

Pendell, Dale
1995 *Pharmak/Poeia: Plant Powers, Poisons, and Herbcraft.* San Francisco: Mercury House.

Perez de Barradas, José
1957 *Plantas magicas americanas.* Madrid: Inst. 'Bernardino de Sahagún.'

Perrine, Daniel M.
1996 *The Chemistry of Mind-Altering Drugs: History, Pharmacology, and Cultural Context.* Washington, DC: American Chemical Society.

Peterson, Nicolas
1979 "Aboriginal Uses of Australian Solanaceae" in: J. G. Hawkes et al. (eds.), *The Biology and Taxonomy of the Solanaceae,* 171–189, London etc.: Academic Press.

Pinkley, Homer V.
1969 "Etymology of *Psychotria* in View of a New Use of the Genus" *Rhodora* 71: 535–540.

Plotkin, Mark J.
1994 *Tales of a Shaman's Apprentice: An Ethnobotanist Searches for New Medicines in the Amazon Rain Forest.* New York: Penguin

Plowman, Timothy, Lars Olof Gyllenhaal, & Jan Erik Lindgren
1971 "*Latua pubiflora*-Magic Plant from Southern Chile" *Botanical Museum Leaflets* 23(2): 61–92.

Polia Meconi, Mario
1988 *Las lagunas de los encantos: medicina tradicional andina del Perú septentrional.* Piura: Central Peruana de Servicios-CEPESER/Club Grau de Piura.

Pope, Harrison G., Jr.
1969 "*Tabernanthe iboga*: An African Narcotic Plant of Social Importance" *Economic Botany* 23: 174–184.

Prance, Ghillian T.
1970 "Notes on the Use of Plant Hallucinogens in Amazonian Brazil" *Economic Botany* 24: 62–68.
1972 "Ethnobotanical Notes from Amazonian Brazil" *Economic Botany* 26: 221–237.

Prance, Ghillian T., David G. Campbell, & Bruce W. Nelson
1977 "The Ethnobotany of the Paumarí Indians" *Economic Botany* 31: 129–139.

Prance, G. T. & A. E. Prance
1970 "Hallucinations in Amazonia" *Garden Journal* 20: 102–107.

Preussel, Ulrike & Hans-Georg
1997 *Engelstrompeten: Brugmansia und Datura.* Stuttgart: Ulmer.

Quezada, Noemí
1989 *Amor y magia amorosa entre los aztecas.* Mexico: UNAM.

Rätsch, Christian
1988 *Lexikon der Zauberpflanzen aus ethnologischer Sicht.* Graz: ADEVA.
1991 *Von den Wurzeln der Kultur: Die Pflanzen der Propheten.* Basel: Sphinx.
1991 *Indianische Heilkräuter* (2 revised edition). Munich: Diederichs.
1992 *The Dictionary of Sacred and Magical Plants.* Santa Barbara etc.: ABC-Clio.
1992 *The Dictionary of Sacred and Magical Plants.* Bridport, England: Prism Press. Originally published as *Lexikon der Zauberpflanzen aus ethnologischer Sicht.* Graz: ADEVA, 1988.
1994 "Die Pflanzen der blühenden Träume: Trancedrogen mexikanischer Schamanen" *Curare* 17(2): 277–314.
1995 *Heilkräuter der Antike in Ägypten, Griechenland und Rom.* Munich: Diederichs Verlag (DG).
1996 *Urbock-Bier jenseits von Hopfen und Malz: Von den Zaubertränken der Götter zu den psychedelischen Bieren der Zukunft.* Aarau, Stuttgart: AT Verlag.
1997 *Enzyklopädie der psychoaktiven Pflanzen.*

Aarau: AT Verlag.
1997 *Plants of Love: Aphrodisiacs in History and a Guide to Their Identification.* Foreword by Albert Hofmann, Berkeley: Ten Speed Press. Originally published as *Pflanzen der Liebe.* Bern: Hallwag, 1990. Second and subsequent editions published by AT Verlag, Aarau, Switzerland.
1998 *Enzyklopädie der psychoaktiven Pflanzen.* Aarau: AT Verlag . English-language edition, *Encyclopedia of Psychoactive Plants,* to be published in 2003 by Inner Traditions, Rochester, Vermont.

Raffauf, Robert F.
1970 *A Handbook of Alkaloids and Alkaloid-containing Plants.* New York: Wiley-Interscience.

Reichel-Dolmatoff, Gerardo
1971 *Amazonian Cosmos: The Sexual and Religious Symbolism of the Tukano Indians.* Chicago and London: The University of Chicago Press.
1975 *The Shaman and the Jaguar: A Study of Narcotic Drugs Among the Indians of Colombia.* Philadelphia: Temple University Press.
1978 *Beyond the Milky Way: Hallucinatory Imagery of the Tukano Indians.* Los Angeles: UCLA Latin American Center Publications.
1985 *Basketry as Metaphor: Arts and Crafts of the Desana Indians of the Northwest Amazon.* Los Angeles Museum of Cultural History.
1987 *Shamanism and Art of the Eastern Tukanoan Indians.* Leiden: Brill.
1996 *The Forest Within: The World-View of the Tukano Amazonian Indians.* Totnes, Devon: Green Books.
1996 *Das schamanische Universum: Schamanismus, Bewußtseins und Ökologie in Südamerika.* Munich: Diederichs.

Reko, Blas Pablo
1996 *On Aztec Botanical Names.* Translated, edited and commented by Jonathan Ott. Berlin: VWB.

Reko, Victor A.
1938 *Magische Gifte: Rausch- und Betäubungsmittel der neuen Welt* (second edition). Stuttgart: Enke (Reprint Berlin: EXpress Edition 1987, VWB 1996).

Richardson, P. Mick
1992 *Flowering Plants: Magic in Bloom* (updated edition). New York, Philadelphia: Chelsea House Publ.

Ripinsky-Naxon, Michael
1989 "Hallucinogens, Shamanism, and the Cultural Process" *Anthropos* 84: 219–224.
1993 *The Nature of Shamanism: Substance and Function of a Religious Metaphor.* Albany: State University of New York Press.
1996 "Psychoactivity and Shamanic States of Consciousness" *Jahrbuch für Ethnomedizin und Bewußtseinsforschung* 4 (1995): 35–43, Berlin: VWB.

Rivier, Laurent & Jan-Erik Lindgren
1972 "'Ayahuasca,' the South American Hallucinogenic Drink: An Ethnobotanical and Chemical Investigation" *Economic Botany* 26: 101–129.

Römpp, Hermann
1950 *Chemische Zaubertränke* (5th edition). Stuttgart: Kosmos-Franckh'sche.

Rosenbohm, Alexandra
1991 *Halluzinogene Drogen im Schamanismus.* Berlin: Reimer.

Roth, Lutz, Max Daunderer, & Kurt Kormann
1994 *Giftpflanzen-Pflanzengifte* (4. edition). Munich: Ecomed.

Rouhier, Alexandre
1927 *La plante qui fait les yeux émerveillés-le Peyotl.* Paris: Gaston Doin.
1996 *Die Hellsehen hervorrufenden Pflanzen.* Berlin: VWB (Reprint from 1927).

Ruck, Carl A. P. et al.
1979 "Entheogens" *Journal of Psychedelic Drugs* 11(1–2): 145–146.

Rudgley, Richard
1994 *Essential Substances: A Cultural History of Intoxicants in Society.* Foreword by William Emboden. New York, Tokyo, London: Kodansha International.
1995 "The Archaic Use of Hallucinogens in Europe: An Archaeology of Altered States" *Addiction* 90: 163–164.

Safford, William E.
1916 "Identity of *Cohoba,* the Narcotic Snuff of Ancient Haiti" *Jornal of the Washington Academy of Sciences* 6: 547–562.
1917 "Narcotic Plants and Stimulants of the Ancient Americans" *Annual Report of the Smithsonian Institution for 1916:* 387–424.
1921 "Syncopsis of the Genus *Datura*" *Journal of the Washington Academy of Sciences* 11(8): 173–189.
1922 "Daturas of the Old World and New" *Annual Report of the Smithsonian Institution for 1920:* 537–567.

Salzman, Emanuel, Jason Salzman, Joanne Salzman, & Gary Lincoff
1996 "In Search of *Mukhomor,* the Mushroom of Immortality" *Shaman's Drum* 41: 36–47.

Samorini, Giorgio
1995 *Gli allucinogeni nel mito: Racconti sull'origine delle piante psicoattive.* Turin: Nautilus.

Schaefer, Stacy & Peter T. Furst (ed.)
1996 *People of the Peyote: Huichol Indian History, Religion, & Survival.* Albuquerque: University of New Mexico Press.

Schenk, Gustav
1948 *Schatten der Nacht.* Hanover: Sponholtz.
1954 *Das Buch der Gifte.* Berlin: Safari.

Schleiffer, Hedwig (ed.)
1973 *Narcotic Plants of the New World Indians: An Anthology of Texts from the 16th Century to Date.* New York: Hafner Press (Macmillan).
1979 *Narcotic Plants of the Old World: An Anthology of Texts from Ancient Times to the Present.* Monticello, NY: Lubrecht & Cramer.

Scholz, Dieter & Dagmar Eigner
1983 "Zur Kenntnis der natürlichen Halluzinogene" *Pharmazie in unserer Zeit* 12(3): 74–79.

Schuldes, Bert Marco
1995 *Psychoaktive Pflanzen. 2. verbesserte und ergänzte Auflage.* Löhrbach: MedienXperimente & Solothurn: Nachtschatten Verlag.

Schultes, Richard E.
1941 *A Contribution to Our Knowledge of Rivea corymbosa: The Narcotic Ololiuqui of the Aztecs.* Cambridge, MA: Botanical Museum of Harvard University.
1954 "A New Narcotic Snuff from the Northwest Amazon" *Botanical Museum Leaflets* 16(9): 241–260.
1963 "Hallucinogenic Plants of the New World" *The Harvard Review* 1(4): 18–32.
1965 "Ein halbes Jahrhundert Ethnobotanik amerikanischer Halluzinogene" *Planta Medica* 13: 125–157.
1966 "The Search for New Natural Hallucinogens" *Lloydia* 29(4): 293–308.
1967 "The Botanical Origins of South American Snuffs" in Daniel H. Efron (ed.), *Ethnopharmacological Search for Psychoactive Drugs,* S. 291–306, Washington, DC: U.S. Government Printing Office.
1969 "Hallucinogens of Plant Origin" *Science* 163: 245–254.
1970 "The Botanical and Chemical Distribution of Hallucinogens" *Annual Review of Plant Physiology* 21: 571–594.
1970 "The Plant Kingdom and Hallucinogens" *Bulletin on Narcotics* 22(1): 25–51.
1972 "The Utilization of Hallucinogens in Primitive Societies-Use, Misuse or Abuse?" in: W. Keup (ed.), *Drug Abuse: Current Concepts and Research,* S. 17–26, Springfield, IL: Charles C. Thomas.
1976 *Hallucinogenic Plants.* Racine, WI: Western.
1977 "Mexico and Colombia: Two Major Centres of Aboriginal Use of Hallucinogens" *Journal of Psychedelic Drugs* 9(2): 173–176.
1979 "Hallucinogenic Plants: Their Earliest Botanical Descriptions" *Journal of Psychedelic Drugs* 11(1–2): 13–24.
1984 "Fifteen Years of Study of Psychoaktive Snuffs of South America: 1967–1982, a Review" *Journal of Ethnopharmacology* 11(1): 17–32.
1988 *Where the Gods Reign: Plants and Peoples of the Colombian Amazon.* Oracle, AZ: Synergetic Press.
1995 "Antiquity of the Use of New World Hallucinogens" *Integration* 5: 9–18.

Schultes, Richard E. & Norman R. Farnsworth
1982 "Ethnomedical, Botanical and Phytochemical Aspects of Natural Hallucinogens" *Botanical Museum Leaflets* 28(2): 123–214.

Schultes, Richard E. & Albert Hofmann
1980 *The Botany and Chemistry of Hallucinogens*. Springfield, IL: Charles C. Thomas.

Schultes, Richard Evans & Bo Holmstedt
1968 "De Plantis Toxicariis e Mundo Novo Tropicale Commentationes II: The Vegetable Ingredients of the Myristicaceous Snuffs of the Northwest Amazon" *Rhodora* 70: 113–160.

Schultes, Richard Evans & Robert F. Raffauf
1990 *The Healing Forest: Medicinal and Toxic Plants of the Northwest Amazonia*. Portland, OR: Dioscorides Press.
1992 *Vine of the Soul: Medicine Men, Their Plants and Rituals in the Colombian Amazonia*. Oracle, AZ: Synergetic Press.

Schultes, Richard E. & Siri von Reis (Ed.)
1995 *Ethnobotany: Evolution of a Discipline*. Portland, OR: Dioscorides Press.

Schurz, Josef
1969 *Vom Bilsenkraut zum LSD*. Stuttgart: Kosmos.

Schwamm, Brigitte
1988 *Atropa belladonna: Eine antike Heilpflanze im modernen Arzneischatz*. Stuttgart: Deutscher Apotheker Verlag.

Sharon, Douglas
1978 *Wizard of the Four Winds: A Shaman's Story*. New York: The Free Press.

Shawcross, W. E.
1983 "Recreational Use of Ergoline Alkaloids from *Argyreia nervosa*" *Journal of Psychoactive Drugs* 15(4): 251–259.

Shellard, E. J.
1974 "The Alkaloids of *Mitragyna* with Special Reference to Those of *M. speciosa*, Korth." *Bulletin of Narcotics* 26: 41–54.

Sherratt, Andrew
1991 "Sacred and Profane Substances: The Ritual Use of Narcotics in Later Neolithic Europe" in: Paul Garwood et al. (ed.), *Sacred and Profane*, 50–64, Oxford University Committee for Archaeology, Monograph No. 32.

Shulgin, Alexander T.
1992 *Controlled Substances: Chemical & Legal Guide to Federal Drug Laws* (second edition). Berkeley: Ronin.

Shulgin, Alexander T. & Claudio Naranjo
1967 "The Chemistry and Psychopharmacology of Nutmeg and of Several Related Phenylisopropylamines" in: D. Efron (ed.), *Ethnopharmacologic Search for Psychoactive Drugs*, S. 202–214, Washington, DC: U.S. Dept. of Health, Education, and Welfare.

Shulgin, Alexander & Ann Shulgin
1991 *PIHKAL: A Chemical Love Story*. Berkeley: Transform Press.
1997 *TIHKAL*. Berkeley: Transform Press.

Siebert, Daniel J.
1994 "*Salvia divinorum* and Salvinorin A: New Pharmacologic Findings" *Journal of Ethnopharmacology* 43: 53–56.

Siegel, Ronald K.
1992 *Fire in the Brain: Clinical Tales of Hallucination*. New York: Dutton.

Siegel, Ronald K. & Louise J. West (ed.)
1975 *Hallucinations*. New York etc.: John Wiley & Co.

Silva, M. & P. Mancinell.
1959 "Chemical Study of *Cestrum parqui*" *Boletin de la Sociedad Chilena de Química* 9: 49–50.

Slotkin, J. S.
1956 *The Peyote Religion: A Study in Indian-White Relations*. Glencoe, IL: The Free Press.

Spitta, Heinrich
1892 *Die Schlaf- und Traumzustände der menschlichen Seele mit besonderer Berücksichtigung ihres Verhältnisses zu den psychischen Alienationen*. Zweite stark vermehrte Auflage. Freiburg i. B.: J. C. B. Mohr (first edition 1877).

Spruce, Richard
1970 *Notes of a Botanist on the Amazon & Andes*. New foreword by R. E. Schultes. New York: Johnson Reprint Corporation (reprint from 1908).

Stafford, Peter
1992 *Psychedelics Encyclopedia* (3. revised edition). Berkeley: Ronin.

Stamets, Paul
1978 *Psilocybe Mushrooms & Their Allies*. Seattle: Homestead.
1996 *Psilocybin Mushrooms of the World*. Berkeley: Ten Speed Press.

Storl, Wolf-Dieter
1988 *Feuer und Asche-Dunkel und Licht: Shiva-Urbild des Menschen*. Freiburg i. B.: Bauer.
1993 *Von Heilkräutern und Pflanzengottheiten*. Braunschweig: Aurum.
1997 *Pflanzendevas-Die Göttin und ihre Pflanzenengel*. Aarau: AT Verlag.

Suwanlert, S.
1975 "A Study of Kratom Eaters in Thailand" *Bulletin of Narcotics* 27: 21–27.

Taylor, Norman
1966 *Narcotics: Nature's Dangerous Gifts*. New York: Laurel Edition. Originally published as *Flight from Reality*. New York: Duell, Sloan and Pearce, 1949.

Torres, Constantino Manuel
1987 *The Iconography of South American Snuff Trays and Related Paraphernalia*. Göteborg: Etnologiska Studier 37.

Torres, Constantino Manuel, David B. Repke, Kelvin Chan, Dennis McKenna, Agustín Llagostera, & Richard Evans Schultes
1991 "Snuff Powders from Pre-Hispanic San Pedro de Atacama: Chemical and Contextual Analysis" *Current Anthropology* 32(5): 640–649.

Turner, D. M.
1996 *Salvinorin: The Psychedelic Essence of Salvia divinorum*. San Francisco: Panther Press. *Der psychodelische Reiseführer*. Solothurn: Nachtschatten Verlag.

Uscátegui M., Nestor
1959 "The Present Distribution of Narcotics and Stimulants Amongst the Indian Tribes of Colombia" *Botanical Museum Leaflets* 18(6): 273–304.

Valdes, Leander J., III.
1994 "*Salvia divinorum* and the Unique Diterpene Hallucinogen, Salvinorin (Divinorin) A" *Journal of Psychoactive Drugs* 26(3): 277–283.

Valdes, Leander J., José L. Diaz, & Ara G. Paul
1983 "Ethnopharmacology of ska María Pastora (*Salvia divinorum* Epling and Játiva-M.)" *Journal of Ethnopharmacology* 7: 287–312.

Van Beek, T. A. et al.
1984 "*Tabernaemontana* (Apocynaceae): A Review of Its Taxonomy, Phytochemistry, Ethnobotany and Pharmacology" *Journal of Ethnopharmacology* 10: 1–156.

Villavicencio, M.
1858 *Geografía de la república del Ecuador*. New York: R. Craigshead.

Völger, Gisela (ed.)
1981 *Rausch und Realität* (2 volumes). Cologne: Rautenstrauch-Joest Museum.

Von Reis Altschul, Siri
1972 *The Genus* Anadenanthera *in Amerindian Cultures*. Cambridge: Botanical Museum, Harvard University.

Vries, Herman de
1989 *Natural Relations*. Nürnberg: Verlag für moderne Kunst.

Wagner, Hildebert
1970 *Rauschgift-Drogen* (second edition). Berlin etc.: Springer.

Wassel, G. M., S. M. El-Difrawy, & A. A. Saeed
1985 "Alkaloids from the Rhizomes of *Phragmites australis* CAV." *Scientia Pharmaceutica* 53: 169–170.

Wassén, S. Henry & Bo Holmstedt
1963 "The Use of Paricá: An Ethnological and Pharmacological Review" *Ethnos* 28(1): 5–45.

Wasson, R. Gordon
1957 "Seeking the Magic Mushroom" *Life* (13 May 1957) 42(19): 100ff.
1958 "The Divine Mushroom: Primitive Religion and Hallucinatory Agents" *Proc. Am. Phil. Soc.* 102: 221–223.
1961 "The Hallucinogenic Fungi of Mexico: An Inquiry into the Origins of the Religious Idea Among Primitive Peoples" *Botanical Museum Leaflets, Harvard University* 19(7): 137–162. [reprinted 1965]
1962 "A New Mexican Psychotropic Drug from the Mint Family" *Botanical Museum Leaflets* 20(3): 77–84.
1963 "The Hallucinogenic Mushrooms of Mexico ﹍nd Psilocybin: A Bibliography" *Botanical Museum Leaflets, Harvard University* 20(2a): 25–73c. [second printing, with corrections and addenda]
1968 *Soma-Divine Mushroom of Immortality*. New York: Harcourt Brace Jovanovich.
1971 "Ololiuqui and the Other Hallucinogens of Mexico" in: *Homenaje a Roberto J. Weitlaner*, 329–348, Mexico: UNAM.
1973 "The Role of 'Flowers' in Nahuatl Culture: A Suggested Interpretation" *Botanical Museum Leaflets* 23(8): 305–324.
1973 "Mushrooms in Japanese Culture" *The Transactions of the Asiatic Society of Japan* (Third Series) 11: 5–25.
1980 *The Wondrous Mushroom: Mycolatry in Mesoamerica*. New York: McGraw-Hill.
1986 "Persephone's Quest" in: R. G. Wasson et al., *Persephone's Quest: Entheogens and the Origins of Religion*, S. 17–81, New Haven and London: Yale University Press.

Wasson, R. Gordon, George and Florence Cowan, & Willard Rhodes
1974 *María Sabina and Her Mazatec Mushroom Velada*. New York and London: Harcourt Brace Jovanovich.

Wasson, R. Gordon, Albert Hofmann, & Carl A. P. Ruck
1978 *The Road to Eleusis: Unveiling the Secret of the Mysteries*. New York: Harcourt Brace Jovanovich.

Wasson, R. Gordon & Valentina P. Wasson
1957 *Mushrooms, Russia, and History*. New York: Pantheon Books.

Watson, Pamela
1983 *This Precious Foliage: A Study of the Aboriginal Psychoactive Drug Pituri*. Sydney: University of Sydney Press (*Oceania Monograph*, 26).

Watson, P. L., O. Luanratana, & W. J. Griffin
1983 "The Ethnopharmacology of Pituri" *Journal of Ethnopharmacology* 8(3): 303–311.

Weil, Andrew
1980 *The Marriage of the Sun and Moon: A Quest for Unity in Consciousness*. Boston: Houghton-Mifflin.
1998 *Natural Mind: An Investigation of Drugs & Higher Consciousness*. Revised edition. Boston: Houghton-Mifflin.

Weil, Andrew & Winifred Rosen
1983 *Chocolate to Morphen: Understanding Mind-Active Drugs*. Boston: Houghton-Mifflin.

Wilbert, Johannes
1987 *Tobacco and Shamanism in South America*. New Haven and London: Yale University Press.

Winkelman, Michael & Walter Andritzky (ed.)
1996 *Sakrale Heilpflanzen, Bewußtsein und Heilung: Transkulturelle und Interdisziplinäre Perspektiven/Jahrbuch für Transkulturelle Medizin und Psychotherapie* 6 (1995), Berlin: VWB.

Zimmer, Heinrich
1984 *Indische Mythen und Symbole*. Cologne: Diederichs.

Index

(prepared by Christian Rätsch)

Italics of numbers refer to captions.